MANUAL OF MEDICAL PROCEDURES

MANUAL OF MEDICAL PROCEDURES

Edited by

PAUL M. SURATT, M.D.

Associate Professor, Department of Internal Medicine,
Pulmonary Allergy Division, University of Virginia School of Medicine,
Charlottesville, Virginia

ROBERT S. GIBSON, M.D.

Assistant Professor, Department of Internal Medicine,
Division of Cardiology, University of Virginia School of Medicine,
Charlottesville, Virginia

with **237** illustrations

Illustrations by

William C. Ober, M.D.
Department of Family Medicine,
University of Virginia Medical Center,
Charlottesville, Virginia

Dianne Witters Ruscher
Crozet, Virginia

The C. V. Mosby Company

ST. LOUIS • TORONTO 1982

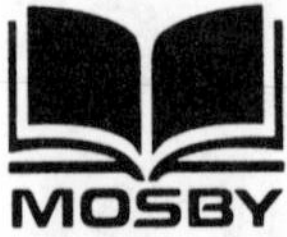

A TRADITION OF PUBLISHING EXCELLENCE

Editor: John Lotz
Manuscript editor: Sandra L. Gilfillan
Design: Nancy Steinmeyer
Production: Mary Stueck

Printed in the United States of America

The C.V. Mosby Company
11830 Westline Industrial Drive, St. Louis, Missouri 63146

Library of Congress Cataloging in Publication Data

Main entry under title:

Manual of medical procedures.

Bibliography: p.
Includes index.
1. Medicine, Clinical—Handbooks, manuals, etc. I. Suratt, Paul M. II. Gibson, Robert S. [DNLM: 1. Internal medicine—Handbooks. 2. Manuals. WX 203 M294]
RC48.M36 616 82-3457
ISBN 0-8016-4850-5 AACR2

AC/D/D 9 8 7 6 5 4 3 2 02/B/276

Contributors

NUZHET O. ATUK, M.D.

Professor of Internal Medicine, Nephrology Division, University of Virginia School of Medicine, Charlottesville, Virginia

BARBARA L. BRAUNSTEIN, M.D.

Chief Resident, Department of Dermatology, University of Virginia School of Medicine, Charlottesville, Virginia

RICHARD S. CRAMPTON, D.M.

Professor of Medicine, Division of Cardiology; Director, Coronary Care Unit, University of Virginia School of Medicine, Charlottesville, Virginia

WILLIAM CUNNINGHAM, M.D.

Fellow in Gastroenterology, Department of Internal Medicine, University of Virginia School of Medicine, Charlottesville, Virginia

JOHN S. DAVIS IV, M.D.

Professor of Internal Medicine, Head of Rheumatology Division, University of Virginia School of Medicine, Charlottesville, Virginia

COSMO A. DIFAZIO, M.D.

Professor of Anesthesiology, University of Virginia School of Medicine, Charlottesville, Virginia

RICHARD F. EDLICH, M.D., Ph.D.

Professor of Plastic Surgery and Biomedical Engineering; Director, Emergency Medical Services, University of Virginia School of Medicine, Charlottesville, Virginia

CARY FISHBURNE, M.D.

Fellow in Pulmonary Disease, Department of Internal Medicine, University of Virginia School of Medicine, Charlottesville, Virginia

ROBERT S. GIBSON, M.D.

Assistant Professor, Department of Internal Medicine, Division of Cardiology, University of Virginia School of Medicine, Charlottesville, Virginia

KENNETH E. GREER, M.D.

Professor of Dermatology, University of Virginia School of Medicine, Charlottesville, Virginia

A. ROSS HILL, M.D.

Fellow in Pulmonary Disease, Department of Internal Medicine, University of Virginia School of Medicine, Charlottesville, Virginia

JOHN W. HOYT, M.D.

Assistant Professor of Anesthesiology; Medical Director, Surgical Intensive Care Unit, University of Virginia School of Medicine, Charlottesville, Virginia

MICHAEL E. JOHNS, M.D.

Associate Professor of Otolaryngology; Director, Head and Neck Oncology Division, University of Virginia School of Medicine, Charlottesville, Virginia

RICHARD P. KEELING, M.D.

Director, Student Health Service, University of Virginia; Assistant Professor of Internal Medicine, Division of Hematology, University of Virginia School of Medicine, Charlottesville, Virginia

JAMES R. KISTNER, M.D.

Assistant Professor of Anesthesiology, University of Virginia School of Medicine, Charlottesville, Virginia

MATTHEW J. LAMBERT III, M.D.

Assistant Professor of Surgery, University of Virginia School of Medicine, Charlottesville, Virginia

BYRD S. LEAVELL, Jr., M.D.

Fellow in Gastroenterology, Department of Internal Medicine, University of Virginia School of Medicine, Charlottesville, Virginia

LINDA L. MARTIN, R.N., M.S.N.

Clinical Nurse Specialist, Department of Nursing, University of Virginia Medical Center, Charlottesville, Virginia

Lt. DOUGLAS L. MAYERS, M.C., U.S.M.C.

U.S. Naval Regional Medical Center, F.P.O. Seattle, Washington

GEORGE R. MINOR, M.D.

Professor of Surgery, University of Virginia School of Medicine, Charlottesville, Virginia

STEVEN A. NEWMAN, M.D.

Assistant Professor of Ophthalmology, University of Virginia School of Medicine, Charlottesville, Virginia

MICHAEL J. OBLINGER, M.D.

Fellow in Gastroenterology, Department of Internal Medicine, University of Virginia School of Medicine, Charlottesville, Virginia

CHARLES A. OSTERMAN, R.N.

Epidemiology Nursing Supervisor, Department of Internal Medicine, Division of Epidemiology, University of Virginia School of Medicine, Charlottesville, Virginia

TED M. PARRIS, M.D.

Senior Resident, Department of Internal Medicine, University of Virginia School of Medicine, Charlottesville, Virginia

JAMES K. POHL, M.D.

Fellow in Pulmonary Division, Department of Internal Medicine, University of Virginia School of Medicine, Charlottesville, Virginia

JOHN C. ROWLINGSON, M.D.

Assistant Professor of Anesthesiology; Director, Pain Clinic, University of Virginia School of Medicine, Charlottesville, Virginia

PAUL M. SURATT, M.D.

Associate Professor, Department of Internal Medicine, Pulmonary Allergy Division, University of Virginia School of Medicine, Charlottesville, Virginia

RICHARD P. WENZEL, M.D.

Professor of Internal Medicine, Division of Infectious Disease, University of Virginia School of Medicine, Charlottesville, Virginia

ARTHUR W. WYKER, Jr., M.D.

Professor of Urology, University of Virginia School of Medicine, Charlottesville, Virginia

Foreword

The advances made in medicine in the past 50 years have been accompanied by a remarkable increase in the number of diagnostic and therapeutic procedures carried out by the physician at the bedside or in the clinic. Most of the procedures are simple, yet all carry significant risks. These risks can be minimized by use of proper technique, awareness of contraindications and potential complications, and appropriate post-procedure care.

The *Manual of Medical Procedures,* prepared by Drs. Suratt and Gibson and their colleagues at the University of Virginia School of Medicine, meets the need for a comprehensive compilation of information on those procedures which are commonly carried out by general and subspecialty internists and family physicians. The step-by-step definition of details of each procedure, with specific recommendations about care before and after the procedure, will prove invaluable for teaching these procedures to students and physicians at all stages of their careers. For more experienced practitioners, the manual will serve as a convenient reference for review. The listing and discussion of complications will be of special value to those responsible for obtaining informed consent for procedures.

This manual will be an important reference and teaching tool for students, physicians, and other members of the health care team, as well as a valuable addition to the working libraries of practitioners at all levels of sophistication.

Edward W. Hook, M.D.

Professor and Chairman,
Department of Internal Medicine,
University of Virginia School of Medicine,
Charlottesville, Virginia

Preface

This book is a manual of procedures that are performed by internal medicine physicians. It has been written specifically for physicians in training but will also serve as a reference for experienced physicians. The book was written because there is no current compact text that describes medical procedures performed by internists. Most medical procedures are taught with the "see one–do one–teach one" method. Although personal instruction is important, this approach tends to perpetuate errors and inadequately deal with the indications and complications associated with each procedure.

All chapters have been written by subspecialists at the University of Virginia Medical Center and are based on both the medical literature and the authors' extensive experience with the procedures. The illustrations were drawn by Dr. William Ober, a practicing physician who has personally performed most of the procedures and who is also an accomplished medical illustrator. An outline format has been used for much of the material to facilitate conciseness and conserve space.

The first two chapters, Aseptic Techniques and Local Anesthesia and Sedation, deal with considerations pertinent to all procedures. The remaining chapters describe what we believe to be the most common important procedures performed by internists. To select these procedures, we relied heavily on the advice of 85 chairmen or spokesmen of internal medicine training programs who were polled by John E. Lotz of The C.V. Mosby Company. Each chapter is divided into several discussions. The General Considerations sections briefly define the procedure and explain how it can be used. They also mention alternative procedures that may be more appropriate for some patients. These are followed by Indications and Contraindications sections. Patient Evaluation and Preparation describes what information or tests should be obtained to determine whether the patient can tolerate the procedure and also lists nursing and medication orders. Next come sections on Personnel and Equipment and Technique. When there are several important technical approaches to a procedure we have described each approach with its advantages and disadvantages. For example, we have described four routes for inserting a balloon flotation (Swan-Ganz) catheter. The Postprocedure Evaluation section lists specific examinations, nursing orders, and laboratory and roentgenographic tests that should be performed following the procedure. Specimen Handling and Specimen Interpretation sections are included when pertinent, for example, in the chapters on thoracentesis, lumbar puncture, and joint aspiration. The Complications section lists complications associated with each procedure, and their frequency is included when known. The last section, References, documents statements in the text and provides sources for further reading.

We wish to thank our authors for their excellent work and patience with us as we continually revised the format of the chapters. We also wish to express our sincere appreciation to our colleagues who critically reviewed portions of the manuscript: Drs. Narinder S. Arora, George A. Beller, Blase Carabello, George B. Craddock, Richard S. Crampton, Thomas J. Gal, Steven K. Goldberg, Dudley F. Rochester, C. Edward Rose, David D. Stone, Munsey S. Wheby, and Edward C. Wilson. Special thanks go to Dr. Edward W. Hook for his encouragement and early support of this project. We wish to thank the chairmen and spokesmen of internal medicine training programs for their thoughtful advice about which procedures to include. We also gratefully acknowledge the continued assistance and advice of John E. Lotz of The C.V. Mosby Company.

Paul M. Suratt
Robert S. Gibson

Contents

PART ONE

ASEPSIS AND ANESTHESIA

CHAPTER 1

Aseptic techniques

■ Charles A. Osterman
Richard P. Wenzel
Paul M. Suratt

■ RECOMMENDATIONS

Percutaneous procedure with no indwelling vascular catheter

1. Wear sterile gloves.
2. Use an iodophor such as a povidone-iodine complex (Betadine) or chlorhexidine, either 4% (undiluted) or 0.5%, in a 70% alcohol solution for an antiseptic agent.
3. Apply the antiseptic at the proposed puncture site and then peripherally in expanding circles with vigorous scrubbing for at least 1 minute.
4. Cover the surrounding unprepared area with draping towels.

Percutaneous procedure with an indwelling vascular catheter

Preparation for catheter insertion

In addition to the steps just described, begin by washing the hands with an antiseptic agent for at least 1 minute and wear a sterile gown, cap, and mask.

Care of the indwelling vascular catheter

1. Daily dressing changes and cleansing the site with an antiseptic are the best ways to prevent infection.[5]
2. Use of antibacterial and antifungal ointments has not been proven beneficial.

■ BACKGROUND DISCUSSION

Handwashing

The two types of organisms colonizing the hand are described as resident and transient. The former survive for long periods and generally do not cause infections. In contrast, the transient flora contain many of the pathogens implicated in nosocomial infections, although they do not survive well on the hands.

In 1938, Price[7] showed that soap and water handwashing for 6 minutes removed 50% of the resident flora, whereas scrubbing with an antiseptic agent reduced the time to 1 minute. In examining transient flora, Lowbury, Lilly, and Bull[6] showed that a 30-second handwash with soap and water reduced experimental contamination from 10^6 to 10^3 organisms, whereas mean counts with antiseptic agents went from 10^6 to 10^2. Recently Sprunt, Redman, and Leidy[8] demonstrated that almost equal results would occur when only friction and water were used to remove transient flora. With the extremely limited data available, the National Center for Disease Control recommends that handwashing with antiseptics be used before performing any invasive procedures.[9]

Repeated use of antiseptics can lead to dermatitis, which may increase skin colonization and shedding of pathogens. Antiseptics are not effective in significantly reducing bacterial counts on hands of people with dermatitis.

Antiseptics[5]

The iodophors (Betadine, Prepodyne, Septo-Dyne, etc.) are effective agents against both gram-negative and gram-positive bacterial organisms, as well as fungal agents, although their activity is transient. Chlorhexidine gluconate (Hibiclens) 4% is rapidly active against gram-negative and gram-positive organisms and has a cumulative and persistent antibacterial effect. Chlorhexidine gluconate 0.5% in 70% isopropanol (Hibitane) offers both the broad-spectrum antimicrobial activity of chlorhexidine and the tuberculocidal and virucidal activity of alcohol. Repeated use of both iodophors and chlorhexidine can lead to skin irritation and dermatitis. Hexachlorophene (pHisoHex) has good cumulative activity against *Staphylococcus aureus*, yet is not very active against the aerobic gram-negative rod organisms that cause 70% of nosocomial infections.

Aseptic technique[1,2]

Sterile disposable gloves should be worn when performing invasive procedures. There are no data, however, on which to base firm conclusions regarding the efficacy of gowns, masks, and caps in reducing infection from these procedures. Data indicate that there are wide variations in efficacy among the masks available, but the best mask can filter out 99% of airborne bacteria and particles for up to 8 hours of continuous use.[3,4]

Care of the indwelling vascular catheter

Although it is popular procedure to keep the area free of obvious dirt and debris, apply antiseptic ointments, and cover the site with a semipermeable bandage, adequate clinical trials supporting the use of antiseptic ointments are lacking. Theoretically the risk of antibacterial agents is that they may select for more resistant pathogens (especially in patients already receiving systemic antibiotics) and organisms that are more difficult to treat, such as fungi.

A study of Jarrard and Freeman[5] in 1977 concluded that thorough antiseptic cleansing of the skin prior to insertion of the central catheter and assiduous care during the insertion are more important than the type of ointments applied to the site once the catheter is in place. They noted that polymyxin B–bacitracin–neomycin (Neosporin), the most widely used antibacterial ointment, selected out for the growth of fungi, particularly *Candida*. Betadine, although more effective against fungi than Neosporin, was less effective against gram-positive organisms and was associated with more gram-positive bacteremias. An attempt to provide Neosporin with fungicidal properties by mixing it with nystatin (Mycostatin) was unsuccessful and failed to supress all skin flora. Jarrard and Freeman suggest that daily subclavian dressing changes along with thorough antiseptic cleansing of the site might reduce the incidence of septicemia associated with catheter use, but cautioned that this may not be practical because of added cost and labor.

REFERENCES

1. Altemier, W.A., Burke, J.F., Pruitt, B.A., and Sandusky, W.R., editors: Manual on control of infection in surgical patients, Philadelphia, 1976, J.B. Lippincott Co.
2. Chlorhexidine and other antiseptics, Med. Letter Drugs Ther. **18:**85-86, Oct. 8, 1976.
3. Dineen, P.: Microbial filtration by surgical masks, Surg. Gyn. Obstet. **133:** 812-814, 1971.
4. Garrow, C., Stephens, L.J., and Ewing, M.R.: Evaluation of surgical masks: the potential of resin-trated wool, Surgery **69:**881-883, 1971.
5. Jarrard, M.M. and Freeman, J.B.: The effects of antibiotics, ointments, and antiseptics on the skin flora beneath subclavian catheter dressings during intravenous hyperalimentation, J. Surg. Res. **22:**521-526, 1977.
6. Lowbury, E.J.L., Lilly, H.A., and Bull, J.P.: Disinfection of hands: removal of transient organisms, Br. Med. J. **II:**230-233, 1964.
7. Price, P.B.: New studies in surgical bacteriology and surgical technique, J.A.M.A. **111:**1993-1996, 1938.
8. Sprunt, K., Redman, W., and Leidy, G.: Antibacterial effectiveness of routine handwashing, Pediatrics **52:**264-271, 1973.
9. Steere, A.C., and Mallison, G.F.: Handwashing practices for hospital personnel, Ann. Intern. Med. **183:**683-690, 1975.

CHAPTER 2

Local anesthesia and sedation

■ Cosmo A. DiFazio

Two major factors make invasive procedures difficult for patients. The first is pain, and the second is fear from not knowing or not completely understanding what is being done. Invasive procedures produce pain and discomfort unless adequate local anesthesia is present. The response to pain will also be further aggravated by fear.

Subcutaneous infiltration of the affected site with a local anesthetic solution will result in an inhibition of excitation of nerve endings and loss of pain perception.[3] The local anesthetic chosen for infiltration anesthesia should be rapid acting and cause as little discomfort as possible. Of the drugs available, lidocaine, mepivacaine, procaine, and bupivacaine best fill these criteria and are widely used. Although the onset of infiltration anesthesia with these agents is almost immediate, the duration of action varies widely, depending on the agent used, concentration used, and whether epinephrine has been added to the injected solution. There is considerable variation of duration from agent to agent (Table 2-1), with procaine being the shortest and bupivacaine the longest acting drug. The concentration used also affects the duration of anesthesia (Table 2-1). A 0.5% lidocaine solution produces a mean duration of anesthesia of 75 minutes, whereas a 1%-solution will produce infiltration anesthesia for 128 minutes. The addition of epinephrine results in decreased absorption from the site injected and prolongation of anesthesia.[3]

Systemic effects from the local anesthetics are directly related to the blood concentration of drug achieved, which in turn is directly related to rapidity of absorption from the site injected. Absorption will vary, depending on the vascularity of

TABLE 2-1. INFILTRATION ANESTHESIA

Agent	Concentration (%)	Duration		
		Plain	Epinephrine added (1:200,00)	Suggested maximum dose (mg/kg)
Procaine	0.5	20 minutes	1 hour	14
Lidocaine	0.5	1 to 1½ hours	3 to 4 hours	7
Lidocaine	1.0	2 hours	6 to 7 hours	7
	1.5	2 to 2½ hours	6 to 7 hours	7
Mepivacaine	0.5	1 hour, 40 minutes	4 hours	7
Bupivacaine	0.25	3 to 3½ hours	6 to 7 hours	2
	0.5	4 to 6 hours	8 to 16 hours	2

the area injected. Epinephrine reduces local tissue blood flow (vascularity) and decreases the likelihood of a systemic toxic reaction. Epinephrine should thus be added to local anesthetic solutions when large volumes (dose) of local anesthetics are to be used. The addition of epinephrine to local anesthetic solutions, however, does result in a solution with a lower pH level, which causes greater local discomfort on injection.

All physicians who use local anesthetics should be aware of maximum safe doses and systemic toxic manifestations of the drug being used. The commonly accepted maximum safe dose of local anesthetic is shown in Table 2-1. These doses, however, need to be significantly decreased if the area being infiltrated is highly vascular (i.e., the nose and hypopharynx), since rapid systemic absorption occurs.

The first major toxic manifestation of high blood levels of local anesthetics is seizures, which may or may not be preceded by a specific drug prodrome. Management of the seizures, if they occur, is best accomplished by the administration of diazepam (Valium)[4] in an intravenous dose of 0.1 to 0.15 mg/kg and careful management of the patient's airway to ensure adequate ventilation.

When local anesthetic concentrations in the blood increase

TABLE 2-2. TOPICAL ANESTHESIA

Agent	Usual concentration (%)	Suggested maximal adult dose (mg)
Lidocaine	2 to 4	200
Cocaine	4 to 10	100
Tetracaine	2	50

to exceedingly high levels (approximately two times that required to produce seizures) cardiorespiratory system toxicity occurs. Respirations become shallow and rapid, and respiratory acidosis develops.[5] Cardiovascular depression also occurs,[6] which is first manifested as hypotension, leading to cardiovascular collapse. Treatment of cardiovascular depression should be directed toward maintenance of respiration and circulation by means of artificial ventilation and vasopressors before collapse occurs. If collapse does occur, cardiopulmonary resuscitation (CPR) should be instituted.

Topical application of local anesthetics is frequently used to produce anesthesia of the nose, hypopharynx, and trachea. The drugs commonly used for this purpose are shown in Table 2-2, along with the suggested maximum doses.[1,2] Generally, the topical application of these drugs in the areas mentioned will result in significantly higher blood levels of drugs than when they are used for subcutaneous infiltration. Such use will therefore have a greater possibility of producing systemic toxicity. The actual blood levels seen are approximately one third to one half those seen when the same drug dose is injected intravenously. Of the topically used local anesthetics, cocaine is unique in that through its effect on blocking norepinephrine reuptake, tachycardia and hypertension frequently result prior to central nervous system excitation as the blood level rises. Cocaine therefore should be used cautiously in the hypertensive patient and in patients who are being treated with monoamine oxidase (MAO) inhibitors. Other factors that require a reduction in dose, regardless of the route of administration, include liver failure, in which the dose of lidocaine, mepivacaine, and bupivacaine must be reduced, and serum cholinesterase deficiencies, in which procaine and tetracaine doses must be reduced to prevent systemic toxicity.

Rapport and sedation of the patient are important whenever extensive interventions are contemplated. Anesthetic agents are used to allay apprehension, produce analgesia where needed, and produce some amnesia for the procedure. In so doing, patient management is facilitated, as is patient acceptance of the procedure. The drug most commonly used is morphine in an intramuscular dose of 0.15 mg/kg or meperidine in an intramuscular dose of 1 mg/kg. Sedation and tranquility can also be produced by barbiturates (1 to 2 mg/kg) or benzodiazapines, such as diazepam (Valium) (0.1 to 0.15 mg/kg IM). The use of narcotic analgesics in patients must be carefully weighed against the potential for inducing hypotension, especially if blood loss has occurred, or if the patient must be moved and allowed to sit or stand. One further potential problem with narcotic use is that these drugs are respiratory depressants and must be used cautiously in patients with evidence of lung disease. The timing for drug administration is also important in that a maximal effect of a drug administerd intramuscularly does not occur for approximately 45 minutes; hence procedures should be scheduled to coincide with peak levels.

REFERENCES

1. Adriani, J., and Campbell, D.: Fatalities following topical application of local anesthetics to mucous membranes (tetracaine, cocaine), J.A.M.A. **162:**1527-1530, 1956.
2. Adriani, J., Zepernick, R., Arens, J., and Authement, E.: The comparative potency and effectiveness of topical anesthetics in man, Clin. Pharmacol. Ther. **5:**49-62, 1964.
3. deJong, R.H.: Local anesthetics, ed. 2, Springfield, Ill., 1977, Charles C Thomas, Publisher.
4. deJong, R.H., and Heavner, J.E.: Diazepam prevents and aborts lidocaine convulsions in monkeys, Anesthesiology **41:**226-230, 1974.
5. Dripps, R.D., and Comroe, J.H.: Clinical studies on morphine, I, The immediate effect of morphine administered intravenously and intramuscularly upon respiration in normal man, Anesthesiology **6:**462-468, 1945.
6. Vandam, L.D.: Clinical pharmacology of narcotic analgesics, Clin. Pharmacol. Ther. **3:**827-838, 1962.

PART TWO

CARDIOVASCULAR PROCEDURES

CHAPTER 3

Pressure monitoring

Robert S. Gibson
James R. Kistner

GENERAL CONSIDERATIONS

The two methods of measuring intravascular pressure require either a water manometer or a strain gauge transducer. Pressure measurements made with a water manometer are often satisfactory for determining central venous pressure. Such measurements tend to produce a mean pressure, since the inertia of the water column prevents the transmission of rapid changes in pressure. Because a continuous phasic display is required for measuring systemic and pulmonary artery pressures and may be desirable for central venous pressures,[4] the strain gauge transducer has largely replaced the water manometer in critical care units. A transducer combined with appropriate electronics and plumbing can provide a continuous reliable display of physiologic pressures. Although increased technology makes available reliable measurements for patient care, the increased complexity creates a greater potential for error.

PRESSURE MONITORING APPARATUS

The complete assembly for pressure monitoring (Fig. 3-1) includes the following: (1) the pressure-sensing catheter, which may be an arterial cannula, central venous pressure catheter, or Swan-Ganz catheter; (2) stiff-walled, noncompliant pressure tubing; (3) a connecting stopcock for blood sampling (sampling stopcock); (4) a flush device (such as the Sorenson Intraflo), which provides continuous irrigation of the catheter with heparinized saline at a rate of 3 ml/hour; (5) a 250- to 500-ml bag of normal saline with one to three units of heparin per milliliter; (6) a pressure bag inflated to 300 mm Hg; (7) standard intravenous tubing to connect the heparin-

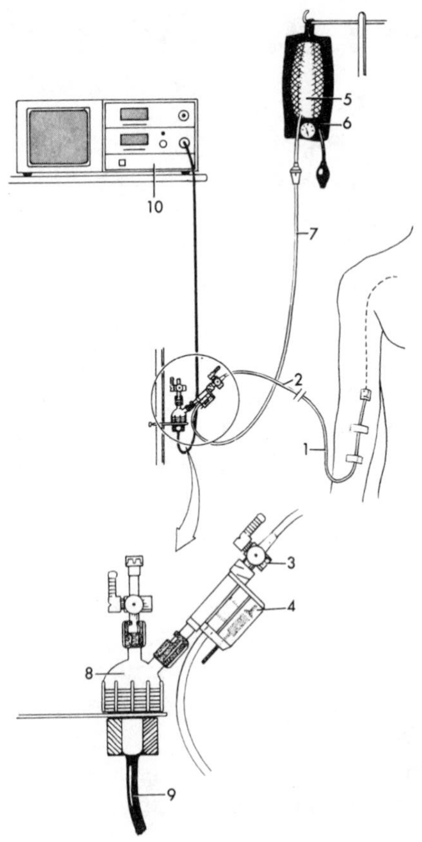

FIG. 3-1. Pressure monitoring system.

ized solution to the flush device; (8) a strain gauge transducer with pressure stopcock; (9) a transducer cable; and (10) the electronic monitor for digital and oscilloscope pressure display.

General guidelines for assembly

1. Use a simple system for all pressure lines. To reproduce pressure variations reliably and avoid distortion, the plumbing system should be short, direct, and free of trapped air bubbles. The catheter–pressure tubing

length must be fairly short (≤4 feet; 122 cm), or it will cause excessive amplification of the transmitted pressure wave.[2] Manifolds and extra stopcocks create unnecessary confusion and serve as good hiding places for air bubbles.

2. Use a continuous flush device to avoid catheter occlusion, small air bubbles, and tiny products of coagulation that will distort the pressure signal.
3. Use a plastic stopcock for blood sampling. Metal stopcocks will leak if they are not periodically cleaned and lubricated or if their washers need replacing.
4. A larger diameter cannula generally gives higher quality tracings. Therefore an 18- to 20-gauge arterial cannula and 7 French Swan-Ganz catheter are preferred over smaller sizes.

Specific guidelines for assembly

1. Connect the plumbing system to the patient catheter after filling the entire system with heparinized saline and removing any air bubbles. The catheter is connected to the pressure tubing, which in turn is connected to the fluid-filled dome that rests on the diaphragm of the transducer (Fig. 3-2). The transducer diaphragm is a thin metal plate that is deformed by pressure waves transmitted through the fluid; beneath it is a mechanism that converts the pressure signal to an electrical signal. The small amperage changes that result are then amplified by the electronic monitor and converted either to a digital display or graphic tracing.
2. Position the pressure stopcock attached to the strain gauge transducer at the atrial level of the patient. In the adult, the atrium is located about 10 cm above the bed or at the midaxillary line.[3] Whichever point is chosen, a line on the patient's chest should be made, so that the same reference point is used for all pressure measurements.
3. Calibrate the transducer. If the electronic monitor has an internal calibration knob (most modern systems do), the calibration constant can be determined by depress-

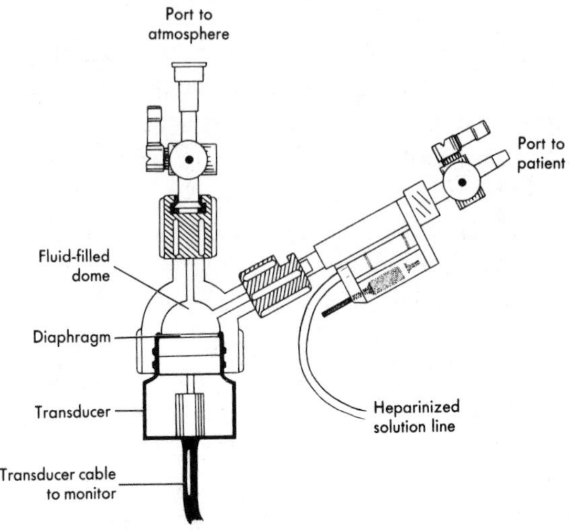

FIG. 3-2. Strain gauge transducer.

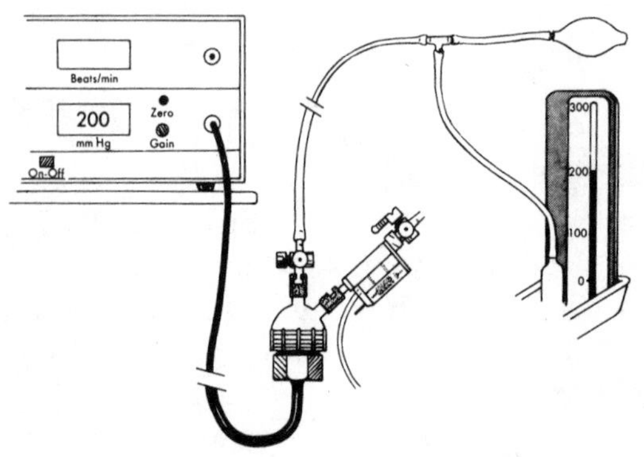

FIG. 3-3. Manometer setup to calibrate transducer.

ing this knob. With older or unchecked modern equipment, use of an external mercury-based calibration standard is advised. Open the transducer to air by turning the pressure stopcock. Adjust the *zero knob* on the electronic monitor, until the digital display reads 0 (this establishes the zero point). Next, using a mercury manometer, pressurize the transducer to 200 mm Hg for arterial readings or 20 mm Hg for venous readings (Fig. 3-3). Last, adjust the *gain knob* on the electronic monitor until the digital display reads 200 (or 20).

NURSING ROUTINE

1. Check to see that the pressure transducer is level with the right atrium before each reading. Optimally, readings should be made with the patient in a horizontal position. Before every reading, the zero point should be checked by opening the transducer to atmospheric pressure.
2. Recalibrate the transducer every 4 hours by using the internal calibration constant. After all calibrations, the oscilloscope gain should be checked. Inappropriate gain settings may make a right atrial trace so pulsatile that it looks similar to a right ventricular trace or may make a phasic pulmonary artery trace almost flat.
3. Recheck the pressure stopcock position, zero point, and calibration when any abrupt change occurs and before any potentially harmful therapy is initiated.

COMMON ERRORS AND ARTIFACTS

1. Respiratory fluctuations. Keep in mind that although atmospheric pressure is used for reference when establishing the zero point and calibrating the transducer, the pressure around the atrium is not truly atmospheric and is affected by intrathoracic pressure. Therefore all pressure measurement should be obtained at end expiration, whether the patient is spontaneously breathing or mechanically ventilated, because the intrathoracic pressure is closest to atmospheric pressure at end expiration. Recall also that the digital display on the monitor may yield an incorrect value, because it is averaging pressure throughout the respiratory cycle. An example of this is depicted in Fig. 3-4. The pulmonary capillary wedge (PCW) pressure varies from 10 to 20 mm Hg, depending on the phase of respiration. The digital display reads 15 mm Hg (average reading), whereas the actual PCW

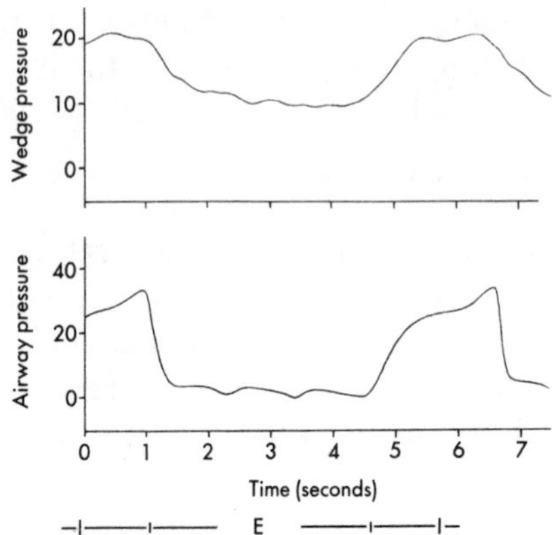

FIG. 3-4. Variation in pulmonary capillary wedge (PCW) pressure due to change in airway pressure (PAW). *I,* Inspiration; *E,* expiration.

pressure at end expiration was 10 mm Hg. To get the most accurate values, PCW and central venous pressure should be taken either from a calibrated strip chart (graphic tracing) or oscilloscope screen.[1]

When evaluating PCW pressure in patients receiving positive end expiratory pressure (PEEP), one must realize that the positive airway and alveolar pressures will, to some extent, increase intrathoracic, pericardial, and atrial pressures.[6,7] This may cause an artificially high PCW pressure. Disconnecting the patient from the ventilator has been advocated by some to minimize this problem but this practice results in a nonsteady state hemodynamic situation with wide swings in venous return and cardiac output. We recommend leaving the patient connected to the ventilator, but recognizing that positive intrathoracic pressure may artificially elevate the measured PCW pressure.

2. Resonance. Resonance refers to a phenomenon caused by a summation of waveforms making up the pressure tracing. It may result from excessive movement of the catheter tip (catheter whip or fling) within the pulmonary artery, resulting in large amplitude changes of cer-

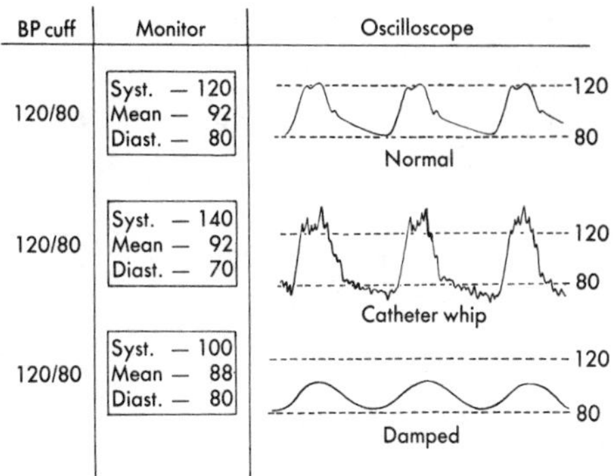

FIG. 3-5. Normal arterial pressure waveform *(top panel)*, catheter fling artifact *(middle panel)*, and overdamping artifact *(bottom panel)*. Cuff blood pressure correlates are shown on left.

tain portions of the pressure tracing. It often leads to transmission of artifactually high systolic pressure and low diastolic pressure to the transducer because of cyclic acceleration and deceleration of the fluid contained within the catheter (Fig. 3-5). Errors of up to 50 mm Hg are possible. Catheter fling artifacts are especially difficult to eliminate in catheterization of the right side of the heart. For arterial pressure measurements using mean pressure instead of systolic pressure will minimize the error.

3. Overdamping. The introduction of even a small amount of blood or a small air bubble in the tubing connecting the intravascular catheter to the pressure transducer often results in overdamping (Fig. 3-5). Systolic pressure reads spuriously low and diastolic pressure spuriously high. The tracing also loses its high frequency characteristics, such as the dicrotic notch, and resembles a sine wave. When damping is observed, the catheter should be flushed and the system, including stopcocks, checked for air bubbles and fibrin debris.
4. Improper catheter tip location in the heart. Positioning a Swan-Ganz catheter tip in a distal pulmonary artery

branch may cause a spuriously high PCW pressure.[5] In such a location, inflation of the balloon may cause occlusion of the catheter tip and result in an artifactually high (up to 15 mm Hg) and damped tracing.

REFERENCES

1. Berryhill, R.E., Benumof, J.L., and Rascher, L.A.: Pulmonary vascular pressure readings at the end of exhalation, Anesthesiology **49:**365-369, 1978.
2. Bruner, J.M.R.: Handbook of blood pressure monitoring, Littleton, Mass., PSG Publishing Co. 1978,
3. Chandraratna, P.A.N.: Determination of zero reference level for left atrial pressure by echocardiography, Am. Heart J. **89**(2):159-162, 1975.
4. Civetta, J.M.: Pulmonary artery pressure determination: electronic superior to manometric, N. Engl. J. Med. **285:**1145-1146, 1971.
5. Meister, S.G., Engle, I.R., Fischer, H.A., et al.: Potential artifacts in measurement of left ventricular pressure with flow-directed catheters, Cathet. Cardiovasc. Diagn. **2:**175, 1976.
6. Quist, J., Pontoppidan, H., and Wilson, R.S.: Hemodynamic responses to mechanical ventilation with PEEP, Anesthesiology **42:**45-55, 1975.
7. Shasby, D.M., Dauber, I.M., Pfister, S., et al.: Swan-Ganz catheter location and left atrial pressure determine the accuracy of the wedge pressure when positive end-expiratory pressure is used, Chest **80:**666-670, 1981.

CHAPTER 4

Venous cutdown

■ **Robert S. Gibson**

■ GENERAL CONSIDERATIONS

Venous cutdown is used to secure entry into the vascular system when percutaneous entry is not possible. It is a reliable and safe technique for administering large volumes of fluid or blood.[2] A saphenous vein cutdown affords rapid vascular access during emergencies.[3,5] The median basilic vein is particularly useful when a central venous pressure (CVP) line, Swan-Ganz catheter, or pacemaker electrode must be inserted in patients with severe pulmonary emphysema, carotid artery disease, or those receiving ventilation therapy.

■ INDICATIONS

Venous cutdown is indicated when percutaneous cannulation techniques are unsuccessful, and access to the venous system is necessary.

■ CONTRAINDICATIONS

1. Phlebitis, previous thrombosis, or vein stripping in the area of intended cutdown.
2. Arterial insufficiency in the area of intended cutdown.

■ PATIENT EVALUATION AND PREPARATION

Explain the procedure to the patient, including its potential complications, and obtain written informed consent.

■ PERSONNEL AND EQUIPMENT

1. A physician skilled in venous cutdown and an assistant.
2. Principal implements.
   a. Venous cutdown: tourniquet, sterile sponges, numbers 11 and 15 scalpel blades, knife handle, two curved and two straight mosquito clamps, one self-

retaining or two small rake retractors, ligatures (3-0 silk), fine-toothed forceps, vein lifter, suture scissors, skin suture, and needle holder.

b. Catheter: Silastic catheter preferred (Deseret Angiocath, or Becton-Dickinson IV Cath) or CVP, Swan-Ganz, or pacemaker catheter.

c. Infusion: intravenous solution, tubing, and stand.

3. Asepsis and sterile field: antiseptic solution; sterile sponges; sterile gloves, mask, and gown; draping towels; and towel clips.
4. Anesthesia: lidocaine (1%, 10 ml), syringe (10 ml), and 23-gauge (1-inch) needle.
5. Dressing: disinfectant ointment, sterile sponges, and adhesive tape (1 inch).

■ TECHNIQUES

Antecubital vein cutdown

1. Place the patient in the supine position with the arm slightly abducted. Immobilize the arm by taping it to an arm board.
2. Locate the basilic vein by applying a tourniquet above the antecubital crease. The basilic vein usually lies 2 to 3 cm above and medial to the epicondyle and runs parallel to the bicipital groove. The basilic vein is preferred because lateral veins (cephalic system) join the subclavian vein at right angles, making passage of a catheter at the shoulder difficult.
3. Prepare the skin and drape a sterile field. Put on sterile gloves and a sterile mask and gown. Prepare the entire antecubital fossae with a disinfectant solution and form a sterile field with draping towels.
4. Anesthetize the skin in the area of the anticipated skin incision. Use 1% lidocaine and a 23-gauge (1-inch) needle. To anesthetize deeper tissue, advance the needle beneath the skin along each side of the vein.
5. Incise the skin and expose the vein (Fig. 4-1, *A*). With the number 15 scalpel, make a 3- or 4-cm transverse skin incision over the vein just above the antecubital

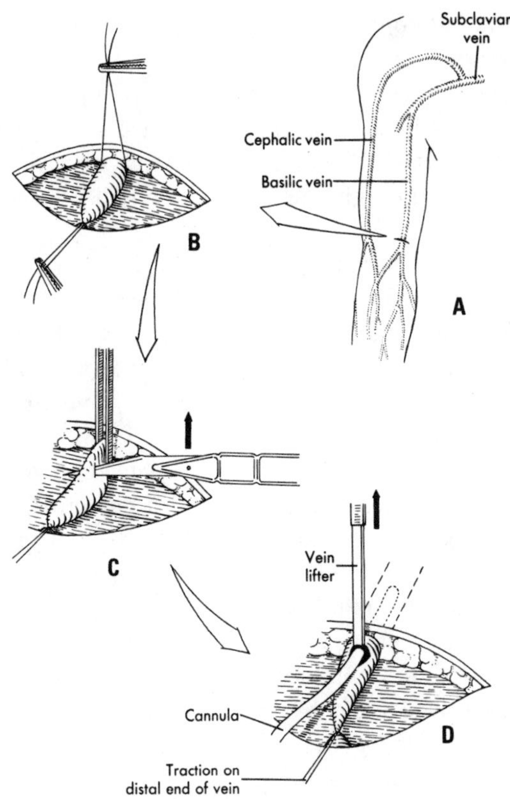

FIG. 4-1. A, Expose antecubital vein. **B,** Place ligature around proximal and distal end of vein. **C,** Perform venotomy. **D,** Insert catheter into vein.

crease and deep enough to expose only the overlying fatty layer. Use a curved mosquito clamp to spread the edges of the incision and to dissect down to the vein. Dissection should be blunt and parallel to the course of the vein so as to lessen the risk of tearing it. Expose 2 or 3 cm of vein.

6. Isolate the vein (Fig. 4-1, *B*). Slide the curved mosquito clamp under the vein and pull a silk ligature back under the vein. Tie the ligature as far distally as possible. Place a second ligature beneath the proximal end of the

vein, but do not tie it. Clip both ligatures with separate straight clamps.

7. Venotomy (Fig. 4-1, *C*). Grasp the vein just distal to the proximal ligature with a fine-tooth forceps and lift the vein upward. Use a number 11 scalpel blade to incise the vein through one third to one half its anterior surface.
8. Catheter insertion (Fig. 4-1, *D*). Place the vein lifter into the proximal venotomy, lift it upward, and expose the lumen of the vein. Slip the venous catheter forward under the vein lifter so that it lies well within the vein. Remove the vein lifter and advance the catheter as far as necessary.
9. Infusion. Attach a 10-ml syringe to the catheter and aspirate to determine whether blood returns and the catheter is in the vein and not lodged against the vessel wall. Remove the syringe and connect the catheter to the intravenous infusion line.
10. Secure the catheter. Tie the proximal ligature around the vein and catheter. It should be tight enough to prevent leakage of blood but not so tight as to constrict the catheter. Tie the distal ligature around the catheter to prevent slippage.
11. Wound closure and dressing. Irrigate the wound with sterile saline and close the incision with 3-0 nylon. Apply a disinfectant ointment and sterile gauze dressing.

Saphenous vein cutdown

Saphenous vein cutdown[3,5] is performed only when very rapid vascular access is needed to administer large volumes of fluid or when the antecubital approach is not feasible.

1. Place the patient in the supine position with the ankle abducted and immobilize the leg.
2. Locate the saphenous vein, which is anterior to the medial malleolus, by applying a tourniquet above the ankle.
3. Prepare the skin with antiseptic solution and drape a sterile field. Put on sterile gloves and a mask and gown.

Prepare the ankle with a disinfectant solution and form a sterile field with draping towels.

4. Anesthetize the vein in the area of the anticipated skin incision. Inject 1% lidocaine into the skin slightly anterior and superior to the medial malleolus. Then, advance the needle beneath the skin along each side of the vein to anesthetize deeper tissues.
5. Incise the skin and expose the vein (Fig. 4-2). Make a superficial 2- or 3-cm transverse skin incision over the vein just above the medial malleolus (Fig. 4-2, *A*). If the

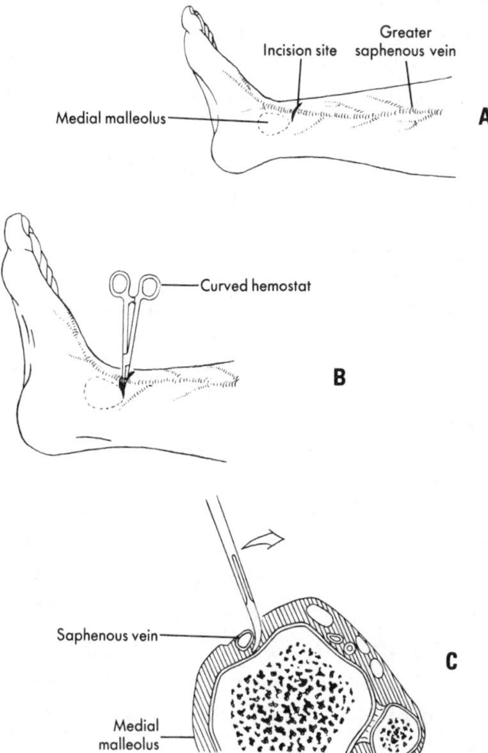

FIG. 4-2. A, Make superficial skin incision just above medial malleolus. **B,** Insert curved mosquito clamp into anterior angle of skin incision. **C,** Curl mosquito clamp under saphenous vein by sweeping it posteriorly. Lift the clamp and vein upward *(arrow)*.

incision is too deep, it will transect the vein. Use a curved mosquito clamp to spread the edges of the incision. Insert a curved mosquito clamp into the anterior angle of the incision (Fig. 4-2, *B*). Push it firmly down to the periosteum. With a sweeping motion, curve the mosquito clamp posteriorly while pressing it against the periosteum (Fig. 4-2, *C*). Curl the clamp completely under the vein and then lift the clamp and vein upward.

6. Isolate the vein. Carefully open the clamp so that the subcutaneous tissue can be spread away from the vein surface. When the vein is exposed, pull a silk ligature back under the vein with the clamp and tie it distally. Slip a second ligature beneath the proximal end of the vein, but do not tie it. Clip both ligatures with separate straight clamps.
7. Follow steps 7 to 11 for antecubital vein cutdown.
8. Stabilize the leg with a leg restraint.

■ POSTPROCEDURE CARE

1. Avoid unnecessary irritating solutions such as high concentrations of potassium chloride.
2. Remove, inspect, and replace the sterile dressing daily.

■ COMPLICATIONS[1,4,6]

1. Damage to adjacent vessels, nerves, and lymphatics.
2. Infection. Infection results from wound contamination and may result in bacteremia. It is prevented by strict asepsis, daily dressing changes, and a short catheter dwell time. An infected catheter should be removed.
3. Phlebitis and thrombosis. The longer the catheter remains in the vein, the higher the frequency of phlebitis. Use of Silastic catheters reportedly decreases this risk.
4. Hematomas. Hematomas may compromise the arterial circulation of the extremity.
5. Inadvertent arterial cannulation. Inadvertent arterial cannulation occurs primarily in patients in shock.

REFERENCES

1. Bogen, J.: Local complications in 167 patients with indwelling venous catheters, Surg. Gynecol. Obstet. **110:**112-114, 1960.
2. Dudrick, S.J., and Daly, J.M.: Performing a safe, successful venous cutdown, Hosp. Physician **10:**34-37, 1974.
3. Kirkham, J.H.: Infusion into the saphenous vein at the ankle, Lancet **2:** 815-817, 1945.
4. Moran, J.M., Atwood, R.P., and Rowe, M.I.: A clinical and bacteriologic study of infections associated with venous cutdown, N. Engl. J. Med. **272:** 554-560, 1965.
5. Randolph, J.: Technique for insertion of a plastic catheter into the saphenous vein, Pediatrics **24:**631-635, 1959.
6. Zinner, S.H. et al.: Risk of infection with intravenous indwelling catheters: effect of application of antibiotic ointment, J. Infect. Dis. **120:**616-619, 1969.

CHAPTER 5

Subclavian vein cannulation

■ Robert S. Gibson

■ GENERAL CONSIDERATIONS

Percutaneous subclavian vein cannulation provides rapid access to a large central vein for the administration of blood or fluids, measurement of central venous pressure (CVP), and for the emergency insertion of a Swan-Ganz or pacemaker catheter. Successful cannulation is possible in 97% of patients, and the complication rate is 0.3% to 9.9%. Compared to internal jugular vein cannulation, subclavian vein cannulation has a slightly higher success rate but a higher frequency of serious complications. Twenty-three different complications and at least sixteen deaths attributable to the procedure have been reported.[1-4]

■ INDICATIONS

1. Rapid administration of blood or fluids in a hypovolemic patient.
2. Total parenteral nutrition. (This is the principal indication in our hospital.)
3. Venous access when peripheral veins are small, thrombosed, or difficult to find.
4. Venous access when the extremities are involved in trauma, burns, or extensive skin lesions.
5. Placement of a temporary cardiac pacemaker, Swan-Ganz catheter, hemodialysis, or plasmapheresis cannula.[5]
6. Central venous pressure monitoring.
7. Administration of medications that cannot be given through peripheral veins, including drugs with potent alpha-constricting properties such as norepinephrine

and high-dose dopamine as well as irritating or hyperosmolar solutions.

■ CONTRAINDICATIONS

1. Anticoagulant therapy or uncorrectable bleeding diathesis.
2. Prior surgery or deforming burns that obcure infraclavicular anatomy.
3. Inability to tolerate a pneumothorax because of severe respiratory disease. The risk of pneumothorax is greatest in patients receiving mechanical ventilation or positive end expiratory pressure (PEEP).

■ ANATOMIC CONSIDERATIONS (Fig. 5-1)

The subclavian vein is a continuation of the axillary vein and is often 2 cm or more in diameter. It is fixed in a constant position by attachments to adjacent fasciae, ligaments, and periosteum beneath the costoclavicular-scalene triangle that is formed by the medial third of the clavicle anteriorly, first rib below, and anterior scalene muscle posteriorly. The subclavian artery and brachial plexus lie superior and posterior to the vein but are separated from it by the anterior scalene muscle. The subclavian vein joins the internal jugular vein to form the innominate vein, which unites with the opposite innominate

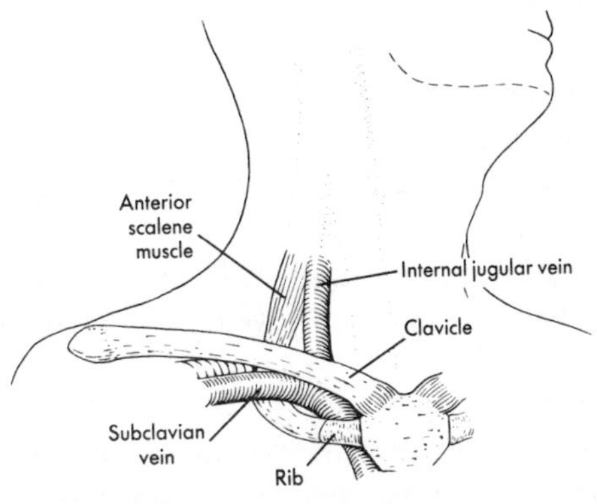

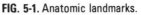

FIG. 5-1. Anatomic landmarks.

to form the superior vena cava behind the right lower half of the manubrium sterni. The phrenic nerve and apical pleura are in contact with the jugular-subclavian junction. No valves are present in the subclavian vein; thus its pressure accurately reflects that of the right atrium. Cannulation of the right subclavian vein is preferred, because puncturing the lower right pleural dome and thoracic duct occurs less frequently compared to left subclavian vein cannulation.

■ PATIENT EVALUATION AND PREPARATION

1. Examine the patient for infraclavicular distortion.
2. Obtain a prothrombin time, partial thromboplastin time, and platelet count.
3. Determine whether the patient can tolerate the Trendelenburg position, which increases venous pressure.
4. Explain the procedure to the patient, including potential complications, and obtain written informed consent.

■ PERSONNEL AND EQUIPMENT

1. A physician skilled in subclavian vein cannulation and an assistant.
2. Principal implements: jugular-subclavian catheter set (14-gauge) (Bard I-CATH) and syringe (6 ml); suture (3-0 silk), needle holder, and suture scissors.
3. Asepsis and sterile field: sterile sponges; antiseptic solution; mask, hair cap, sterile gown, and gloves; and draping towels and towel clips.
4. Anesthesia: a syringe (3 ml) and 23-gauge (1-inch) needle; lidocaine (1%, 10 ml).
5. Infusion: intravenous solution, connecting tubing, and stand.
6. Dressing: sterile sponges; disinfectant ointment; tincture of benzoin; and adhesive tape (1 inch and 3 inch).

■ TECHNIQUE

1. Place the patient in the Trendelenburg position to distend the subclavian vein and lessen the risk of air embolism during cannula insertion. Place a rolled sheet

under the patient's shoulders. Turn the patient's head to the opposite side.

2. Select a site for venipuncture (Fig. 5-1). Usually this is beneath and slightly medial to the midpoint of the clavicle.
3. Prepare the skin and drape a sterile field. Put on a mask, hair cap, sterile gloves, and gown. Prepare the right infraclavicular and suprasternal area with antiseptic solution and form a sterile field with draping towels.
4. Anesthetize the skin and subcutaneous tissue overlying the site of the anticipated venipuncture. Insert the needle slightly medial to the midpoint of, and 1 to 2 cm caudal to, the clavicle, so that the needle will pass under the clavicle.
5. Insert the cannulation needle and intracatheter (Fig. 5-2). Detach the needle from the 14-gauge intracatheter set and connect it to a 6-ml syringe. With the index finger of the left hand in the sternal notch and the thumb along the clavicle, insert the needle through the skin and subcutaneous tissue at the same point used to infiltrate the anesthetic. Advance the needle gently forward while maintaining slight suction. Advance the needle parallel to the anterior chest wall and

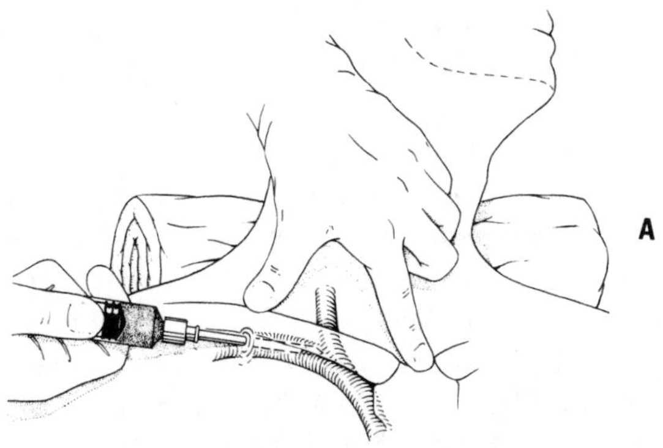

FIG. 5-2. A, Insert cannulation needle. Aim for suprasternal notch. Advance needle as close to underside of clavicle as possible; aspirate.

Continued.

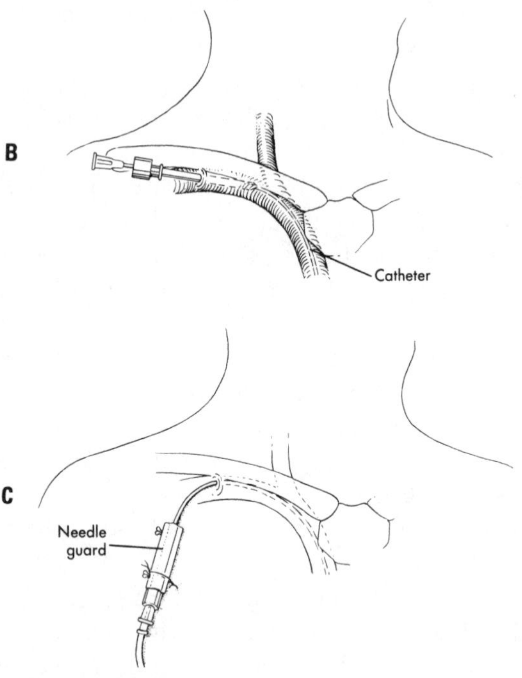

FIG. 5-2, cont'd. B, When venous blood returns freely, remove syringe and slide intracatheter through needle into subclavian vein. **C,** Attach needle guard and lock.

as close to the underside of the clavicle as possible, aiming for the left index finger in the suprasternal notch until blood flows into the syringe. If no blood returns after the needle is fully advanced, withdraw the needle slowly with continuous aspiration. If venipuncture is unsuccessful, remove the needle and reevaluate the landmarks. Once venous blood has been freely aspirated, advanced the needle another 2 or 3 mm, so that its entire beveled tip lies within the vein lumen. Detach the syringe from the needle (occluding its hub with a finger to reduce the risk of air embolism) and then insert the intracatheter through the needle (Fig. 5-2, *B*). Advance the catheter into the superior vena cava.

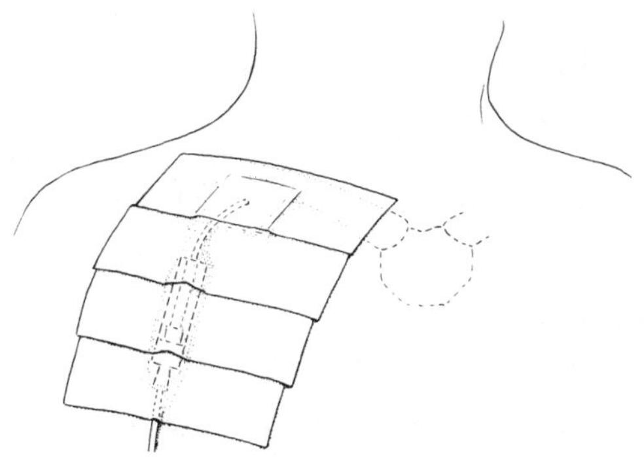

FIG. 5-3. Apply dressing.

6. Remove the cannulation needle carefully from the vein and skin by withdrawing both the needle and catheter as a unit. Do not withdraw the catheter through a stationary needle, since this may shear off the catheter. Attach the needle guard (Fig. 5-2, *C*).
7. Infusion. Connect the proximal catheter to the intravenous tubing set using Luer-Lok connections. Lower the intravenous bottle below the level of the heart to observe whether blood flows back into the tubing. Do not infuse hypertonic solutions (i.e., hyperalimentation solutions) until proper catheter position has been confirmed with a chest roentgenogram.
8. Secure the catheter to the skin with 3-0 silk sutures.
9. Dressing. Apply antiseptic ointment to the puncture site and tincture of benzoin to the surrounding skin. Apply a sterile gauze dressing and tape it securely (Fig. 5-3).
10. Place the patient and bed in a head-up position.

■ POSTPROCEDURE CARE

1. Auscultate both lung fields for symmetric breath sounds.
2. Obtain a chest roentgenogram to check catheter position and look for a pneumothorax.

3. Remove, inspect, and replace the sterile dressing daily. When the subclavian line is used for hyperalimentation, change the dressing three times a week.
4. If fever develops, culture blood peripherally and through the catheter. If no other source is found, remove the catheter.

■ COMPLICATIONS[1-3]

Nonspecific complications of central venous cannulation

1. Infection. Infection results from wound contamination either during insertion or dressing change. It may be associated with bacteremia. Piro[4] cultured catheter tips after removal and found a 9% frequency of positive cultures; 5% were pathogens and the rest were contaminants. Infection is preventable by strict asepsis and short catheter dwell time. An infected catheter should be removed.
2. Phlebitis and thrombosis. Phlebitis and thrombosis are uncommon in large central veins.
3. Air embolism. There are at least seven reported cases of air embolus, in which four patients died.[1] It can occur during insertion of the catheter or long after, when the connections of the catheter are disengaged and air is sucked into the venous system because of negative intrathoracic pressure. The risk of this complication can be minimized by using the Trendelenburg position during the cannulation procedure and Luer-Lok connections.
4. Mediastinal fluid infusion or hydrothorax. Mediastinal fluid infusion or hydrothorax occurs when the cannula is inserted extraluminally and can be prevented by lowering the infusion set below heart level and looking for blood return.
5. Catheter shearing and embolism.

Specific complications of subclavian vein cannulation

1. Pneumothorax. The frequency of pleural puncture varies from 0.5% to 2%, but is higher with unskilled

operators. It can be fatal, especially in patients with severe respiratory disease. A pneumothorax can be partial, total, or of the tension type. Small pneumothoraces may resolve by themselves, but generally chest tube thoracostomy is indicated (Chapter 41). Positive airway pressure should be avoided during needle insertion by removing the patient from the ventilator.

2. Subclavian or innominate artery puncture. The frequency of this complication is as high as 3%. It can be life threatening in the patient with a bleeding dyscrasia. Because of anatomic factors already mentioned, digital compression of the artery after puncture is often useless.
3. Hemothorax. A hemothorax occurs from venous or arterial bleeding through a pleural tear.
4. Hematoma from the puncture site. A hematoma from the puncture site can result from local venous or arterial bleeding.
5. Myocardial perforation. Myocardial perforation occurs when a long rigid polyethylene catheter is advanced to the right-side heart chambers. At least two cases of pericardial tamponade have been reported from this complication.[1]
6. Cannula advancing up the internal jugular vein. This is not always a preventable complication. However, the risk may be lessened by turning the patient's head to the ipsilateral side during cannula advancement, so that the acuteness of the subclavian–internal jugular vein angle is increased. Because of the possibility of this complication, do not infuse vasopressors or hyperalimentation solutions until proper catheter position is confirmed by a chest roentgenogram.
7. Rare complications include pain in the precordial or scapular area; nerve injury (brachial plexus, phrenic, vagus, and recurrent laryngeal nerves); puncture of the trachea, thymus, thyroid gland, and thoracic duct; kinking, knotting, or plugging of the catheter; innominate vein perforation; or subclavian or innominate vein thrombosis.

REFERENCES

1. Borja, A.R.: Current status of infraclavicular subclavian vein catheterization, Ann. Thorac. Surg. **13**:615-624, 1972.
2. Defalgue, R.J.: Subclavian venipuncture: a review, Anesth. Analg. **47**:677-682, 1968.
3. Linos, D.A., Mucha, P., and Van Heerden, J.A.: Subclavian vein: a golden route, Mayo Clin. Proc. **55**:315-321, 1980.
4. Piro, D.F.: Central venous pressure monitoring by percutaneous infraclavicular subclavian vein catheterization, S.D. J. Med. **22**:94-97, 1969.
5. Udall, P.R., Dyck, R.F., Woods, F. et al.: A subclavian cannula for temporary vascular access for hemodialysis or plasmapheresis, Dialysis Transplant. **8**:963-965, 1979.

CHAPTER 6

Internal jugular vein cannulation

Robert S. Gibson
James R. Kistner

GENERAL CONSIDERATIONS

Percutaneous internal jugular vein cannulation provides access to a large central vein for the administration of blood or fluids, measurement of central venous pressure (CVP), and insertion of a Swan-Ganz or pacemaker catheter. Successful cannulation is possible in greater than 90% of patients with a complication rate of 2% to 6%.* Compared to subclavian vein cannulation, it has a lower frequency of serious complications but also a slightly lower success rate.[7] Skill and past experience of the operator may determine whether internal jugular vein cannulation is preferred over subclavian vein cannulation. Compared to venous cutdown, it has a higher success rate and a lower risk of thrombophlebitis.[8,10]

INDICATIONS

1. Rapid administration of blood or fluids in a hypovolemic patient.
2. Need for venous access when peripheral veins are small, thrombosed, or difficult to find.
3. Need for venous access when extremities are involved in trauma, burns, or extensive skin lesions.
4. Placement of temporary cardiac pacemaker or Swan-Ganz catheter.
5. CVP monitoring.[4,13]
6. Administration of medications that cannot be given through peripheral veins. These include drugs with

*References 2, 7, 8, 10, 11, 18, 20.

potent alpha-constricting properties, such as norepinephrine and high-dose dopamine, as well as highly irritating or hyperosmolar solutions.

7. Total parenteral nutrition. Although an internal jugular cannula is acceptable for central hyperalimentation, a subclavian cannula is more stable and easier to dress. This is particularly true in patients with tracheostomies.

■ CONTRAINDICATIONS

1. Uncorrectable bleeding diathesis.
2. Prior surgery or deforming burns that obscure neck anatomy.
3. Carotid artery disease such as plaques in the ipsilateral artery or high-grade obstruction of the contralateral artery. If the carotid artery is inadvertently punctured, a plaque may be dislodged and embolize. Furthermore, therapeutic compression of the carotid artery after puncture may cause neurologic symptoms in patients with a high-grade contralateral carotid stenosis.
4. Inability to tolerate a pneumothorax because of severe respiratory disease. The risk of pneumothorax is greatest in patients receiving mechanical ventilation or positive end expiratory pressure (PEEP).

■ ANATOMIC CONSIDERATIONS (Fig. 6-1)

The internal jugular vein courses down the neck and lies anterolateral to the carotid artery. It runs under the apex of the triangle formed by the two heads of the sternocleidomastoid muscle and joins the subclavian vein behind the clavicle. Its anatomy is relatively constant regardless of body habitus. The right internal jugular vein is preferred because of a higher rate of successful cannulation and a lower risk of puncturing the lower right pleural dome and thoracic duct.

■ PATIENT EVALUATION AND PREPARATION

1. Examine the patient for neck distortion.
2. Obtain a prothrombin time, partial thromboplastin time, and platelet count.

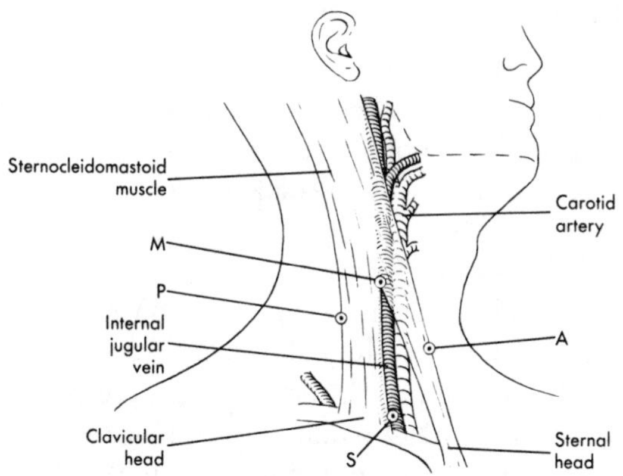

FIG. 6-1. Anatomic landmarks. Common approaches to venipuncture are anterior *(A)*, medial *(M)*, posterior *(P)*, and suprasternal *(S)*.

3. Determine whether the patient can tolerate the Trendelenburg position, which increases venous pressure.
4. Explain the procedure to the patient, including its potential complications, and obtain written informed consent.

■ PERSONNEL AND EQUIPMENT

1. A physician skilled in internal jugular vein cannulation and an assistant.
2. Principal implements: a 21-gauge (1½-inch) seeking needle and syringe (6 ml), 14-gauge subclavian-jugular catheter set (Bard I-CATH) and syringe (6 ml), 3-0 silk, needle holder, and suture scissors.
3. Asepsis and sterile field: sterile sponges; antiseptic solution; sterile gloves and a sterile mask and gown; and draping towels and towel clips.
4. Anesthesia: a syringe (3 ml), 23-gauge (1-inch) needle, and lidocaine (1%, 10 ml).
5. Infusion: intravenous solution, connecting tubing, and stand.
6. Dressing: sterile sponges, disinfectant ointment, tincture of benzoin, and adhesive tape (1 inch and 3 inches).

■ TECHNIQUES

The 18 published techniques for internal jugular vein cannulation can be grouped into four general approaches: anterior, medial, posterior, and supraclavicular (Fig. 6-1). The most widely reported are the medial and posterior approaches.

Medial approach

1. Place the patient in the Trendelenburg position to distend the jugular vein and lessen the risk of air embolism during cannula insertion. Turn the patient's head to the left and place a rolled sheet under the shoulders.
2. Select a site for venipuncture. Locate the right internal jugular vein and carotid artery. Have the patient lift the head from the bed to define the sternal and clavicular heads of the sternocleidomastoid muscle. Mark the apex of the triangle between the two heads (Fig. 6-1). This point should be approximately three finger breadths above the clavicle. Palpate the carotid artery medial to this point to verify its position.
3. Prepare the skin and drape a sterile field. Put on sterile gloves and a sterile mask and gown. Prepare the neck with an antiseptic solution. Form a sterile field with draping towels.
4. Anesthetize the skin overlying the site of anticipated venipuncture. Use 1% lidocaine and a 23-gauge needle. Insert the needle at the apex of the triangle formed by the sternal and clavicular heads of the sternocleidomastoid muscle.
5. Insert the "seeking" needle (Fig. 6-2). Use a 1½-inch 21-gauge needle attached to a 6-ml syringe. Insert the needle at a 30-degree angle to the skin, aiming it at the ipsilateral nipple, and advance it caudally. Maintain syringe suction until dark red blood flows into the syringe, indicating that the vein has been entered. If blood does not return, redirect the needle 5 to 10 degrees medially. When the vein is entered, note the angle and depth of the needle and then remove the needle and syringe, without letting the skin under the left hand move, since

this would change the underlying anatomy.

6. Insert the cannulation needle and intracatheter (Fig. 6-3, *A* and *B*). Use a 14-gauge needle attached to a 6-ml syringe. Insert the needle at the same angle and depth into the vein. Maintain syringe suction until dark red blood flows into the syringe (Fig. 6-3, *A*). Detach the syringe from the needle (occluding its hub with a fin-

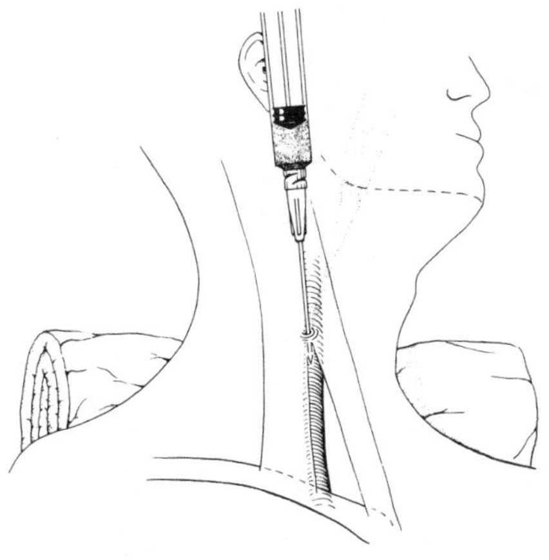

FIG. 6-2. Insert "seeking" needle. Aim for ipsilateral nipple, aspirate.

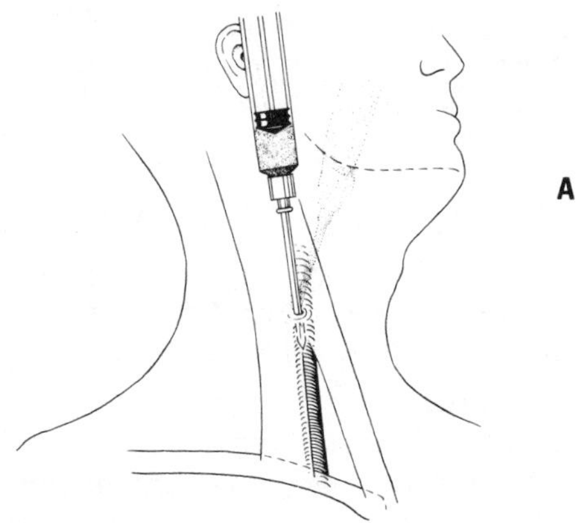

FIG. 6-3. A, Insert cannulation needle at same angle and depth, aspirate.

Continued.

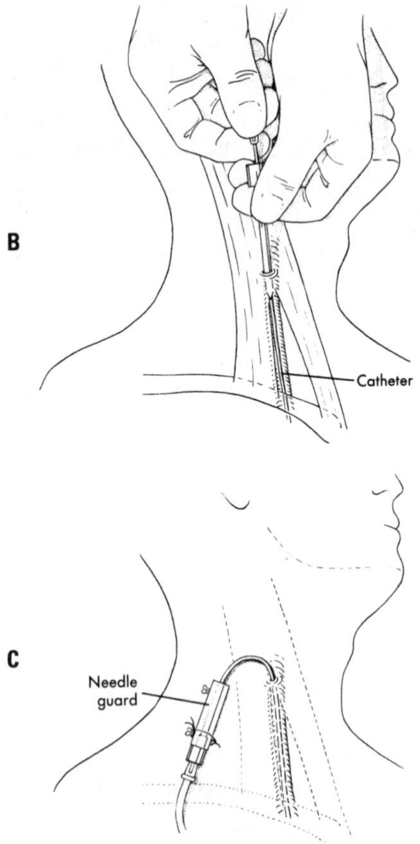

FIG. 6-3, cont'd. B, When venous blood returns freely, remove syringe and slide intracatheter through needle into internal jugular vein. **C,** Withdraw needle from vein; attach needle guard and lock.

ger to reduce the risk of air embolism) and then insert the intracatheter through the needle. Advance the catheter into the internal jugular vein and superior vena cava (Fig. 6-3, *B*).

7. Remove the cannulation needle carefully from the vein by withdrawing both the needle and catheter together as a unit. Do not withdraw the catheter through a stationary needle, since this may shear off the catheter. Attach the needle guard (Fig. 6-3, *C*).

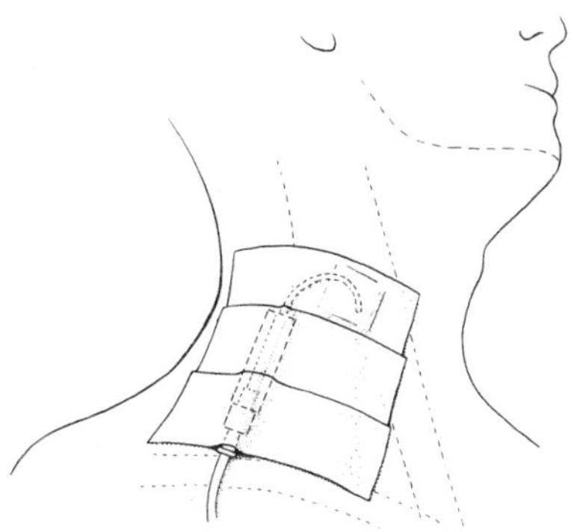

FIG. 6-4. Apply dressing.

8. Infusion. Connect the proximal catheter to the intravenous tubing set using Luer-Lok connections. Document blood return up the catheter by lowering the intravenous bottle below the level of the heart. Do not infuse hypertonic solutions (e.g., hyperalimentation solutions) until proper catheter position has been confirmed with a chest roentgenogram.
9. Secure the catheter to the skin with 3-0 silk sutures.
10. Dressing. Apply disinfectant ointment to the puncture site and tincture of benzoin to the surrounding skin. Apply a sterile gauze dressing and tape it securely. The catheter may be taped along the anterior border of the ear or curved down onto the chest so that the major portion of the dressing is off the neck (Fig. 6-4).
11. Place the patient and bed in a head-up position.

Posterior approach

1. Place the patient in the Trendelenburg position to distend the vein and lessen the risk of air embolism. Turn the patient's head to the left and place a rolled sheet under the shoulders.
2. Locate the right internal jugular vein and carotid artery. Have the patient lift the head up from the bed to define the lateral (posterior) border of the sternocleidomastoid muscle. The point of puncture should be approximately

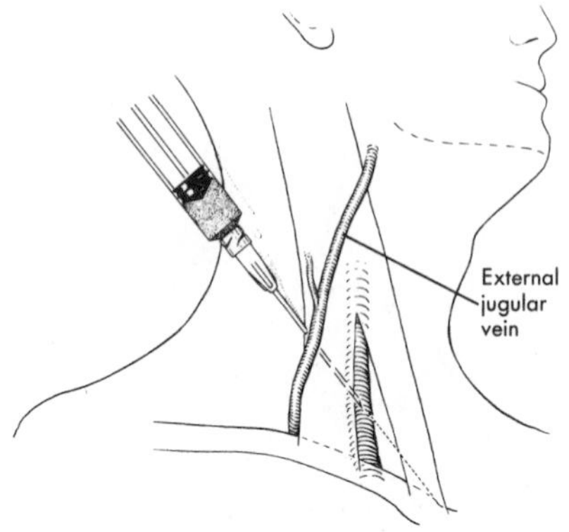

FIG. 6-5. Insert "seeking" needle. Aim for suprasternal notch, aspirate.

5 cm above the clavicle or just above where the external jugular vein crosses the muscle (Fig. 6-1). Palpate medial to this point to verify the position of the carotid artery.

3. Follow step 3 of the medial approach.
4. Follow step 4 of the medial approach, except insert the needle 5 cm above the clavicle at the posterior border of the sternocleidomastoid muscle (Fig. 6-1).
5. Insert the "seeking" needle using a 21-gauge needle attached to a 6-ml syringe (Fig. 6-5). Insert the needle at a 30-degree angle to the skin and advance it caudally. Aim the needle at the suprasternal notch. Maintain syringe suction until dark red blood flows into the syringe, indicating that the vein has been entered. If blood does not return after the needle is fully advanced, withdraw it slowly, and occasionally blood will then flow into the syringe. If the vein has still not been entered, remove the needle, reevaluate the landmarks, and try again. When venous blood is aspirated, note the angle and depth of the needle and then remove the needle and syringe.
6. Follow steps 6 to 11 in the medial approach, except insert the cannulation needle and intracatheter as indi-

cated in Fig. 6-5 and aim the needle at the suprasternal notch.

■ POSTPROCEDURE CARE

1. Auscultate both lung fields for symmetric breath sounds.
2. Obtain a chest roentgenogram to confirm proper catheter position and look for a pneumothorax.
3. Check for a hematoma.
4. Remove, inspect, and replace the sterile dressing daily.

■ COMPLICATIONS

Nonspecific complications of central venous cannulation

1. Infection. Infection results from wound contamination either during insertion or dressing change. It may be associated with bacteremia. It is preventable by strict asepsis and short catheter dwell time. An infected catheter should be removed.
2. Phlebitis and thrombosis. Phlebitis and thrombosis are uncommon in large central veins.
3. Air embolism. Air embolism can occur during insertion of the catheter or long after, when the connections of the catheter are disengaged and air is sucked into the venous system because of negative intrathoracic pressure. The risk of this complication can be minimized by using the Trendelenburg position during the cannulation procedure and Luer-Lok connections.
4. Mediastinal fluid infusion or hydrothorax.[15] Mediastinal fluid infusion or a hydrothorax occurs when the cannula is inserted extraluminally and can be prevented by lowering the infusion set below heart level and by looking for blood return.
5. Catheter shearing and embolism.

Specific complications of internal jugular puncture

1. Pneumothorax. The frequency of pleural puncture is less than 1%,[8,10,18] but when it occurs the results can be serious.[1,5] Positive airway pressure should be avoided

during needle insertion by removing the patient from the ventilator.

2. Carotid artery puncture. Carotid artery puncture occurs in 1% to 5%[2,8,10] of procedures. It rarely causes problems and should be treated by compression for at least 5 to 10 minutes. Serious problems, including hematomas requiring surgical removal or tracheal compression, have been reported.[3,17]
3. Thoracic duct injury. Thoracic duct injury can occur if the left jugular vein is used. Chylothorax requiring surgical treatment has been reported.[9,14]
4. Nerve damage. The Horner syndrome, phrenic nerve injury, vagal injury, and brachial plexus damage have been reported.[19]
5. Puncture of the trachea and an endotracheal tube cuff.[1]
6. Neck tenderness. Neck tenderness occurs in as many as 34% of the patients and is treated symptomatically.
7. Failure of cannulation or catheter malposition. Successful cannulation cannot be accomplished in 3% to 7%* of patients, and the catheter is not placed in a satisfactory central vein in 1% to 6%.[6,9,12,16]

REFERENCES

1. Arnold, S., Feathers, R.S., and Gibbs, E.: Bilateral pneumothoraces and subcutaneous emphysema: a complication of internal jugular puncture, Br. Med. J. **1**:211-212, 1973.
2. Brinkman, A.J., and Costley, D.O.: Internal jugular venipuncture, J.A.M.A. **223**:182-183, 1973.
3. Brown, C.S., and Wallace, C.I.: Chronic hematoma: a complication of percutaneous catheterization of the internal jugular vein, Anesthesiology **45**:368-369, 1976.
4. Cohn, J.N., Tristani, F.E., and Khatri, I.M.: Studies in clinical shock and hypotension: relationship between left and right ventricular function, J. Clin. Invest. **48**:2008-2018, 1969.
5. Cook, I.L., and Ducket, C.W.: Tension pneumothorax following internal jugular cannulation and general anesthesia, Anesthesiology **45**:554-555, 1976.
6. Daily, P.O., Griepp, R.B., and Shumway, N.E.: Percutaneous internal jugular vein cannulation, Arch. Surg. **101**:534-536, 1970.
7. Defalgue, R.J.: Percutaneous catheterization of the internal jugular vein, Anesth. Analg. **53**:116-121, 1974.

*References 2, 8, 10, 18, 20.

8. English, I.C., Frew, R.M., Pigott, J.I., et al.: Percutaneous catheterization of the internal jugular vein, Anesthesia **24:**521-531, 1969.
9. Fisher, J., Lundstrom, J., and Ottander, H.G.: Central venous cannulation: a radiological determination of catheter positions and immediate intrathoracic complications, Acta. Anaesthesiol. Scand. **21:**45-49, 1977.
10. Jernigan, W.R., Gardner, W.C., Mahr, M.E. et al.: Use of the internal jugular vein for placement of central venous catheter, Surg. Gynecol. Obstet. **130:**520-524, 1970.
11. Kaplan, J.A., and Miller, E.D.: Internal jugular vein catheterization, Anesthesiol. Rev., May, 1976, pp. 21-23.
12. Kellnor, G.A., and Smart, J.F.: Percutaneous placement of catheters to monitor "central venous pressure," Anesthesiology **36:**515-516, 1972.
13. Kelman, G.R.: Interpretation of CVP measurements, Anaesthesia **26:**209-215, 1971.
14. Khalil, K.G., Parker, F.B., Mukherjee, N. et al.: Thoracic duct injury: a complication of jugular vein catheterization, J.A.M.A. **221:**908-909, 1972.
15. Koch, M.J.: Bilateral "IV hydrothorax," N. Engl. J. Med. **286:**218, 1972.
16. McConnel, R.Y., and Fox, R.T.: Experience with percutaneous internal jugular-innominate catheterization, Calif. Med. **117:**1-6, 1972.
17. McEnany, M.I., and Austen, W.G.: Life threatening hemorrhage from inadvertent cervical arteriotomy, Ann. Thorac. Surg. **24:**233-236, 1977.
18. Mosert, J.W., Kenny, G.M., and Murphy, G.P.: Safe placement of central venous catheter into internal jugular veins, Arch. Surg. **101:**431-432, 1970.
19. Parikh, R.K.: Horner's syndrome: a complication of percutaneous catheterization of the internal jugular vein, Anesthesia **27:**327-329, 1972.
20. Vaughan, R.W., and Weygandt, G.R.: Reliable percutaneous central venous pressure measurement, Anesth. Analg. **52:**709-716, 1973.

CHAPTER 7

Arterial cannulation

■ **Robert S. Gibson**

■ GENERAL CONSIDERATIONS

Arterial cannulation is the most accurate method of measuring blood pressure. Indirect determinations by sphygmomanometers, Doppler instruments, or plethysmographs may underestimate blood pressure in patients who are massively obese, hypothermic, hypotensive, severely hypertensive, or peripherally vasoconstricted.[5,13]

■ INDICATIONS

1. Hypotension. It is well-documented[5,13] that in shock, indirect determination of blood pressure by sphygmomanometer may underestimate the true blood pressure by more than 60 mm Hg.
2. Accelerated hypertension with evidence of progressive vascular damage. The clinical syndrome of accelerated or "malignant" hypertension[8] includes (1) the presence of progressive central nervous system symptoms such as headache, nausea, vomiting, and visual difficulties, which may progress to seizures and coma; (2) proteinuria and cellular elements in the urine, including red blood cells and casts; (3) funduscopic findings such as fresh hemorrhage, exudates, and papilledema; (4) left-side ventricular failure; and (5) evidence of acute destruction of blood vessels with red blood cell injury and microangiopathic hemolytic anemia. The magnitude of blood pressure elevation, for example, diastolic blood pressures of greater than 130 mm Hg, should not be used as a criterion for accelerated hypertension because the clinical syndrome can occur at lower blood pressures, and some patients with essential hypertension may have chronically elevated blood pressure without apparent vascular damage.

3. To monitor the effects of potent vasoactive agents such as intravenous nitroprusside, trimethaphan, nitroglycerin, epinephrine, norepinephrine, and moderate or high doses of isoproterenol and dopamine.
4. During major abdominal, thoracic, or vacular surgery in patients with significant cardiovascular diseases.[10]
5. Rarely in patients with limited vascular access who require frequent blood gas analysis.
6. To measure cardiac output by the Fick oxygen method.

■ CONTRAINDICATIONS

1. Inadequate collateral circulation.[1,11]
2. Inadequate monitoring of equipment or inadequate nursing support. A tubing disconnection can be fatal (Chapter 3).
3. Severe aortoiliac atherosclerosis when using the femoral artery. A subintimal dissection is common in this situation.

■ ANATOMIC CONSIDERATIONS AND CHOICE OF VESSEL (Fig. 7-1)

1. *Radial artery.* We prefer this artery because it is easily cannulated and stabilized, and the collateral circulation is usually adequate and easy to check. At the wrist, the radial artery lies just lateral to the tendon of the flexor carpi radialis at the base of the thenar eminence. The presence of collateral circulation to the hand from the ulnar artery should be checked with an Allen test.[1,11]
2. *Dorsalis pedis artery.* This artery is a reasonable alternative to radial artery cannulation; however, it may be absent in 5% to 12% of normal patients.[3,14] It is the distal continuation of the anterior tibial artery and can be palpated between the extensor hallucis longus and the extensor digitorum longus on the dorsum of the foot. The presence of collateral flow to the foot from the lateral palmar artery via the posterior tibial artery should be checked.[14]
3. *Femoral artery.* The femoral artery is the easiest artery

to cannulate, but has a greater risk of serious vascular complications. With experience, however, prolonged femoral artery cannulation can be accomplished without major complications.[6] The artery begins below the inguinal ligament as the continuation of the external iliac artery. It can be palpated midway between the pubic symphysis and the anterosuperior iliac spine. The femoral artery (A) lies between the laterally located femoral nerve (N) and the medially located femoral vein (V). A useful mnemonic for these structures is "NAV." Prior to cannulation, the vascular integrity of the extremity should be assessed.[6]

4. *Ulnar artery*. Occasionally, the regular Allen test demonstrates radial artery dominance.[8] In this instance, it may

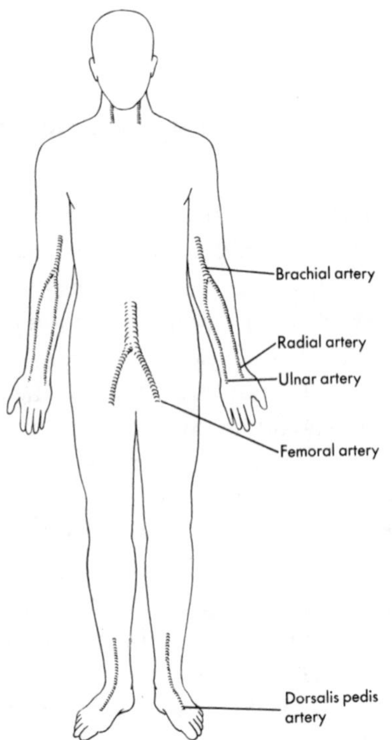

FIG. 7-1. Choice of vessel.

be preferable to cannulate the ulnar artery. At the wrist, the ulnar artery lies between the tendons of the flexor carpi ulnaris and the flexor digitorum superficialis at the base of the hypothenar eminence.

5. *Brachial artery*. We rarely use this artery for cannulation because of its propensity to develop vasospasm. In one series, the brachial artery was shown to have a 17% frequency of obstruction after cardiac catheterization.[2] It is also subject to high bifurcations and, occasionally, a double brachial artery may envelope the median nerve. Generally, it lies lateral to the basilic vein and the median nerve at the elbow. Its pulsation can be felt just above the antecubital fossa at the medial insertion of the biceps tendon.

■ PATIENT EVALUATION AND PREPARATION

1. Evaluate collateral or distal circulation. If the radial artery is chosen, perform an Allen test[1,11] (Fig. 7-2). Simultaneously occlude the radial and ulnar arteries with the thumbs, while having the patient repeatedly clench a fist until the hand blanches. Then, allow the patient's hand to remain in an open relaxed position. While compressing the radial artery, release the ulnar artery and observe the color of the hand. Prevent the patient from overextending the wrist, otherwise an abnormal result will be produced by occlusion of the transpalmar arch under the flexor retinaculum.[7] Adequate collateral circu-

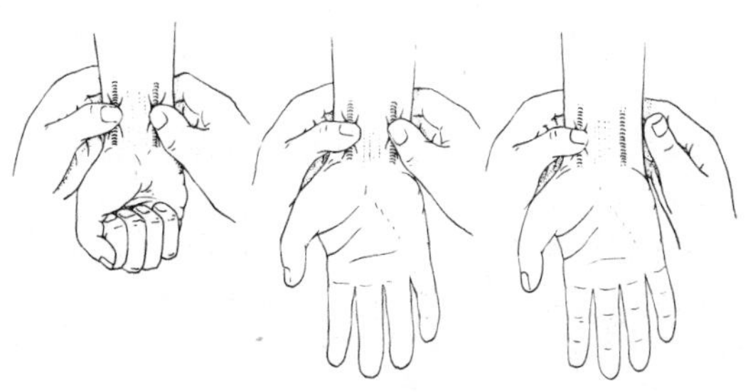

FIG. 7-2. Perform Allen test to evaluate collateral circulation.

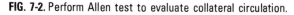

lation is demonstrated by the appearance of an erythematous flush within 5 to 10 seconds. If the hand does not regain its color within 10 seconds, we consider it unsafe to cannulate the radial artery. Repeat the test but release the radial artery instead of the ulnar artery. If a palmar flush appears within 10 seconds and the ulnar pulsation is easily felt, consider ulnar artery cannulation. If the dorsalis pedis artery is chosen,[14] occlude both the dorsalis pedis and posterior tibialis artery (behind the medial malleolus) and blanch the great toe by having an assistant compress it. On release of the posterior tibialis artery, if the great toe does not flush within 10 seconds, do not proceed with cannulation. If the femoral artery is chosen, evaluate the vascular integrity of the extremity by eliciting symptoms of claudication, auscultating for bruits, and checking the strength of the distal pulses.

2. Assemble and calibrate the pressure monitoring equipment (Chapter 3).
3. Explain the procedure to the patient, including potential complications, and obtain written, informed consent.

■ PERSONNEL AND EQUIPMENT

1. A physician skilled in arterial cannulation and an assistant.
2. Principal implements.
   a. Arterial access and catheter. For radial, ulnar, and dorsalis pedis arteries: 18- or 20-gauge nontapered Teflon catheter (Deseret Angiocath, Becton-Dickinson IV Cath, or Critikon Cathlon IV), suture scissors, skin suture, and a needle holder. For the femoral artery: a Potts-Cournand needle with a cutting obturator, a 4 to 6 French percutaneous catheter introducer set (UMI or Cordis), a number 11 scalpel blade and knife handle, one straight mosquito clamp, suture scissors, a skin suture, and a needle holder. If the Seldinger technique is not employed, use a 5-inch 18-gauge Teflon catheter.
   b. Pressure monitoring: arterial pressure transducer and cable, calibrated oscilloscope, nondistensible

pressure tubing, and three-way stopcock (Chapter 3).

   c. Flushing apparatus: the catheter should be flushed with heparinized saline (1 to 3 units/ml) at least every 30 minutes. A device is available to do this automatically (Sorenson Intraflo) (Chapter 3).

3. Asepsis and sterile field: antiseptic solution, sterile sponges, a mask, hair cap, sterile gloves and gown, draping towels, and towel clips.
4. Anesthesia: lidocaine (1%, 10 ml), syringe (10 ml), and 23-gauge (1-inch) needle.
5. Dressing: antiseptic ointment, sterile sponges, adhesive tape or Elastoplast, and an arm board or ankle restraint.

■ TECHNIQUES

Radial artery cannulation

1. Position the nondominant hand by hyperextending it over a wrist roll (pack of sponges). Immobilize the hand and lower arm by taping both to an arm board (Fig. 7-3).
2. Determine the course of the radial artery by palpation. The puncture site is just proximal to where the vessel enters the carpal tunnel.
3. Put on a mask, hair cap, and sterile gloves and gown. Prepare the skin with an antiseptic solution and form a sterile field with draping towels.

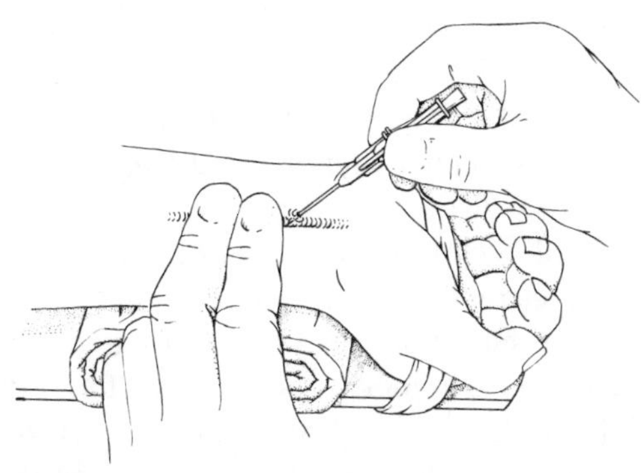

FIG. 7-3. Hyperextend hand over wrist roll; immobilize hand and lower arm.

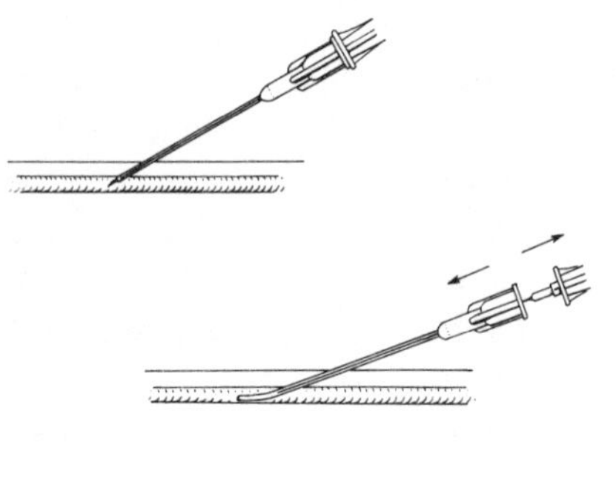

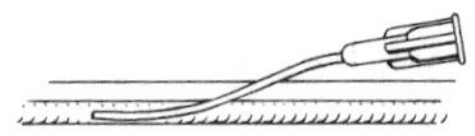

FIG. 7-4. Insert angiocatheter through skin; cannulate artery.

4. Anesthetize the skin but do not obscure the artery by injecting an excessive amount of anesthetic.
5. Insert the angiocatheter through the skin at a 30- to 45-degree angle to the skin and advance it parallel to the course of the artery (Fig. 7-4). When blood begins to drip from the needle hub, depress the needle slightly so that the angle between the skin and needle is 15 degrees. Withdraw the needle while threading the outer catheter into the vessel lumen and off the needle. The catheter should advance easily; if it does not, it is not in the vessel lumen and may be dissecting the intima. Withdraw the needle and catheter and begin again. A catheter that develops kinks at its end should be discarded. If blood should stop dripping after entering the vessel, the needle has penetrated the back wall. Remove the needle and slowly pull back the catheter until a spurt of blood occurs and then advance the catheter up the artery.
6. Attach pressure tubing. Attach a syringe to the catheter and aspirate to remove any clot and to confirm good blood flow. Detach the syringe and connect the catheter to the pressure tubing and functioning irrigation system (Chapter 3).

7. Secure the catheter to the skin with a silk ligature. Secure the connection between the catheter hub and the pressure tubing with ½-inch adhesive tape to prevent accidental disconnections.
8. Dressing. Take the wrist out of the hyperextended position to avoid median nerve damage. Clean the area and apply a disinfectant ointment to the puncture site. Place a sterile dressing and secure it with 1-inch (2.5-cm) adhesive tape. Position the arm so that it is comfortable for the patient. Limit movement of the wrist by splinting the dorsal aspect to maintain catheter stability.

Ulnar and dorsalis pedis artery cannulation

We use the same technique and equipment to cannulate these vessels as for the radial artery.

Percutaneous femoral artery cannulation

1. Place the patient in a supine position and rotate the foot outward. This maneuver will open the inguinal triangle and often separates the femoral artery from the vein and avoids simultaneous puncture of both vessels.
2. Palpate the femoral pulse and determine the site for arterial puncture (Fig. 7-1). This should be well below the inguinal ligament, since hemorrhage and hematoma formation may occur in the retroperitoneal space from puncture of the back wall of the femoral artery. A safe puncture site is usually 1 or 2 inches (2.5 to 5 cm) below the inguinal crease.
3. Put on a mask, hair cap, sterile gloves, and gown. Prepare the skin with an antiseptic solution and form a sterile field with draping towels.
4. Anesthetize the skin and subcutaneous tissue.
5. Make a small skin incision (nick) through the dermis over the arterial pulsation with a number 11 scalpel blade. Use a straight mosquito clamp for deeper blunt dissection to facilitate passage of the catheter through the subcutaneous tissue.
6. Insert the Potts-Cournand needle through the skin

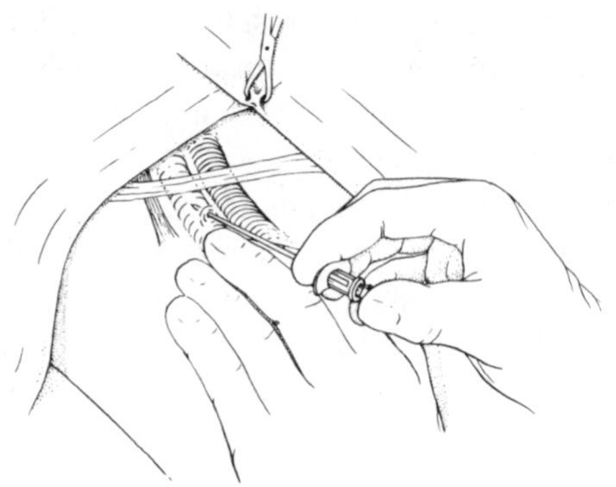

FIG. 7-5. Insert Potts-Cournand needle into femoral artery.

nick and subcutaneous channel at a 60-degree angle to the skin (Fig. 7-5). Advance both the needle and cutting obturator until a "give" is felt. This indicates penetration into the artery. If a "give" is not felt, advance to the hilt or until resistance is felt. Remove the obturator and, if necessary, slowly withdraw the needle until arterial blood spurts from the needle hub. Place a gloved thumb over the needle hub to prevent loss of more than a few milliliters of blood.

7. Insert the catheter, using the Seldinger technique (Fig. 7-6). Depress the hub of the Potts-Cournand needle slightly and insert the soft flexible end of the guidewire through the lumen of the needle (Fig. 7-6, *A*). Gently advance the guidewire approximately 15 cm. If resistance is encountered, remove the guidewire from the artery and needle and use a 3-mm J-tip wire (USCI 007054) to bypass the obstruction. Remove the needle, leaving the guidewire in the artery (Fig. 7-6, *B*). Slide the vessel dilator and catheter over the guidewire and advance them as a unit to skin level (Fig. 7-6, *C*). If the guidewire does not protrude out from the distal end of the dilator catheter, withdraw it from the artery so that it does. Firmly rotate the dilator-catheter unit close to the skin, while advancing both over the guidewire,

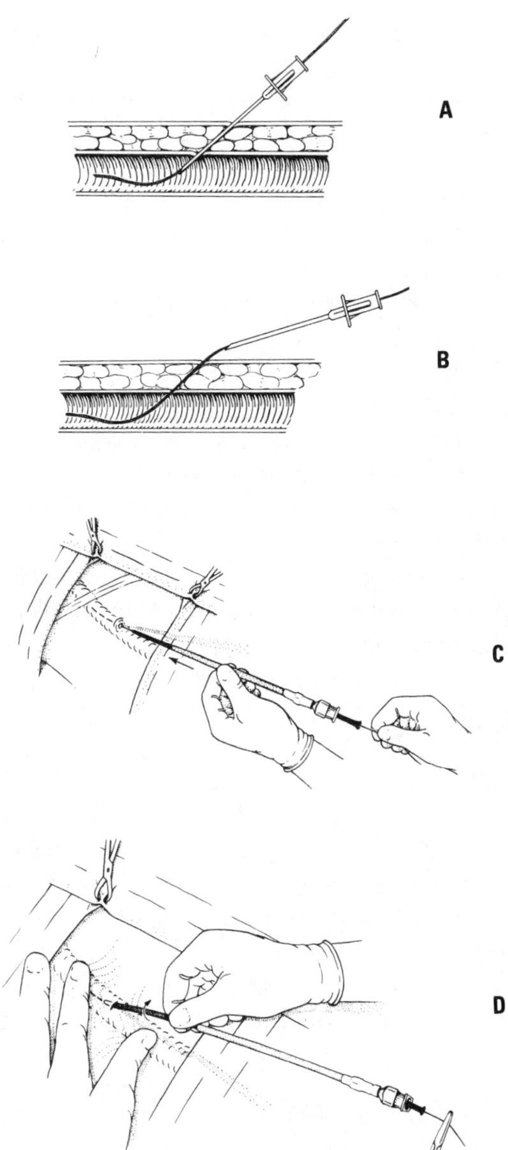

FIG. 7-6. A, Insert guidewire through Potts-Cournand needle. **B,** Remove Potts-Cournand needle from artery. **C,** Advance vessel dilator and catheter over guidewire to skin level. **D,** Cannulate artery by rotating dilator-catheter unit close to the skin, while advancing both over the guidewire.

through the subcutaneous channel, and into the arterial lumen (Fig. 7-6, *D*). The dilator-catheter unit should be advanced until its distal end reaches skin level. Remove both the guidewire and dilator through the catheter.

8. Attach pressure tubing. Attach a syringe to the catheter and aspirate to remove any clot and to confirm good blood flow. Detach the syringe and connect the catheter to the pressure tubing and functioning irrigation system (Chapter 3).
9. Secure the catheter to the skin with a silk ligature to prevent slipping. Secure the connection between the catheter hub and the pressure tubing with ½-inch adhesive tape to prevent accidental disconnections. Position the leg comfortably and limit movement with an ankle restraint.
10. Dressing. Cleanse the area and apply disinfectant ointment to the puncture site. Apply tincture of benzoin to the surrounding skin. Apply a sterile dressing and secure it with 3-inch adhesive tape or Elastoplast.

■ CATHETER REMOVAL

Withdraw the catheter and apply firm, digital pressure to the puncture site for at least 10 to 15 minutes. The pulse at and/or distal to the puncture site should be palpable after 1 or 2 minutes of compression to ensure that the vessel is not being occluded by the compression. It may be necessary to apply digital pressure for more than 15 minutes if the patient has aortic regurgitation, hypertension, or a bleeding diathesis. When the bleeding is stopped, apply a nonconstricting bandage.

■ POSTPROCEDURE CARE

1. Keep the arterial line patent by using an irrigation system (Sorenson Intraflo device) and a continuous infusion of heparinized saline. This minimizes thrombus formation and helps prolong catheter function.
2. Observe the patient for signs of arterial insufficiency,

local infection, and hematoma. If any of these complications occur, remove the catheter immediately.

3. Remove, inspect, and replace the sterile dressing daily.

COMPLICATIONS[4,9,12]

1. Thombosis and occlusion of the vessel occur in 0.5% to 38% of procedures and increases with the duration of cannulation. This complication can be minimized by using small-diameter, nontapered Teflon catheters. A Fogarty embolectomy catheter can be used to remove thrombi.
2. Arterial spasm and occlusion of the vessel occur in approximately 8% of procedures. The frequency of this complication is higher for brachial artery cannulation.
3. Digital ischemia. Digital ischemia results from diminished flow to the hand or foot and is most commonly seen in patients in shock or who have poor collateral circulation. Finger ischemia is minimized by documenting a normal response to the Allen test. If shock exists, the benefits of the procedure should be weighed against the possible complications of ischemia.
4. Hematoma due to bleeding at the puncture site occurs in 9% to 83% of procedures. It is caused by a faulty insertion technique or inadequate application of local pressure following catheter removal. If large, a hematoma may compromise the arterial circulation of the extremity.
5. Pain at the cannula insertion site occurs in 17% of procedures.
6. Arterial embolism. A clot formed at the site of the cannula insertion may embolize to the distal extremity in 0.5% to 30% of procedures. Retrograde flushing of the cannula may embolize the clot proximally. Cerebral emboli may occur but are very rare. Continuous irrigation with heparinized solutions to maintain catheter patency minimizes the risk of clot embolism.
7. Infection. Infection results from wound contamination, occurs with a frequency of up to 4%, and may result in

bacteremia. It is minimized by strict asepsis, daily dressing changes, and a short catheter dwell time.

8. Bleeding from the arterial line. Massive bleeding may result if a tubing disconnection occurs. It can be fatal. All tubing connections should be taped, and the patient should not be left unattended.

9. Arteriovenous fistula, skin necrosis due to interference of blood flow by the catheter, aneurysm formation, and subintimal dissection are all very rare.

REFERENCES

1. Allen, E.V.: Thromboangiitis obliterans: methods of diagnosis of chronic occlusive arterial lesions distal to the wrist, Am. J. Med. Sci. **178:**237-244, 1929.
2. Barnes, R.W. et al.: Complications of brachial artery catheterization: prospective evaluation with the Doppler ultrasonic velocity detector, Chest **66:**363-367, 1974.
3. Barnhorst, B.A., and Boener, H.B.: Prevalence of generally absent pedal pulses, N. Engl. J. Med. **278:**264-265, 1968.
4. Bedford, R.F., and Wollman, H.: Complications of percutaneous radial-artery cannulation: an objective prospective study in man, Anesthesiology **38:**228-236, 1973.
5. Cohn, J.N.: Blood pressure measurement in shock: mechanism of inaccuracy in auscultatory and palpatory methods, J.A.M.A. **199:**972-976, 1967.
6. Ersoz, C.J. et al.: Prolonged femoral artery catheterization for intensive care, Anesth. Analg. **49:**160-164, 1973.
7. Greenhow, D.E.: Incorrect performance of Allen's test, Anesthesiology **37:**356-357, 1972.
8. Kaplan, J.A.: Hemodynamic monitoring. In Kaplan, J.A., editor: Cardiac anesthesia, New York, 1979, Grune & Stratton, Inc.
9. Kim, J.M., Arakawa, K., and Bliss, J.: Arterial cannulation: factors in the development of occlusion, Anesth. Analg. **54:**836-841, 1975.
10. Mundth, E.D. and Austen, W.G.: Postoperative intensive care in the cardiac surgical patient, Prog. Cardiovasc. Dis. **11:**229-261, 1968.
11. Ryan, J.R. et al.: Arterial dynamics of radial artery cannulation, Anesth. Analg. **52:**1017-1025, 1973.
12. Stamm, W.E., et al.: Indwelling arterial catheters as a source of nosocomial bacteremia, N. Engl. J. Med. **292:**1099-1102, 1975.
13. Van Bergen, F.H. et al.: Comparison of indirect and direct methods of measuring blood pressure, Circulation **10:**481-490, 1954.
14. Youngberg, J.A., and Miller, E.D.: Evaluation of percutaneous cannulation of the dorsalis pedis artery, Anesthesiology **44:**80-83, 1976.

CHAPTER 8

Swan-Ganz catheter insertion

Robert S. Gibson
James R. Kistner

GENERAL CONSIDERATIONS

The Swan-Ganz balloon-tipped catheter is very useful in measuring central venous pressure (CVP), pulmonary artery (PA) pressure, pulmonary capillary wedge (PCW) pressure, and cardiac output.[31,32] The PCW pressure equals left-sided atrial pressure and is therefore a sensitive indicator of the presence of pulmonary congestion and left-sided congestive heart failure.[8,15,20,30] Relying on CVP measurements alone as a guide to left ventricular function is hazardous in patients with severe cardiovascular disease.[30] Several investigators[15,20] have observed large changes in PCW pressure with almost no change in the CVP. For critically ill patients, precise hemodynamic monitoring should be available at all times so that dangerous physiologic changes can be detected early and corrected.

INDICATIONS

1. To monitor hemodynamic effects of potent inotropic or vasodilator therapy for severe left-sided heart failure.[4,5,9]
2. To distinguish cardiogenic from noncardiogenic pulmonary edema.[26]
3. To diagnose acute mitral regurgitation or ventricular septal rupture in a patient with an acute myocardial infarction and a new systolic murmur.[6,23,34]
4. To diagnose pulmonary arterial hypertension.
5. To diagnose pericardial tamponade or constrictive pericarditis.[21,33]

6. To diagnose right ventricular infarction.[21]
7. To monitor hemodynamic effects of fluid therapy in patients with right-sided heart failure when it is due to severe obstructive lung disease, adult respiratory distress syndrome, or pulmonary embolism.[22,30]
8. To assess prognosis and guide therapy in patients with bacteremic shock.[35]
9. During major abdominal, thoracic, or vascular surgery in patients with significant cardiovascular disease.[17]

■ CONTRAINDICATIONS

1. Lack of special pressure-monitoring apparatus (Chapter 3).
2. Lack of good nursing coverage.
3. Same as for venous cutdown and internal jugular and subclavian vein cannulation (Chapters 4 to 6).

■ PATIENT EVALUATION AND PREPARATION

1. Obtain prothrombin time, partial thromboplastin time, and platelet count.
2. Explain the procedure to the patient, including its potential complications, and obtain written informed consent.
3. Assemble and calibrate the pressure monitoring equipment. The pressure transducer should be positioned at the right atrial or midheart level. Calibration, both on the digital display and oscilloscope, should be checked by the physician (Chapter 3).

■ PERSONNEL AND EQUIPMENT

1. A physician skilled in right-sided heart catheterization, an assistant, and a nurse or hemodynamic technician capable of assembling reliable equipment.
2. Principal implements.
   a. Venous access for brachial route: cutdown set (Chapter 4).
   b. Venous access for subclavian or jugular route: 17-gauge needle and syringe (6 ml), percutaneous

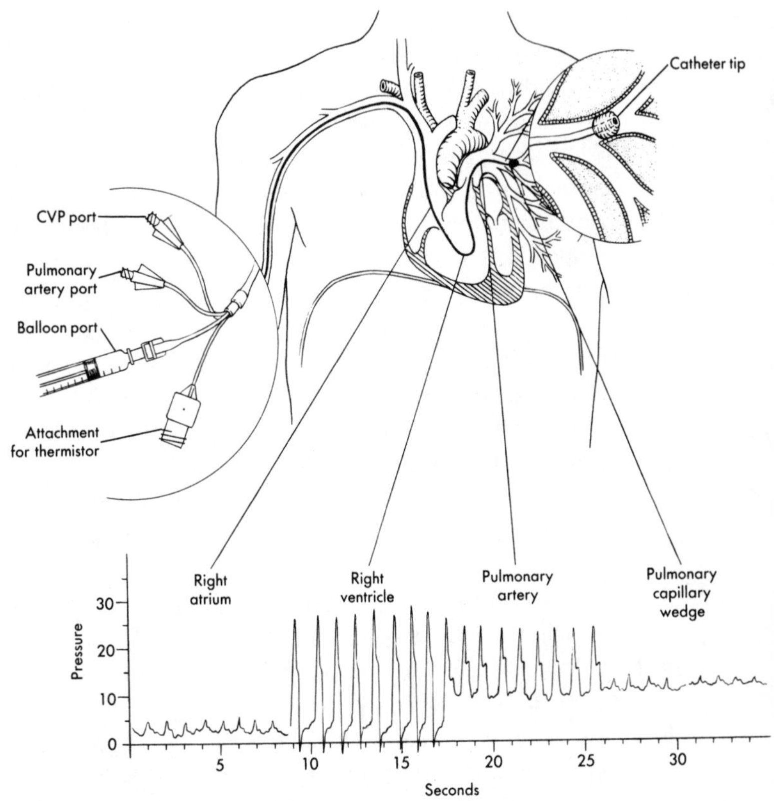

FIG. 8-1. Swan-Ganz catheter placement. Swan-Ganz catheter (7 French) depicting CVP port, PA and balloon port, and attachment for thermistor. During advancement through right side of heart, characteristic pressure tracings are recorded from right atrial, right ventricular, PA, and PCW positions.

catheter introducer set (UMI or Cordis), which includes a Teflon sheath, vessel dilator, and guidewire; number 11 scalpel blade; knife handle; curved mosquito clamp; sponges; suture scissors; skin suture; and needle holder.

c. Swan-Ganz catheter: the standard 5 French catheter has one pressure lumen located at the tip for PA pressure recording. The 7 French catheter (Fig. 8-1), which we recommend, and the 5 French pediatric catheter have a distal port (PA pressure lumen), proximal port (CVP lumen, located 30 cm from the tip), balloon port, and an optional thermistor (located behind the inflatable balloon) for cardiac output measurement.

d. Monitoring system: electrocardiograph, (ECG), pressure recorder, pressure transducer, and cable, and nondistensible connecting tubing and three-way stopcock (Chapter 3).

e. Flushing apparatus: the catheter should be flushed with heparinized saline (1 to 3 units/ml) at least every 30 minutes. A device is available to do this automatically (Sorenson Intraflo) (Chapter 3).

f. Standby fluoroscopy: in most cases, positioning of the catheter does not require fluoroscopy.

3. Disinfection and sterile field: disinfectant solution; sterile sponges; sterile gloves and gown; mask and hair cap; and draping towels and towel clips.
4. Anesthesia: lidocaine (1%, 10 ml); syringe (10 ml); and 23-gauge (1-inch) needle.
5. Dressing: disinfectant ointment; sterile sponges; and adhesive tape (1 inch and 3 inches).
6. Resuscitation: cardiac defibrillator; suction apparatus; oxygen; airways; and preloaded syringes of atropine (1 mg) and lidocaine (100 mg). When there is manipulation of catheters in the heart, the defibrillator must be plugged in, turned on, and ready for rapid use.

■ TECHNIQUES

The Swan-Ganz catheter can be inserted through a venous cutdown or percutaneously, using a modified Seldinger technique. The following steps are undertaken with either approach:

1. Test the balloon for leaks by injecting air while holding the balloon under water. The 5 French catheter holds a maximum of 0.8 ml of air and the 7 French catheter, 1.5 ml of air. In patients with intracardiac shunts, carbon dioxide should be used for balloon inflation because of the risk of gas embolism.

2. Assemble the pressure monitoring apparatus as described in Chapter 3.
3. Flush all tubing and the catheter with heparinized saline.
4. Begin ECG monitoring of the patient.

Insertion through antecubital vein

1. Follow steps 1 to 7 of the venous cutdown technique in Chapter 4.
2. Insert the catheter (Chapter 4, Fig. 4-1, *D*). Place the vein lifter into the proximal venotomy, lift upward, and expose the lumen of the vein. Slip the Swan-Ganz catheter forward underneath the vein lifter, so that it lies well within the vein. Remove the vein lifter and advance the catheter until the tip has reached the superior vena cava, approximately 35 to 40 cm from the right and 45 to 50 cm from the left antecubital fossa. The colored bands on the catheter are 10 cm apart.
3. Connect the catheter to the pressure recording assembly (Chapter 3). Attach the CVP and PA lumens to the Intraflo device by means of the nondistensible connecting tubing. Periodically flush each lumen with heparinized saline to maintain patency. Attach the Intraflo device to the pressure recorder.
4. Advance the catheter through the right-side heart chambers (Fig. 8-1). Inflate the balloon with the recommended volume of air. Advance the catheter through the right atrium, right ventricle, and PA while observing the ECG and pressure tracing, until a damped PCW pressure trace is obtained (Fig. 8-1, bottom). During passage of the catheter through the right side of the heart, measure and record pressures from the right atrial, right ventricular, PA, and PCW positions. Once a tracing resembling the PCW pressure is obtained, deflate the balloon. A phasic PA trace should be seen, confirming proper position. Proper position can also be confirmed by fluoroscopy and finding fully saturated blood in the wedged catheter. If premature ventricular contractions (PVCs) are elicited during catheter advancement, de-

flate the balloon and withdraw the catheter back into the right atrium. The catheter has probably coiled within the right ventricle. If further attempts to advance the catheter are unsuccessful because of PVCs, administer lidocaine (75 to 100 mg) and consider fluoroscopic guidance. If an intracardiac shunt is suspected, obtain blood samples for oxygen analysis from the superior vena cava, right atrium, right ventricle, and PA.

5. Secure the catheter and apply the dressing as for steps 10 and 11 of the venous cutdown technique in Chapter 4.

Insertion through right internal jugular vein

1. Follow steps 1 to 5 of the internal jugular cannulation technique in Chapter 6.
2. Insert a 17-gauge needle attached to a 6-ml syringe into the vein (Chapter 6, Fig. 6-3, *A*). Insert the needle at a 30-degree angle to the skin and advance it caudally. Aim the needle at the ipsilateral nipple. Maintain syringe suction until dark red blood flows into the syringe, indicating that the vein has been entered. If the vein is not immediately entered, the needle should be redirected 5 to 10 degrees more medially. When venous blood is aspirated, advance the needle another 2 or 3 mm to ensure that the beveled tip is well within the vein lumen.
3. Insert the catheter (Fig. 8-2). Remove the syringe and slide the guidewire through the needle into the vein (Fig. 8-2, *A*). Remove the needle and replace it with the vessel dilator and sheath after first nicking the skin with a number 11 scalpel blade (Fig. 8-2, *B*). Remove the guidewire; then remove the vessel dilator and leave the venous sheath in the vein. Slide the Swan-Ganz catheter through the venous sheath into the superior vena cava (approximately 10 to 15 cm) (Fig. 8-2, *C*).
4. Connect the catheter to the pressure recording assembly (Chapter 3) and advance it through the right side of the heart as for step 4 of insertion through the antecubital vein.

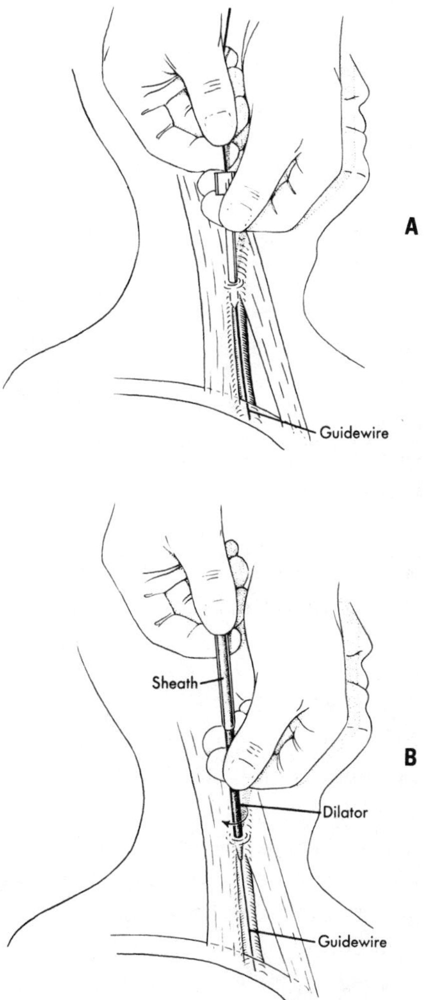

FIG. 8-2. A, Slide guidewire through needle and advance it into internal jugular vein. **B,** Insert vessel dilator and sheath into vein over guidewire.

Continued.

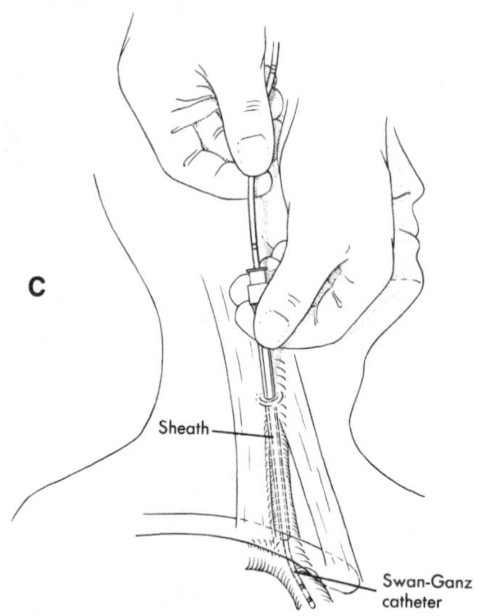

FIG. 8-2, cont'd. C, Insert Swan-Ganz catheter through vessel sheath into superior vena cava.

5. Secure the catheter and apply a dressing, following steps 9 and 10 of the internal jugular vein cannulation technique in Chapter 6.

Insertion through subclavian vein

1. Follow steps 1 to 4 of the infraclavicular subclavian vein cannulation technique in Chapter 5.
2. Insert the cannulation needle (Chapter 5, Fig. 5-2). Use a 17-gauge intracatheter needle attached to a 6-ml syringe. With the index finger of the left hand in the sternal notch and the thumb along the clavicle, insert the needle through the skin and subcutaneous tissue at the same point used to infiltrate the anesthetic. Advance the needle parallel to and as close to the underside of the clavicle as possible. Maintain suction on the syringe until dark red blood flows into it, indicating that the subclavian vein has been entered. When venous blood is aspirated, advance the needle another 2 or 3 mm to ensure that its beveled tip is well within the vein lumen.

3. Insert the catheter using the Seldinger technique explained in step 3 of insertion through the internal jugular vein.
4. Connect the catheter to the pressure recording assembly (Chapter 3) and advance it through the right side of the heart, as in steps 3 and 4 of insertion through the antecubital vein.
5. Secure the catheter and apply a dressing as explained in steps 8 and 9 of the subclavian vein cannulation technique (Chapter 5).

■ POSTPROCEDURE CARE

1. Auscultate both lung fields for symmetric breath sounds.
2. Obtain a chest roentgenogram to check catheter position[2] and look for a pneumothorax.
3. Check for a hematoma.
4. Remove, inspect, and replace the sterile dressing daily.
5. Catheter care.
   a. Balloon inflation. Inflate the balloon only when measuring PCW pressure and leave it inflated for a maximum of 30 to 60 seconds to prevent pulmonary infarction. To minimize the risk of balloon rupture, do not put more than the recommended volume of air in the balloon port.
   b. Infusion. Continue constant infusion of heparinized saline by means of the Intraflo device. Flush the catheter every 30 minutes.
   c. Pressure measurements. Be sure that the pressure transducer is at the right atrial or midheart level. Calibrate the transducer and measure pulmonary vascular pressures at end exhalation to minimize errors created by changes in intrapleural pressure during the respiratory cycle (Chapter 3).
   d. Adjust the catheter position as necessary. The catheter has a tendency to soften at body temperature; consequently the transcardiac loop may shorten and permit distal catheter migration. This may cause the

catheter to become wedged in a distal PA branch vessel. If unrecognized, pulmonary infarction will occur. If the phasic PA pressure trace (Fig. 8-1, *bottom*) begins to resemble the PCW trace, withdraw the catheter until the PA trace is again observed.

e. PA pressure damping. When the PA phasic pressure trace becomes damped there may be clotting in the catheter, forward migration and wedging of the catheter, or the catheter may be in the right atrium. To regain phasic pressures, first try to remove air bubbles from the connecting tubing and transducer by aspirating and then flushing the catheter. If blood cannot be aspirated from the catheter, yet flushes easily, suspect a ball-valve thrombus at the catheter tip. If there is a ball-valve thrombus, patency may be reestablished by filling the lumen with 5000 units of heparin for 15 to 30 minutes and then initiating a continuous drip of heparin (5 units/1-ml saline). The next step to reestablish an undamped tracing is to withdraw it gradually, 5 cm at a time, while constantly monitoring the pressure waveform.
f. Obtain daily chest roentgenograms to check for pulmonary infarction and catheter migration.

■ COMPLICATIONS DUE TO VASCULAR ACCESS

The complications of venous cutdown and subclavian and internal jugular vein cannulation are the same as those given in Chapters 4 to 6.

■ COMPLICATIONS DUE TO THE SWAN-GANZ CATHETER

1. Arrhythmias.[1,3,10,14] Although there is a 50% frequency of at least one premature ventricular contraction during intracardiac catheter passage, it is unusual for serious ventricular arrhythmias to occur. If, however, the balloon is inflated while the catheter is in the right ventricle, the catheter tip may become lodged under a papillary muscle or trabeculation, resulting in ventricular tachycardia or ventricular fibrillation. Premature ventricular contractions can also occur if the catheter "re-

coils" from the PA back into the sensitive right ventricular outflow tract. Atrial fibrillation, atrial flutter, and complete heart block may also occur with Swan-Ganz catheter insertion.

2. Catheter coiling and knotting.[19] Catheter coiling or knotting is more likely with the smaller 5 French catheters, which are very flexible. It occurs when an excessive length of catheter is advanced without noting the pressure tracing and when the catheter is advanced too rapidly and fluoroscopy is unavailable. The catheter should not be advanced farther than 15 cm once it enters the right ventricle if it does not pass into the PA. Ventricular arrhythmias associated with right atrial pressure waveform suggest this complication.
3. Valve damage.[16,25] Both the tricuspid and pulmonary valves can be damaged if the catheter is withdrawn with the balloon inflated. Moreover, endocardial or intimal trauma may result from the pumping of the heart against a mobile indwelling catheter. Pulmonary regurgitation and systolic nonejection clicks can be produced by the catheter.
4. Endocarditis.[13,27] Catheter trauma to the tricuspid and pulmonary valve and the right ventricular endocardium can result in aseptic thrombotic vegetations in 3% to 17% of the patients. These lesions pose potential risks of embolization and infection.
5. Thromboembolism.[12] Thromboembolism is due to clot formation on the catheter or endocardial vegetations. The risk of this complication may be reduced by a constant infusion of heparinized saline by means of the Intraflo device.
6. Pulmonary infarction.[7] Ischemic pulmonary damage occurs in 7% of the cases. It is due to persistent undetected wedging of the catheter tip in a peripheral PA (75%) or catheter-related thromboembolism (25%). To lessen this risk, the balloon should be inflated only during pressure recording and then for only 30 to 60 seconds. Skilled nursing personnel capable of monitoring the PA pressure tracing on the oscilloscope is mandatory.

7. PA rupture.[11,18] Excessive inflation of the balloon can damage the PA wall and lead to production of hemoptysis or hemorrhage. Although rare, PA rupture can be fatal.
8. PA perforation. PA perforation can occur from catheter advancement with the balloon deflated or catheter migration.
9. Balloon rupture. Balloon rupture is in not uncommon when the catheter has been left in place for more than a few days or when the balloon is inflated with more than the recommended volume of air. It is diagnosed when injected air cannot be withdrawn.
10. Gas embolism. Gas embolism may result from balloon rupture. Small volumes of air injected into the PA will be of no consequence. In patients with intracardiac shunts, carbon dioxide should be used for inflation, and great care must be taken to avoid balloon rupture and the possibility of systemic gas embolism.
11. Hemoptysis from flushing the catheter in the wedge position.[24] Pulmonary wedge injections of 5 to 8 ml of solution in an effort to cause transpulmonary transmission of echocardiographic contrast can result in PA rupture with hemoptysis.
12. Cardiac tamponade. Cardiac tamponade is generally due to right ventricular perforation. It may occur when the catheter is advanced with the balloon deflated.
13. Inaccurate diagnosis from a malfunctioning catheter.[24,28] Malfunction of the catheter or balloon can cause inaccuracies in the PCW pressure and incorrect treatment of the patient. Eccentric inflation of the balloon, with the catheter tip impinging on the PA wall can cause "pseudowedging" of the catheter and erroneous estimation of the PCW pressure. Be sure that the PCW pressure is less than the mean PA pressure and comparable to the PA diastolic pressure. Incorrect blood sampling from the PA catheter can also cause errors in measuring cardiac output by the Fick technique.[29]

REFERENCES

1. Abernathy, W.S.: Complete heart block caused by the Swan-Ganz catheter, Chest **65:**349, 1974.
2. Benumof, J.L. et al.: Where pulmonary artery catheters go: intrathoracic distribution, Anesthesiology **46:**336-338, 1977.
3. Braunwald, E., and Swan, H.J.C.: Cooperative study on cardiac catheterization, Circulation **37-38**(Suppl. 3):27-35, 1968.
4. Chatterjee, K. et al.: Effects of vasodilator therapy for severe pump failure in acute myocardial infarction on short-term and late prognosis, Circulation **53:**797-802, 1976.
5. Chatterjee, K., and Parmley, W.W.: The role of vasodilator therapy in heart failure, Prog. Cardiovasc. Dis. **19:**301-325, 1977.
6. Falcone, M.W., Ronan, J.A., Jr., and Roberts, W.C.: Silent mitral regurgitation complicating silent myocardial infarction: hemodynamic and morphologic documentation, Chest **62:**226-228, 1972.
7. Foote, G.A., Schabel, S.I., and Hodges, M.: Pulmonary complications of the flow-directed balloon-tipped catheter, N. Engl. J. Med. **290:**927-931, 1974.
8. Forrester, J.S.: Filling pressures in the right and left sides of the heart in acute myocardial infarction, N. Engl. J. Med. **285:**190-193, 1971.
9. Forrester, J.S. et al.: Medical therapy of acute myocardial infarction by application of hemodynamic subsets, N. Engl. J. Med. **295:**1356-1362 and 1404-1413, 1976.
10. Geha, D.G., Davis, N.J., and Lappas, D.G.: Persistent atrial arrhythmias associated with placement of a Swan-Ganz catheter, Anesthesiology **39:**651-653, 1973.
11. Golden, M.S. et al.: Fatal pulmonary hemorrhage complicating use of a flow-directed balloon-tipped catheter in a patient receiving anticoagulant therapy, Am. J. Cardiol. **32:**865-867, 1973.
12. Goodman, D.J. et al.: Thromboembolic complications with the indwelling balloon-tipped pulmonary arterial catheter, N. Engl. J. Med. **291:**777, 1974.
13. Greene, J.F., and Cummings, K.C.: Aseptic thrombotic endocardial vegetations: a complication of indwelling pulmonary artery catheters, J.A.M.A. **225:**1525-1526, 1973.
14. Gupta, P.K., and Haft, J.I.: Complete heart block complicating cardiac catheterization, Chest **61:**185-187, 1972.
15. Humphrey, C.B. et al.: An analysis of direct and indirect measurement of left atrial filling pressure, J. Thorac. Cardiovasc. Surg. **71:**643-647, 1976.
16. Isner, J.M., Horton, J., and Ronan, J.A., Jr.: Systolic click from a Swan-Ganz catheter, Am. J. Cardiol. **43:**1046-1048, 1979.
17. Katz, J.D. et al.: Pulmonary artery flow-guided catheters in the perioperative period, J.A.M.A. **237:**2832-2834, 1977.
18. Lapin, E.S., and Murray, J.A.: Hemoptysis with flow-directed cardiac catheterization, J.A.M.A. **220:**1246, 1972.
19. Lipp, H., O'Donoghue, K., and Resnekov, L.: Intracardiac knotting of a flow directed balloon catheter, N. Engl. J. Med. **284:**220, 1971.
20. Loeb, H.S. et al.: Relationship between central venous and left ventricu-

lar filling pressures prior to and during treatment of shock, Am. J. Cardiol. **23:**125, 1969.
21. Lorell, B. et al.: Right ventricular infarction: clinical diagnosis and differentiation from cardiac tamponade and pericardial constriction, Am. J. Cardiol. **43:**465-471, 1979.
22. Lozman, J. et al.: Correlation of pulmonary wedge and left atrial pressure: a study in the patient receiving positive end–expiratory pressure ventilation, Arch. Surg. **109:**270-277, 1974.
23. Meister, S.G., and Helfaut, R.H.: Rapid bedside differentiation of ruptured interventricular septrum from acute mitral insufficiency, N. Engl. J. Med. **287:**1024-1025, 1972.
24. Meltzer, R. et al.: Hemoptysis after flushing Swan-Ganz catheters in the wedge position, N. Engl. J. Med. **304:**1171, 1981.
25. O'Toole, J.D. et al.: Pulmonary-valve injury and insufficiency during pulmonary-artery catheterization, N. Engl. J. Med. **301:**1167-1168, 1979.
26. Overland, E.S., and Severinghaus, J.W.: Noncardiac pulmonary edema, Adv. Int. Med. **23:**307-326, 1978.
27. Pace, N.L., and Horton, W.: Indwelling pulmonary artery catheters: their relationship to aseptic thrombotic endocardial vegetations, J.A.M.A. **233:** 893-895, 1975.
28. Shin, B. et al.: Problems with measurements using the Swan-Ganz catheter, Anesthesiology **43:**474-476, 1975.
29. Suter, P.M. et al.: Errors in data derived from pulmonary artery blood gas values, Crit. Care Med. **3:**175-181, 1975.
30. Swan, H.J.C.: Central venous pressure monitoring is an outmoded procedure of limited practical value. In Gelfinger, F., et al., editors: Controversy in internal medicine, vol. 1, Phildelphia, 1974, W.B. Saunders Co.
31. Swan, H.J.C., and Ganz, W. et al.: Catheterization of the heart in man with use of a flow-directed balloon-tipped catheter, N. Engl. J. Med. **283:** 447-451, 1970.
32. Swan, H.J.C., and Ganz, W.: Use of balloon flotation catheters in critically ill patients, Surg. Clin. North Am. **55:**501-520, 1975.
33. Weeks, K.R. et al.: Bedside hemodynamic monitoring: its value in the diagnosis of tamponade complicating cardiac surgery, J. Thorac. Cardiovasc. Surg. **71:**250-252, 1976.
34. Wei, J.Y., Hutchins, G.M., and Bulkley, B.H.: Papillary muscle rupture in fatal acute myocardial infarction, Ann. Int. Med. **90:**149-152, 1979.
35. Weil, M.H., and Nishjima, H.: Cardiac output in bacterial shock, Am. J. Med. **64:**920-922, 1978.

CHAPTER 9

Pericardiocentesis and intrapericardial catheter insertion

■ Robert S. Gibson

■ GENERAL CONSIDERATIONS

Pericardiocentesis is a method of removing fluid from the pericardial space for diagnostic studies or to relieve cardiac tamponade. It is a risky procedure and should only be performed by skilled operators because the frequency of serious complications is higher than with cardiac catheterization and coronary angiography.

By inserting an intrapericardial catheter, pericardial fluid can be removed continuously as it reaccumulates. This technique may be useful in patients with recurrent tamponade, hemorrhagic uremic pericarditis, malignant pericardial effusions, and purulent pericarditis.[11] In selected patients, this procedure may allow time for a specific therapeutic intervention to take effect and thus make repeated pericardiocentesis, pericardiotomy, or pericardiectomy unnecessary. In others, it may be a valuable temporary measure, permitting stabilization of a critically ill patient.

■ THERAPEUTIC INDICATIONS

1. Cardiac tamponade. In many patients, cardiac tamponade can be managed successfully by pericardiocentesis alone. In tamponade due to trauma, aortic dissection, or after thoracic surgical procedures, pericardiocentesis should be combined with surgical exploration. An intrapericardial drainage catheter should be inserted if the effusion or tamponade is likely to recur rapidly.[11]

2. Instillation of drugs such as antineoplastic agents[2,10] or corticosteroids.[4]

■ DIAGNOSTIC INDICATION

A specific diagnosis can be established in 25% to 30% of the cases of *pericardial effusion*.[8] The yield is highest in carcinomatous[12] and infectious pericarditis.[1,7] The approach to *pericardial effusion associated with elevated venous pressure* may also include measurement of intravascular and intrapericardial pressure before and after fluid removal.[8] *Simple tamponade* is diagnosed when elevated venous pressure equals the level of intrapericardial pressure and falls after removal of fluid to normal levels. *Visceral constrictive pericarditis* is indicated by failure of elevated venous pressure to fall significantly when the increased intrapericardial pressure has been reduced to normal and by equilibration of diastolic pressure in all of the cardiac chambers. *Congestive heart failure* or *fluid overload* is diagnosed when intrapericardial pressures are not sufficiently elevated to explain the elevated venous pressure and when diastolic pressure levels in the chambers on the left side of the heart are higher than those on the right side. Last, *superior vena cava obstruction* is indicated when right atrial pressure is lower than jugular venous pressure.

■ CONTRAINDICATIONS

There are no absolute contraindications to pericardiocentesis to relieve cardiac tamponade. The single relative contraindication to diagnostic pericardiocentesis is the presence of an uncorrectable bleeding diathesis.

■ CHOICE OF PUNCTURE SITE

The subxiphoid approach is preferred, because in this region, the lung does not cover the heart. When a left pleural effusion is present, this approach ensures that pericardial rather than pleural fluid is drained. Additionally, the subxiphoid approach often yields fluid when the effusion is small, since the volume of pericardial fluid is likely to be greatest on the inferior heart surface. The apical approach is used when the subxiphoid route is unsuccessful or the maximum volume of fluid lies at the cardiac apex. Apical pericardiocentesis is often preferred over the subxiphoid approach in the presence of marked pulmonary hypertension.

Two-dimensional echocardiography may assist the physician in choosing between the subxiphoid or apical approach, since proximity to adjacent structures can be assessed and the maximum volume and distribution of pericardial fluid precisely determined.[5,8,9]

PATIENT EVALUATION AND PREPARATION

1. Perform echocardiography to document the pericardial effusion. Pericardial fluid may spontaneously regress, and estimating the size of the effusion is helpful in predicting the likelihood of a successful pericardiocentesis.[5,8,9]
2. Obtain prothrombin time, partial thromboplastin time, platelet count, hematocrit, and serum electrolytes.
3. Explain the procedure to the patient, including its potential complications, and obtain written informed consent.
4. Insert an intravenous line.
5. Take the patient to the coronary care unit or cardiac catheterization laboratory so that the maximum amount of electrocardiographic and hemodynamic information can be obtained. Measurement of intracardiac pressures with a Swan-Ganz catheter before and after fluid removal may be desirable.[8]

PERSONNEL AND EQUIPMENT

1. A physician skilled in pericardiocentesis and an assistant.
2. Principal implements.
   a. Pericardiocentesis: two 4-inch (18- and 20-gauge) spinal needles; two syringes (10 ml, 50 ml); three-way stopcock; rubber connecting tubing for stopcock drainage; Kelly clamp; battery-powered ECG machine; sterile alligator clip; and collecting basin.
   b. Fluid collection and analysis: graduated collecting

basin (1000 ml); sterile culture tube; cytology specimen bottle; and hematocrit and blood chemistry tubes.

c. Indwelling pericardial drainage: Seldinger needle (number 18); Teflon-coated spring guidewire with flexible 3-mm J-tip (USCI 007054); 8 French vessel dilator (Cordis 501-200); 8 French femoral-ventricular "pigtail" angiographic catheter, with 12 side holes and end hole (Cordis 523-850); and vacuum drainage container.

3. Disinfection and sterile field: disinfectant solution; sterile sponges; sterile gloves, mask, hair cap, and gown; draping towels and towel clips; biopsy towels.
4. Anesthesia: lidocaine (1%, 10 ml); syringe (10 ml); 23-gauge (1-inch) needle.
5. Dressing: disinfectant ointment; sterile sponges; and adhesive tape (1 inch).
6. Resuscitation: cardiac defibrillator; suction apparatus; oxygen; airways; and preloaded syringes with atropine (1 mg) and lidocaine (100 mg).

■ TECHNIQUES

Subxiphoid approach

1. Place the patient in a semirecumbent position. This position allows the heart to recede posteriorly away from the chest wall. If pericardiocentesis is performed with the patient supine, the operator can expect to encounter the myocardium more frequently than fluid.
2. Attach the ECG limb leads to the patient.
3. Locate the left xiphocostal angle.
4. Prepare the skin and drape a sterile field. Put on sterile gloves, mask, hair cap, and gown. Prepare the upper abdomen and lower chest with disinfectant solution. Place a biopsy towel on the patient's chest with the hole centered over the left xiphocostal angle. Form a complete sterile field with draping towels.
5. Anesthetize the left xiphocostal site. Use 1% lidocaine and a 23-gauge (1-inch) needle to inject the skin at the

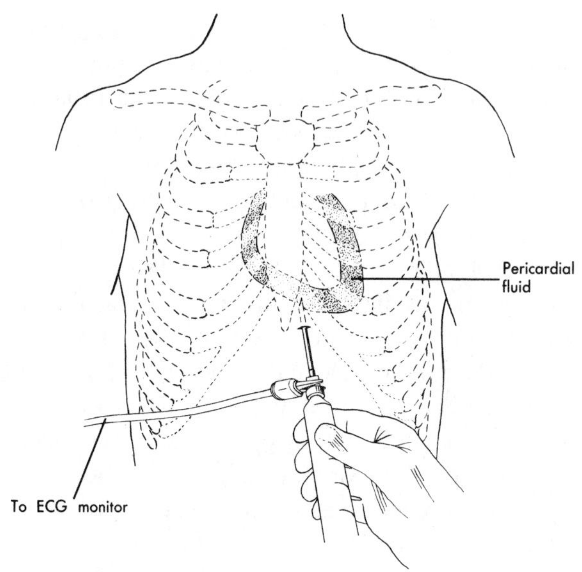

FIG. 9-1. Subxiphoid pericardiocentesis.

left xiphocostal angle. To anesthetize deeper tissues, advance the needle beneath the costal arch toward the suprasternal notch until either the pericardial cavity is entered or to the hilt. Aspirate carefully. If pericardial fluid returns, withdraw the needle until no additional fluid returns. Inject lidocaine slowly (total 3 to 5 ml) while withdrawing the needle.

6. Insert the pericardiocentesis needle. Connect the ECG lead V_1 to the metal pericardiocentesis needle with a sterile alligator clip (Fig. 9-1). Use a battery-powered ECG for electrical safety. Place a 10-ml syringe on the needle. Insert the needle through the anesthetized skin. Once the needle is beneath the left costal arch, monitor lead V_1 on the ECG. Slowly advance the needle toward the suprasternal notch (aspirating during advancement) until pericardial fluid is obtained or either a ventricular or an atrial epicardial injury current is seen on the ECG.[3,6] A sudden "give" may be felt with pericardial

puncture. If the needle penetrates the epicardium, the ECG may show increased P wave amplitude, ST segment elevation, or ectopic beats. If epicardial injury is seen, withdraw and reposition the needle so that inadvertent myocardial puncture can be avoided. If pericardial fluid cannot be obtained, redirect the needle toward the left shoulder.

7. Removal and analysis of fluid. Place a Kelly clamp around the needle at its junction with the skin. Remove the 10-ml syringe and attach a 50-ml syringe with a stopcock to the needle and withdraw the fluid. If bloody fluid that clots is withdrawn and if the hematocrit of the fluid is similar to that of peripheral venous blood, suspect myocardial puncture. Place aliquots of fluid in specimen tubes for cell count, protein, glucose, culture, gram stain, and cytologic examination.
8. Withdraw the needle and apply a dressing over the puncture site.

Apical approach

1. Place the patient on the left side in a semirecumbent position, so that there is still easy access to the cardiac apex. With female patients, tape the left breast to the left side of the thorax so that it is outside the field of operation.
2. Attach ECG limb leads to the patient.
3. Locate the apical impulse and the border of cardiac dullness.
4. Prepare the skin and drape a sterile field. Put on sterile gloves and a mask, hair cap, and gown. Prepare the left side of the chest with disinfectant solution. Place a biopsy towel on the patient's chest with the hole centered over the cardiac apex. Form a complete sterile field with draping towels.
5. Anesthetize the apical site as described in step 5 of the subxiphoid approach, but in the skin over the cardiac apex. Advance the needle over the top of a rib.
6. Insert the pericardiocentesis needle as described in step

6 of the subxiphoid approach, but through the skin over the cardiac apex. Advance the needle over the top of a rib.

7. Follow steps 7 and 8 of the subxiphoid approach.

INSERTION OF INTRAPERICARDIAL DRAINAGE CATHETER

1. Follow steps 1 to 5 of the subxiphoid approach.
2. Insert the pericardial catheter (Fig. 9-2). Connect the ECG lead V_1 to the number 18 Seldinger needle with a sterile alligator clip. Place a 10-ml syringe on the needle. Insert the needle through anesthetized skin. Once the needle is beneath the left costal arch, begin to monitor the lead V_1 on the ECG. Slowly advance the needle toward the suprasternal notch (aspirating during advancement) until pericardial fluid is obtained or an epicardial injury current is seen on the ECG (Fig. 9-2, *A*). When intrapericardial needle position is confirmed by fluid withdrawal, remove the syringe and insert the J-tip guidewire through the lumen of the needle. It is very important that the operator inserts the flexible end of the guidewire and that the assistant controls the guidewire so that it does not spring out of the sterile field. Advance the guidewire approximately 10 cm into the pericardial cavity (Fig. 9-2, *B*). Withdraw the needle over the guidewire while maintaining the intrapericardial position of the guidewire. Insert a number 8 French vessel dilator over the guidewire to enlarge the tract into the pericardial cavity and then remove it. Insert a number 8 French femoral-ventricular "pigtail" catheter over the guidewire and into the pericardial space (Fig. 9-2, *C*). Remove the guidewire. Connect a 10-ml syringe to the catheter and confirm the intrapericardial catheter position by fluid withdrawal.
3. Drainage of fluid. Attach the catheter by means of a three-way stopcock and connecting tubing to a closed sterile container with vacuum drainage. Use fluoroscopy to position the catheter in a dependent portion of the pericardial space for optimal drainage of fluid. To facili-

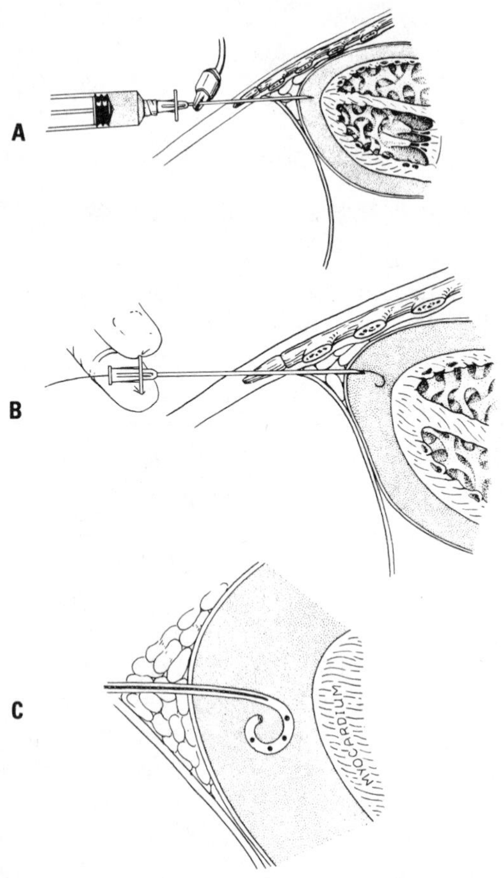

FIG. 9-2. A, Advance needle into pericardial space. **B,** Advance J-tip guidewire into pericardial space. **C,** Insert "pigtail" catheter over guidewire and into pericardial space.

tate evacuation of the pericardial fluid, the patient's position may be periodically changed from side to side to upright and supine.

4. Apply disinfectant ointment and a sterile dressing to the point of the entrance of the catheter.

■ POSTPROCEDURE CARE

1. Obtain a chest roentgenogram. Check the size of the cardiac silhouette and for a pneumothorax. If an in-

dwelling drainage catheter was inserted, check the catheter position.

2. Monitor the heart rate, blood pressure, central venous pressure, and respiratory rate. Check for paradoxical pulse. Observe for complications.
3. If an indwelling drainage catheter was inserted, flush the catheter aseptically every 1 or 2 hours with 2 to 4 ml of heparinized saline. Use a three-way stopcock as a flushing port. Record the amount of drainage every 2 to 4 hours. Remove, inspect, and replace the sterile dressing daily.

COMPLICATIONS[8]

1. Hemopericardium. A hemopericardium usually results from chamber perforation or coronary artery laceration, particularly in patients with platelet counts less than 50,000 mm^3. Therapy includes immediate pericardiocentesis for relief of tamponade and insertion of an intrapericardial drainage catheter. If hemopericardium persists, prompt surgical exploration is necessary to locate the bleeding site.
2. Arrhythmias. A wide variety of arrhythmias may occur if the exploring needle pierces the atrial or ventricular myocardium. Most arrhythmias stop when the needle is withdrawn.
3. Pneumothorax. Any pneumothorax greater than 20% should be decompressed with a chest tube (Chapter 41). A patient requiring mechanical ventilation should have a chest tube regardless of the pneumothorax size.
4. Perforation or laceration of adjacent structures such as the internal mammary artery, stomach, or liver. Immediate surgical consultation is advised.
5. Contamination of the pleural, mediastinal, or peritoneal space from purulent pericardial effusions may occur as the needle is withdrawn. Broad-spectrum antimicrobial therapy should be administered based on a Gram stain and culture of the fluid.
6. Purulent pericarditis following insertion of an intrapericardial drainage catheter.

7. Injection of air into a cardiac chamber. This can occur when air is instilled into the pericardial space for diagnostic purposes. Since echocardiography provides more reliable information about heart size and pericardial wall thickness, this procedure should no longer be performed.
8. Vasovagal reactions with hypotension and/or bradycardia. The patient should be placed in the Trendelenburg position and given intravenous atropine and fluid.

REFERENCES

1. Agner, R.C., and Gallis, H.A.: Pericarditis: differential diagnostic considerations, Arch. Intern. Med. **139:**407-412, 1979.
2. Biran, S. et al.: The management of pericardial effusion in cancer patients, Chest **71:**182-186, 1977.
3. Bishop, L.H., Jr., Estes, E.H., Jr., and McIntosh, H.D.: Electrocardiogram as a safeguard in pericardiocentesis, J.A.M.A. **162:**264-265, 1956.
4. Buselmeiser, T.J. et al.: Uremic pericardial effusion: treatment by catheter drainage and local nonabsorbable steroid administration, Nephron **16:** 371-380, 1976.
5. Horowitz, M.S. et al.: Sensitivity and specificity of echocardiographic diagnosis of pericardial effusion. Circulation **50:**239-247, 1974.
6. Kerber, R.E., Ridges, J.D., and Harrison, D.C.: Electrocardiographic indications of atrial puncture during pericardiocentesis, N. Engl. J. Med. **282:**1142-1143, 1970.
7. Klacsmann, P.G., Bulkley, B.H., and Hutchins, G.M.: The changed spectrum of purulent pericarditis, Am. J. Med. **63:**666-673, 1977.
8. Krikorian, J.G., and Hancock, E.W.: Pericardiocentesis, Am. J. Med. **65:** 808-814, 1978.
9. Tajik, A.J.: Echocardiography in pericardial effusion, Am. J. Med. **63:**29, 1977.
10. Theologides, A.: Neoplastic cardiac tamponade, Semin. Oncol. **5**(2):181-192, 1978.
11. Wei, J.Y., Taylor, G.J., and Achuff, S.C.: Recurrent cardiac tamponade and large pericardial effusions: management with an indwelling pericardial catheter, Am. J. Cardiol. **42:**281-282, 1978.
12. Zipf, R.E., and Johnson, W.W.: The role of cytology in the evaluation of pericardial effusions, Chest **62:**593-596, 1972.

CHAPTER 10

Temporary transvenous pacemaker insertion

■ Robert S. Gibson

■ GENERAL CONSIDERATIONS

Temporary transvenous cardiac pacing is a technique that permits sustained electrical stimulation of the right side of the heart by a percutaneously applied endocardial electrode. It is used primarily to control heart rate in patients with symptomatic bradycardia, threatened complete heart block, and various other acute rhythm disturbances associated with signs of cardiac or cerebral insufficiency.[6,7,9,17] Temporary pacing is also employed for diagnostic purposes* and occasionally for standby management in certain patients during acute myocardial infarction, cardiac catheterization, and surgery.[11,12,15,16] The veins used for temporary pacing, in order of preference, are subclavian, jugular, femoral, and brachial. The subclavian and jugular veins are reusable, allow neck and arm motion and early ambulation, and offer the advantage of speed of insertion during emergencies when fluoroscopy is unavailable. Although the femoral approach is a quick and easy means of pacemaker insertion, the high incidence of venous thrombosis, especially in the hemodynamically compromised patient, weakens its appeal.[14] The transbrachial approach is the easiest approach for the uninitiated, but sacrifices a vessel that may require eventual reuse and is associated with a high incidence of electrode displacement and myocardial perforation during arm motion.[1]

*References 2, 4, 5, 8, 18.

■ CHOICE OF ATRIAL OR VENTRICULAR STIMULATION

The chamber to pace is chosen on the basis of the patient's underlying rhythm, the integrity of atrioventricular nodal conduction, the desired hemodynamic effect, and the technical expertise of the operator. Atrial pacing or sequential atrial-ventricular pacing is more physiologic than ventricular pacing because synchronized atrioventricular systole is preserved. Atrial pacing, however, is complicated by the fact that a stable electrode position is difficult to maintain, since the smooth atrial sac offers no trabeculae into which the electrode can be inserted. Because a great deal of expertise is required for sequential atrioventricular pacing, this method is rarely used in emergency situations. For most patients, conventional ventricular pacing suffices.

■ THERAPEUTIC INDICATIONS[6,7,9,17*]

1. Symptomatic bradycardias from the following:
   a. Sinus node dysfunction, including sinus arrest, sinoatrial block, sinus bradycardia, or "brady-tachy" syndrome (V).
   b. Atrial fibrillation or flutter with high-grade atrioventricular block (V).
   c. High-grade second-degree atrioventricular block (V).
   d. Complete heart block (V).
   e. Drug-induced bradycardia with a necessary drug (A-V).
   f. Nodal bradycardia (V).
   g. Ventricular asystole (V).
2. Symptomatic tachycardias from the following:
   a. Paroxysmal atrial tachycardia (A).
   b. Ectopic atrial tachycardia (A).
   c. Atrial flutter (A).
   d. Intermittent ventricular tachycardia (A-V).
   e. Intermittent ventricular fibrillation (A-V).
3. Malfunction of a permanent pacemaker (V).
4. Carotid sinus syncope (A-V).

*The preferred site of catheter electrode placement is indicated as follows: A, atrium; V, ventricle; A-V, atrium or ventricle.

DIAGNOSTIC INDICATIONS*†

1. HIS bundle function studies (A-V).
2. Sinus node function studies (A).
3. Rhythm identification of arrhythmia analysis (A-V).
4. To provoke coronary insufficiency or detect subclinical left ventricular failure (A).
5. In cardiodynamic studies testing pacing effect for selection of optimal rate and mode of pacing (A-V).

PROPHYLACTIC OR STANDBY MANAGEMENT[11,12,15,16*]

1. During acute myocardial infarction with onset of the following:
   a. Mobitz type II atrioventricular block (V).
   b. Second- or third-degree atrioventricular block due to intra-HIS or infra-HIS block (V). This may include Mobitz type I block, if associated with anterior infarction and complete heart block.
   c. Right bundle branch block with either abnormal right or left axis deviation (V).
   d. Alternating right bundle branch block and left bundle branch block (V).
   e. Left bundle branch block with prolonged PR interval (V).
2. During cardiac catheterization with the following preexisting conditions:
   a. Right bundle branch block (V).
   b. Left bundle branch block (V).
3. During surgery with the following preexisting conditions:
   a. Severe bradycardia (heart rate ≤ 40 per minute) (V).
   b. Sinus bradycardia (heart rate ≤ 60 per minute) with impaired sinoatrial node response to treadmill exercise and/or intravenous atropine (sinus rate increase ≤ 90 per minute after 1.5-mg bolus) (V).
   c. Mobitz type II atrioventricular block or complete

*The preferred site of catheter electrode placement is indicated as follows: A, atrium; V, ventricle; A-V, atrium or ventricle.
†References 2, 4, 5, 8, 18.

heart block unless the permanent pacemaker is already in place (V).

d. Chronic bifascicular heart block associated with unexplained syncope, unstable angina, or recent myocardial infarction (V).

■ CONTRAINDICATIONS

1. Anticoagulant therapy or uncorrectable bleeding diathesis for the subclavian, femoral, or jugular vein approach.
2. Inability to tolerate a pneumothorax because of severe respiratory disease for the subclavian or jugular vein approach.
3. Prior surgery or deforming burns that obscure the neck anatomy for the subclavian or jugular vein approach.
4. Carotid artery disease such as plaques in the ipsilateral artery or high-grade obstruction of the contralateral artery for the jugular vein approach. If the carotid artery in inadvertently punctured, a plaque may be dislodged and embolize. Furthermore, therapeutic compression of the carotid artery after puncture may cause neurologic symptoms in patients with a high-grade contralateral carotid stenosis.

■ PATIENT EVALUATION AND PREPARATION

1. Initiate continuous cardiac rhythm monitoring of the patient.
2. Obtain a 12-lead electrocardiogram and, if possible, chest roentgenogram.
3. Obtain prothrombin time, partial thromboplastin time, and a platelet count.
4. Insert an intravenous line.
5. Explain the procedure to the patient, including its potential complications, and obtain written informed consent.
6. Place the patient on fluoroscopy table. Positioning of the pacing electrode using fluoroscopic control is relatively rapid and more secure, but electrocardiographic positioning can be used in emergency situations when

fluoroscopy is unavailable. Generally, the pacing threshold is lower and more stable when the electrode is guided into place fluoroscopically.

■ PERSONNEL AND EQUIPMENT

1. A physician skilled in pacemaker insertion, a radiology technician familiar with cardiac fluoroscopy, and a nurse capable of accurately reporting the patient's rhythm during the procedure.
2. Principal implements.
   a. Venous access. Subclavian or jugular route: 17-gauge needle and syringe (6 ml); catheter introducer set (UMI or Cordis)*; number 11 scalpel blade and knife handle; and straight mosquito clamp. Femoral route: Potts-Cournand needle; catheter introducer set (UMI or Cordis)*; number 11 scalpel blade and knife handle; and straight mosquito clamp. Brachial route: cutdown set (Chapter 4).
   b. Pacemaker assembly: bipolar pacing electrode (numbers 5 to 7 French) and a battery-powered pulse generator.
   c. Portable fluoroscope and lead aprons.
3. Disinfection and sterile field: antiseptic solution; sterile sponges, a mask, hair cap, gown, and gloves; draping towels; and towel clips.
4. Anesthesia: lidocaine (1%, 10 ml), syringe (10 ml), and 23-gauge (1-inch) needle.
5. Dressing: disinfectant ointment, sterile sponges, tincture of benzoin, and adhesive tape (1 inch, 3 inches) or Elastoplast (3 inches).
6. Resuscitation: cardiac defibrillator, suction apparatus, oxygen, airways, and preloaded syringe of lidocaine (100 mg). When there is manipulation of catheters in the heart, the defibrillator must be plugged in, turned on, and ready for rapid use.

*Includes guidewire, vessel dilator, and sheath. Choose the size appropriate for the pacing catheter.

■ TECHNIQUES

Subclavian vein insertion

1. Place the patient in the Trendelenburg position with a rolled sheet under the shoulders. Turn the patient's head to the opposite side.
2. Select a site for venipuncture (Chapter 5).
3. Put on a mask, haircap, sterile gloves, and gown. Put on a lead apron underneath the sterile gown.
4. Prepare and drape a sterile field.
5. Anesthetize the skin and subcutaneous tissue overlying the site of proposed venipuncture.
6. Perform a venipuncture. Use a subclavian venipuncture technique (Chapter 5, step 5) but use a 17-gauge needle. After venous blood has been freely aspirated, detach the syringe from the needle and occlude its hub with a finger to reduce the risk of air embolism.
7. Cannulate the vein. This is accomplished by using a modified Seldinger technique. First, insert the flexible end of the guidewire into the vein through the needle (Fig. 10-1, *A*). Withdraw the needle over the guidewire. Advance the introducer (sheath and dilator) over the guidewire, through the skin and subcutaneous tissue, and into the vein with a twisting motion (Fig. 10-1, *B*). Sufficient wire must be left externally so that it will protrude from the hub end of the introducer. Remove the guidewire and dilator, leaving the sheath in the vein (Fig. 10-1, *C*). Attach the syringe and aspirate venous blood.
8. Insert a pacing electrode. Place a 45-degree curve in the distal 5 cm of the electrode catheter. Detach the syringe from the introducing sheath and advance the electrode catheter through the sheath in the vein (Fig. 10-2). Leave the sheath in the vein.
9. Fluoroscopic positioning of pacing electrode. Advance the electrode catheter through the superior vena cava into the right atrium. Position the catheter tip against the lateral wall of the right atrium and form a **J** loop (Fig. 10-3, *A*). This position, or one at the junction of

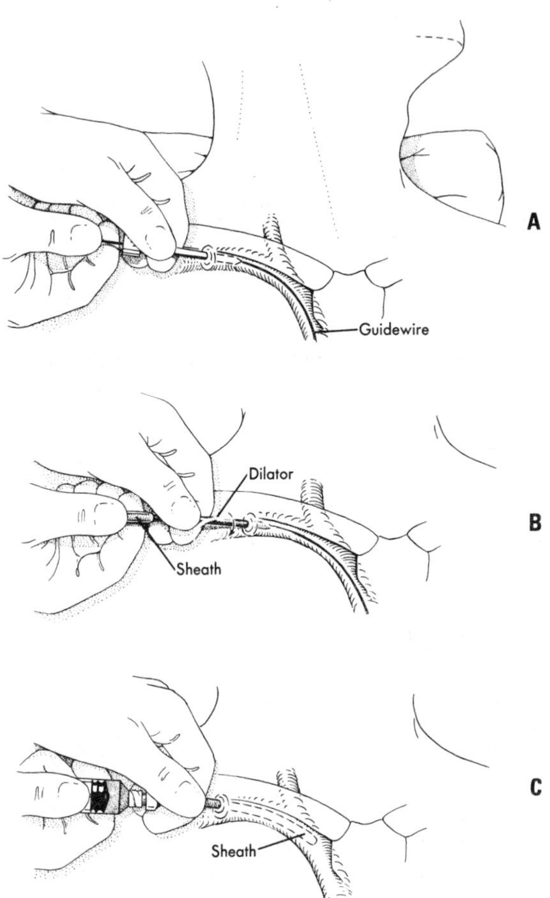

FIG. 10-1. A, Insert guidewire through needle into vein. Withdraw needle. **B,** Advance vessel dilator and sheath over guidewire into vein. **C,** Remove guidewire and dilator, leaving vessel sheath in vein. Attach syringe and aspirate.

the upper right atrium and superior vena cava, is satisfactory for rapid atrial pacing of supraventricular rhythms. For ventricular pacing, rotate the catheter in a counterclockwise direction and simultaneously advance it across the tricuspid valve into the right ventricle (Fig. 10-3, *B*). Rotate the catheter so that its tip

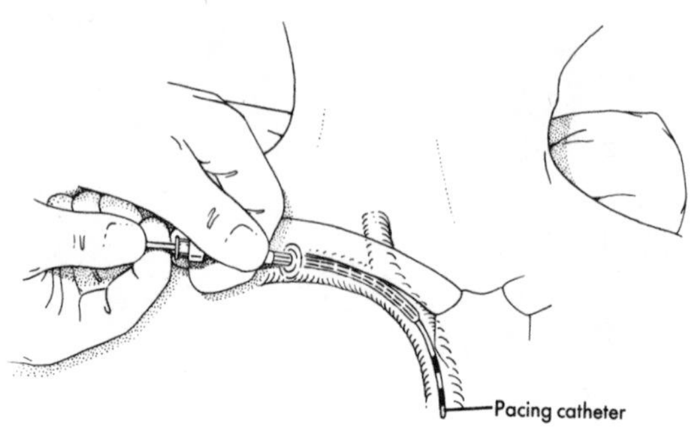

FIG. 10-2. Advance pacing catheter through sheath into vein.

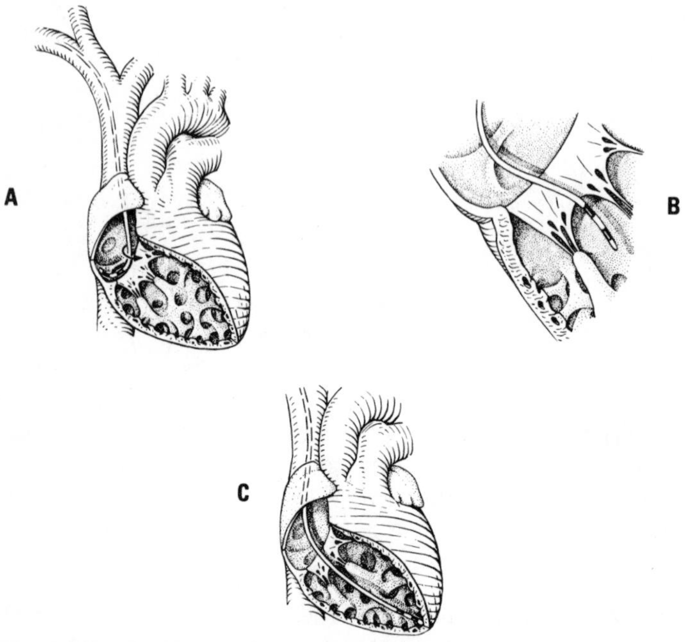

FIG. 10-3. A, Advance pacing catheter to right atrium. Form J loop against lateral wall of right atrium. **B,** Rotate pacing catheter in counterclockwise direction and simultaneously advance it across tricuspid valve into right ventricle. **C,** Advance pacing catheter tip to right ventricular apex and wedge it into a trabecula.

points inferiorly. Advance the catheter tip to the right ventricular apex and gently wedge it into a trabeculae (Fig. 10-3, *C*). Determine electrode stability fluoroscopically; wide swings of the tip during systole, heavy breathing, cough, the Valsalva maneuver, and body movement indicate improper position. The final electrode position should have the tip lodged in the right ventricular apex with slight tension on it. Excessive tension (i.e., too much buckling in the right ventricle) may cause ventricular perforation. Constant monitoring of the ECG is imperative during electrode manipulation. When there is excessive irritability, multiple extrasystole, or ventricular tachycardia, the catheter should be withdrawn to the right atrium or superior vena cava and a fresh approach made after abnormal electrical activity has subsided.

10. Establish cardiac pacing. The pulse generator should initially be turned to "off," and set on the "demand" mode with a rate of 70 and a current output of 0 milliamperes (mamp). Connect the *distal electrode* to the negative terminal of the pulse generator and the *proximal electrode* to the positive terminal. Turn the pulse generator "on" and set its rate slightly faster than the patient's rate. Slowly increase the current output until the ECG monitor confirms ventricular pacing. When the need to pace is urgent (i.e., ventricular asystole), the current is turned as high as necessary to secure immediate capture. This should be maintained, even at 15 to 25 mamp, to sustain pacing until the catheter is finally positioned. The pacing spike should be followed immediately by a wide QRS complex. Perform a 12-lead ECG to document the left bundle branch block pattern; if a right bundle branch pattern is observed, the electrode position is incorrect.
11. Establish a pacing threshold. Slowly decrease the generator output while monitoring the patient's rhythm. The output level at which ventricular pacing ceases is the stimulation threshold and should be less than 1

mamp, preferably 0.5 mamp. Resume pacing at an output 2 mamp above threshold.

12. Secure the pacing catheter. Once placement has been completed, the venous sheath is carefully withdrawn over the catheter, wiped free of blood, and pulled back to the electrode bifurcation. The catheter is then secured by suturing it at the skin entrance point.
13. Apply a dressing. Apply disinfectant ointment to the skin puncture site. Form two small loops of sterile catheter adjacent to the puncture site. Cover the puncture site and catheter loops with sterile dressing. Apply tincture of benzoin to the skin and tape the dressing securely.
14. Place the pulse generator in a cloth pouch and tie it loosely around the patient's neck.

Internal jugular vein insertion

1. Place the patient in the Trendelenburg position with a rolled sheet under the shoulders. Turn the patient's head to the opposite side.
2. Select a site for venipuncture (Chapter 6, step 2).
3. Put on a mask, hair cap, sterile gloves, and gown. Put on a lead apron underneath the sterile gown.
4. Prepare and drape a sterile field.
5. Anesthetize the skin and subcutaneous tissue overlying the site of proposed venipuncture.
6. Perform a venipuncture. Use an internal jugular venipuncture technique (Chapter 6, steps 5 and 6), but use a 17-gauge needle for vein cannulation. After venous blood has been freely aspirated, detach the syringe from the needle and occlude its hub with a finger to reduce the risk of air embolism.
7. Follow steps 7 to 14 of the subclavian vein insertion technique.

Femoral vein insertion

1. Place the patient in a supine position with the leg abducted.

2. Identify the anatomic landmarks for femoral venipuncture. The point of entry is just medial to the femoral artery pulse and approximately 1 or 2 inches (2.5 to 5 cm) below the inguinal crease (Chapter 7, Fig. 7-1).
3. Shave the groin.
4. Put on a mask, hair cap, sterile gloves, and gown. Put on a lead apron underneath the sterile gown.
5. Prepare and drape a sterile field.
6. Anesthetize the skin and subcutaneous tissue overlying the site of proposed venipuncture.
7. Perform a venipuncture. Make a small nick in the skin with a number 11 scalpel blade. Form a channel through the subcutaneous tissue by blunt dissection with a straight mosquito clamp. Insert the Potts-Cournand needle (with cutting obturator in place) through the skin nick at a 60-degree angle. Advance the needle until blood drips out of the needle hub (Fig. 10-4). Remove the obturator and attach a syringe to the needle. Aspirate to confirm venous blood return. Detach the syringe with the right hand, while holding the needle with the left hand to maintain venous access. Hold the thumb over the hub to prevent excessive blood loss.

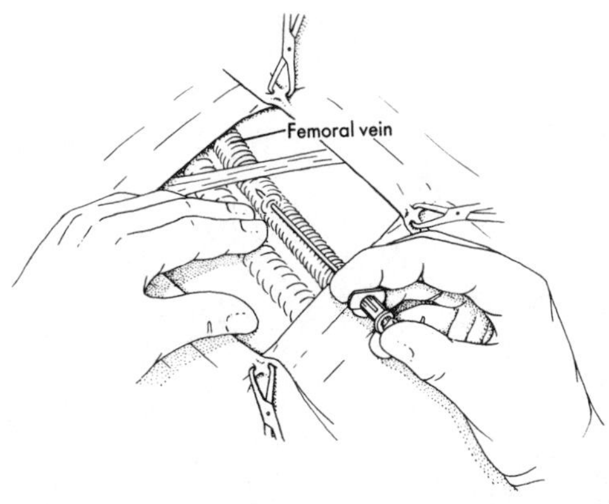

FIG. 10-4. Puncture vein with Potts-Cournand needle.

8. Cannulate the vein. Use the Seldinger technique as previously described (Fig. 10-1).
9. Insert a pacing electrode. Refer to step 8 of the subclavian vein insertion (Fig. 10-2).
10. Fluoroscopic positioning of the pacing electrode. Advance the electrode catheter up the inferior vena cava into the right atrium. In the right atrium, the catheter often catches on the upper rim of the tricuspid valve and promptly deflects into the apex of the right ventricle. If it does not, the catheter should be manipulated up and down until the tip catches a crevice in the lateral right atrial wall, and the catheter can be bent into a loop (Fig. 10-5, *A*). If ventricular placement is desired, the loop is then rotated clockwise so that the catheter tip lies medially and in the plane of the tricuspid valve (Fig. 10-5, *B*). The catheter is then withdrawn gradually until the tip is seen to make a slight movement toward the left side of the heart. This usually occurs as

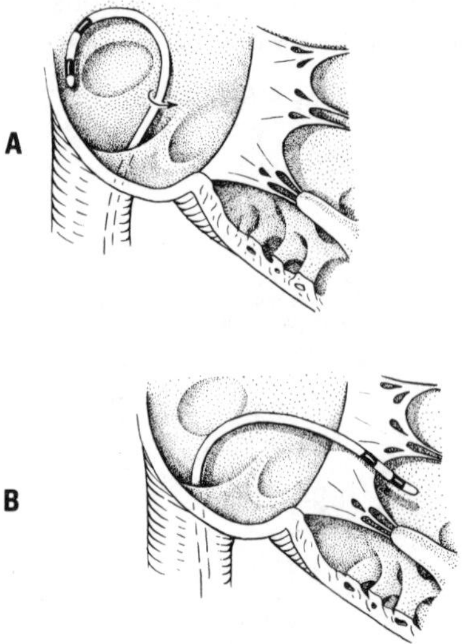

FIG. 10-5. A, Form J loop against lateral right atrial wall. **B,** Rotate pacing catheter so that its tip lies medially and in plane of tricuspid valve.

the tip slips through the tricuspid valve. The catheter is then rapidly advanced and gently wedged into a trabecula at the right ventricular apex. Determine electrode stability as previously described.

11. Establish cardiac pacing. Follow step 10 of the subclavian vein insertion.
12. Establish a pacing threshold. Follow step 11 of the subclavian vein insertion.
13. Secure the pacing catheter. Follow step 12 of the subclavian vein insertion, but limit movement of the lower extremity with a leg restraint.
14. Apply a dressing. The pulse generator should be securely taped to the anterior thigh.

Brachial vein insertion

1. Place the patient in the supine position with the arm slightly abducted. Immobilize the arm by taping it to an arm board.
2. Select a site for the venipuncture (Chapter 4, step 2).
3. Put on a mask, hair cap, sterile gloves, and gown. Put on a lead apron underneath the sterile gown.
4. Prepare and drape a sterile field.
5. Anesthetize the skin and subcutaneous tissue overlying the site of the proposed venipuncture.
6. Perform a venous cutdown and cannulate the vein (Chapter 4, steps 5 to 8).
7. Fluoroscopic positioning of the pacing electrode. Advance the electrode catheter toward the heart, through the superior vena cava and into the right atrium. Not infrequently, when the brachial vein is used, there is some holdup at shoulder level, which is usually due to the catheter passing down the lateral thoracic vein. This can be circumvented by withdrawing and turning the catheter tip toward the head. Once past this point, the tip should be rotated until it points toward the feet so that passage into the superior vena cava can be accomplished. The catheter tip is then positioned against the lateral wall of the right atrium so that it forms a J

loop (Fig. 10-3, *A, above*). This position, or one at the junction of the upper right atrium and superior vena cava, is satisfactory for rapid atrial pacing of supraventricular rhythms. For ventricular pacing, rotate the catheter in a *counterclockwise* direction and simultaneously advance it across the tricuspid valve into the right ventricle (Fig. 10-3, *B, above*). Rotate the catheter so that its tip points inferiorly and advance it to the right ventricular apex (Fig. 10-3, *C*). Gently wedge the tip into a trabecula. Determine electrode stability as described.

8. Establish cardiac pacing. (See step 10 of the subclavian vein insertion.)
9. Establish a pacing threshold. (See step 11 of the subclavian vein insertion.)
10. Secure the pacing catheter. Tie the proximal ligature around the vein and the catheter tight enough to prevent leakage of blood. Tie the distal ligature around the catheter to prevent slippage.
11. Close the wound and apply a dressing. Irrigate the wound with sterile saline and close the incision with 3-0 nylon. Apply a disinfectant ointment to the suture line. Form one or two small loops of sterile catheter adjacent to the suture line. Cover the wound and catheter loops with sterile dressing and tape securely. The pulse generator should be securely taped to the forearm.

■ POSTPROCEDURE CARE

1. Obtain a portable PA and lateral chest roentgenogram to confirm proper electrode position and as a baseline for possible future displacement. A well-positioned ventricular electrode, seen in the frontal plane, arises from the lower right side of the heart, makes a slight upward arc across the vertebral column, and dips inferiorly toward the left. In the lateral view, the catheter tip points *anteriorly* and lies inferior to the lower border of the sternum. If the tip points posteriorly, it may be lodged in the coronary sinus. When rapid pacing of the atrium is

to be performed, it is imperative that the catheter tip be positioned in an area of the atrium where the risk of displacement into the ventricle is minimal. Check the catheter tip frequently to ensure its safe position in the atrium.

2. Monitor pacemaker function continuously. Choose an appropriate ECG lead so that the pace spikes and QRS complexes are well seen.
3. Avoid electrical hazards. All monitoring equipment, when not battery powered, should be properly grounded. Insulate the exposed pacemaker terminals and electrodes from stray currents by covering them with a rubber glove. Unplug an electric bed, obtain all electrocardiograms with a battery-operated machine, and do not allow the patient to use an electric razor.
4. Check the stimulation threshold daily.
5. Inspect the venipuncture site and change the dressings daily. Remove old crusts with peroxide and keep the site as clean and dry as possible.
6. Management of ectopic rhythms. Persistent ectopic ventricular beats that result from catheter irritation may be ignored if they are infrequent and the patient has a stable rhythm. They usually disappear within a few hours. If they continue and are frequent, multifocal, or associated with a recent myocardial injury or tachyrhythmia, they should be suppressed by overdrive pacing or lidocaine administration.

■ COMPLICATIONS

Nonspecific complications of vascular access

See Chapters 4 to 6.

Specific complications of pacemaker use*

1. Myocardial perforation. Perforation of the right ventricular wall complicates 1% to 3% of temporary pacemaker insertions and has caused death. It results from continuous or intermittent pressure of the catheter on the thin

*References 1, 3, 10, 13, 14.

right ventricular apex or anterior wall. The incidence is increased by use of a stiff electrode and excessive motion of the extremity if the femoral or brachial routes are used. Perforation frequently is signaled by loss of pacing, particularly when extrusion of the stimulating tip is complete and myocardial or epicardial contact is lost. It should be considered in the differential diagnosis of a postinsertion friction rub and the patient watched closely for confirmatory evidence. Sometimes perforation may not be evident clinically when neither loss of pacing nor noticeable pericardial bleeding occur. Acute pericardial tamponade is rare. A greater problem is posed by the patient with a slow blood leak and no evident electrode displacement on chest roentgenograms or loss of pacing function, whose condition deteriorates into increasing congestive heart failure or shock. When suspected, echocardiography may be diagnostic.

2. Pacing failure without loss of pacing artifact. Threshold elevation due to intracardiac electrode displacement, myocardial perforation and inflammation or, necrosis at the catheter tip are the usual causes. Minor electrode displacement results in intermittent pacing failure (cessation of ventricular response), shifting threshold levels, and, possibly, a change in the QRS axis. Often, pacing can be restored with greater current output (e.g., 5 to 10 mamp). If a reasonable increase in output fails to restore regular pacing, the electrode should be repositioned. Rarely, battery depletion with enough residual current output to produce a pacemaker artifact, but not enough to meet threshold requirements, causes this problem.
3. Pacing failure with loss of pacing artifact. This may be caused by partial or total disruption of the exteriorized electrode assembly (disconnected, broken, or short-circuited wires), battery failure, or pulse generator malfunction. If the electrodes are intact and a fresh battery and pulse generator do not restore normal pacing, a reduction of sensitivity of the sensor circuit to screen out

excessive stimuli (while remaining sensitive to contractions) may correct this problem.

4. Pacemaker runaway. Instability of the electronic circuitry may result in a pacemaker rate over 120 beats per minute, which is called "runaway pacemaker." This is probably the most dangerous of all pacemaker malfunctions and can result in congestive heart failure, hypotension, ventricular fibrillation, and death. Fortunately, its incidence has decreased with newer instruments.
5. Diaphragmatic stimulation. This may be due to catheter displacement into the right atrium or superior vena cava with stimulation of the right phrenic nerve or myocardial perforation with direct stimulation of the left diaphragmatic leaf. Diaphragmatic stimulation can also occur if the right ventricle rests on the diaphragm and the electrode tip is directed posteriorly rather than anteriorly. Withdrawal of the electrode tip into the right ventricle or appropriate repositioning of the tip restores normal stimulation.

REFERENCES

1. Austin, J.L., Preis, L.K., and Crampton, R.S. et al.: An analysis of malfunction and complications of temporary pacing, Am. J. Cardiol. **45:**459, 1980.
2. Benchimol, A., and Liggett, M.S.: Cardiac hemodynamics during stimulation of the right atrium, right ventricle, and left ventricle in normal and abnormal hearts, Circulation **33:**933-944, 1966.
3. Bramowitz, A.D., Smith, J.W., and Eber, I.M. et al.: Runaway pacemaker: a persisting problem, J.A.M.A. **228:**340-341, 1974.
4. Chandry, K.R., Orifus, L.S., and Ogawa, S.: Uses and limitations of HIS bundle electrocardiography, Cardiovasc. Med. **3:**1039-1041, 1978.
5. Cheng, T.O.: Atrial pacing: its diagnostic and therapeutic applications, Prog. Cardiovasc. Dis. **14:**230-247, 1971.
6. Escher, D.J., Furman, S., Fisher, J.D., and Ginsti, R.: Temporary pacing in the treatment of arrhythmias. In Watanabe, Y., editor: Cardiac pacing, Amsterdam, 1977, Excerpta Medica.
7. Escher, D.J., and Furman, S.: Emergency treatment of cardiac arrhythmias: emphasis on use of electrical pacing, J.A.M.A. **214:**2028-2034, 1970.
8. Evans, T.R., Callowhill, E.S., and Kirkler, D.M.: Clinical values of test of sinoatrial function, PACE **1:**2-7, 1978.
9. Fontaine, G., and Marcus, F.I.: Current status of pacemaker therapy of arrhythmias, Curr. Probl. Cardiol. **5**(4):1-45, 1980.

10. Furman, S., and Escher, D.J.: Temporary transvenous pacing. In Furmans, S., and Escher, D.J., editors: Principles and techniques of cardiac pacing, New York, 1970, Harper Row, Publishers, Inc.
11. Hindman, M.G., Wagner, G.S., nd JaRo, M. et al.: The clinical significance of bundle branch block complicating acute myocardial infarction, II. Indications for temporary and permanent pacemaker insertion, Circulation **58:**689-699, 1978.
12. Kimbiris, D., Dreifus, L.S., and Linhart, J.W.: Complete heart block occurrence during cardiac catheterization in patients with pre-existing bundle branch block, Chest **65:**95-97, 1974.
13. Lumia, F.J., and Rios, J.C.: Temporary transvenous pacemaker therapy: an analysis of complications, Chest **64:**604-608, 1973.
14. Nolewajka, A.J., Goddard, M.D., and Brown, I.C.: Temporary transvenous pacing and femoral vein thrombosis, Circulation **62:**646-650, 1980.
15. Pastore, J.O., Yurchak, P.M., and Janis, K.M. et al.: The risk of advanced heart block in surgical patients with right bundle branch block and left axis deviation, Circulation **57:**677-680, 1978.
16. Rose, S.D., Corman, L.C., and Mason, D.I.: Cardiac risk factors in patients undergoing noncardiac surgery, Med. Clin. North Am. **63:**1271-1288, 1979.
17. Schwartz, K.M., MacLean, W.A.H., and Waldo, A.L.: Treatment of life threatening cardiac arrhythmias. In Rackley, E.C., editor: Cardiovascular clinics, Philadelphia, 1981, F.A. Davis Co.
18. Wellens, H.J.J.: Value and limitations of programmed electrical stimulation of the heart in the study and treatment of tachycardias, Circulation **57:**845-853, 1977.

CHAPTER 11

Cardioversion: synchronized transthoracic direct current shock

■ Robert S. Gibson
Richard S. Crampton

■ GENERAL CONSIDERATIONS

Transthoracic synchronized cardioversion is a method of delivering a direct current electric shock to the heart via a pair of electrodes placed on the chest wall to terminate supraventricular and ventricular tachycardias. Delivery of the shock is controlled by synchronizing the capacitor's discharge to the R wave of the QRS complex to avoid the ventricular vulnerable period and hence accidentally fibrillating the ventricles. The electric shock transiently depolarizes the majority of automatic pacemaker and myocardial cells and abolishes the arrhythmia. Then, the sinoatrial node or subsidiary pacemaker in the atrium, atrioventricular junction, or ventricle regains control of cardiac rhythm.

■ INDICATIONS[2,3,8]

Urgent cardioversion

1. Supraventricular tachycardia, atrial flutter, and atrial fibrillation associated with hypotension, systemic hypoperfusion, congestive heart failure, or myocardial ischemia.
2. Ventricular tachycardia associated with a palpable pulse that fails to convert to sinus rhythm with lidocaine.

Elective cardioversion

Cardioversion may be elected for supraventricular tachycardia, atrial flutter, and atrial fibrillation, which fail to convert to sinus rhythm with digitalis, propranolol, edrophonium, phenylephrine, quinidine, or verapamil. Generally, sinus rhythm is preferable to arrhythmias because of enhanced cardiac output and lower frequency of embolism.

■ CONTRAINDICATIONS

1. Digitalis intoxication. Ventricular fibrillation may be produced despite synchronization of the direct current shock at a safe point in the cardiac cycle.[7,8,13] Rapid atrial stimulation with a temporary pacing electrode may convert supraventricular arrhythmias with little or no danger.[4,9] Likewise, ventricular arrhythmias occasionally convert with impulses delivered via a pacing electrode (Chapter 10).
2. Underlying conduction system disease. Complete atrioventricular block is an absolute contraindication, since cardioversion will not provide hemodynamic benefit. Furthermore, cardioversion may produce asystole.[8,11] If advanced second-degree atrioventricular block or bradycardia is present, a prophylactic temporary pacemaker should be inserted before attempting cardioversion in anticipation of a very slow rate after direct current shock (Chapter 10). This protective measure with a pacing electrode is also applicable in the tachycardia phase of the bradycardia-tachycardia syndrome, if indications for cardioversion are present.
3. Patients who have not been able to maintain a satisfactory heart rate when in sinus rhythm.[8]
4. Atrial fibrillation of several years duration.[8]
5. When previous cardioversion has been followed by prompt return to atrial fibrillation, despite adequate prophylactic doses of quinidine.[8]
6. Recent valvular heart surgery.[9] A patient in whom tachyarrhythmias develop immediately after valve replacement often does not maintain sinus rhythm even if it is restored electrically. Therefore if the patient is tolerating the tachyarrhythmia without difficulty, cardioversion should be postponed for 10 to 14 days after the

operation. In most cardiovascular surgical units, atrial electrodes are available for terminating tachyarrhythmias (Chapter 10).

7. Cardiac enlargement, especially when the left atrium is greatly enlarged.[5]

■ PATIENT EVALUATION AND PREPARATION

1. Evaluate the patient for hyperthyroidism, digitalis intake, hypoxemia, recent psychologic stress, anemia, hypokalemia, hyperkalemia, hypocalcemia, hypomagnesemia, or other autonomic or metabolic disturbances that contribute to or cause arrhythmias.
2. Explain the procedure fully to the patient, including its potential complications, and obtain signed informed consent.
3. Consider prophylactic anticoagulation.[1,2,12] Administration of warfarin for 2 to 4 weeks before cardioversion may prevent systemic embolization. Although no controlled randomized studies justify prophylactic anticoagulation, it is nevertheless recommended for patients in atrial fibrillation with a history of embolism, mitral stenosis, congestive heart failure, or left atrial enlargement.
4. Discontinue digitalis. Digoxin should be stopped 24 hours before cardioversion and perhaps 48 to 72 hours in the elderly. Longer acting preparations like digitoxin should be discontinued for 2 to 5 days. If digitalis intoxication is suspected, obtain the appropriate serum glycoside level.
5. Administer quinidine (300 mg every 6 hours) for 2 days before the cardioversion to ascertain whether it can be tolerated, obtain adequate blood and tissue levels for preventing a recurrence of atrial fibrillation, and convert the 10% to 15% of patients who will respond to this drug alone.[12] In addition, quinidine reduces the necessary number of shocks, decreases by about 40% the energy required to restore normal sinus rhythm, and diminishes the incidence of postcardioversion arrhythmias. In a

small number of sensitive individuals, treatment with quinidine induces ventricular tachycardia and, occasionally, ventricular fibrillation. These arrhythmias may be aggravated by direct current shock.

6. Do not permit the patient to eat or drink for at least 6 hours before the procedure.
7. Place the patient in a special care unit where cardiac rhythm can be continuously monitored. Obtain a 12-lead electrocardiogram (ECG) to document the rhythm. Tracings from ECG recorders that provide three simultaneous leads are preferred.
8. Insert an intravenous line.
9. Place a cardiac resuscitation backboard beneath the patient's chest.

■ PERSONNEL AND EQUIPMENT

1. A physician skilled in electric cardioversion and a nurse capable of setting up the capacitor-synchronizer unit. Although an anesthetist is not strictly necessary, we prefer to have one present in case the patient is slow to awaken or, rarely, if the patient should require airway management, such as endotracheal intubation.
2. Principal implements: direct-current cardioverter with oscilloscope monitor, synchronization mode, selection switch for energy levels, electrode paddles and electrode jelly. Saline soaked pads cause electric spark arcs if too wet and increased resistance to current flow if too dry.
3. Drugs for sedation: amnesia or anesthesia during cardioversion is achieved with diazepam (Valium), thiopental sodium (Pentothal), or methohexital sodium (Brevital).
4. Resuscitation: backboard, suction apparatus, oxygen, airways, hand-held ventilation bag, and syringes preloaded with atropine (1 mg) and lidocaine (100 mg).

■ TECHNIQUE[10]

1. Place the patient supine on the cardiac resuscitation board.

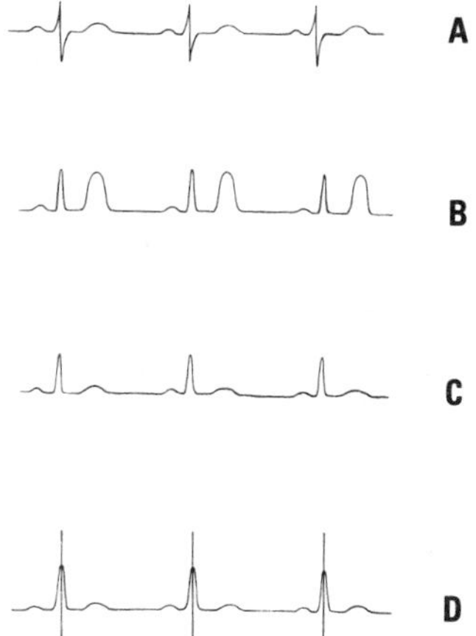

FIG. 11-1. A, Equiphasic QRS complexes. **B,** Large T waves. **C,** Proper lead position, demonstrating major QRS deflection and low-voltage T wave. **D,** Synchronizing signal falls on R wave.

2. Attach the ECG monitoring leads to the patient's chest. Position the leads so as to obtain a large R or Q wave deflection on the ECG. Avoid positions that record equiphasic QRS complexes (Fig. 11-1, *A*) or large T waves (Fig. 11-1, *B*). Whenever possible, choose lead positions that record a major QRS deflection and a low-voltage T wave (Fig. 11-1, *C*).
3. Turn the cardioversion and synchronizer switch on. Ascertain that the synchronizing signal falls on the R wave (Fig. 11-1, *D*). Adjust the R wave sensor so that the shock will fall during or just at the end of the QRS complex, but not in the S-T segment or on the T wave.
4. Remove the oxygen and its apparatus or any other potentially combustible and flammable substances from the vicinity.
5. Administer the sedative drug slowly, monitoring heart rate, respirations, and blood pressure.
6. Reduce transthoracic resistance by applying electrode paste to the paddles. Gauze pads soaked in saline should not be used. They can lead to dangerous current

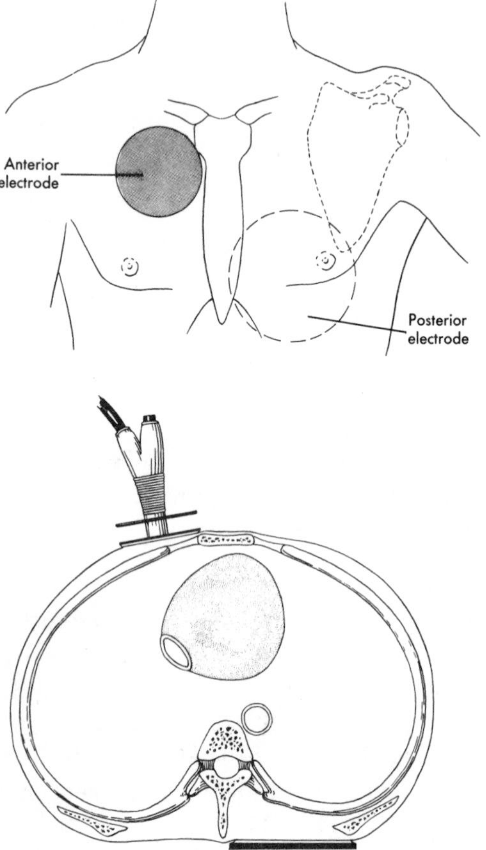

FIG. 11-2. Anteroposterior paddle electrode position.

arcs if too wet and increased resistance to current flow if too dry.

7. Depending on the type of cardioverter and types of electrodes available, two positions are conventionally used for placing the chest electrodes: the anteroposterior (Fig. 11-2) and anteroapical (Fig. 11-3) positions. In the anteroposterior orientation, the anterior electrode is placed lateral to the right edge of the sternum and the posterior electrode between the spine and left scapula

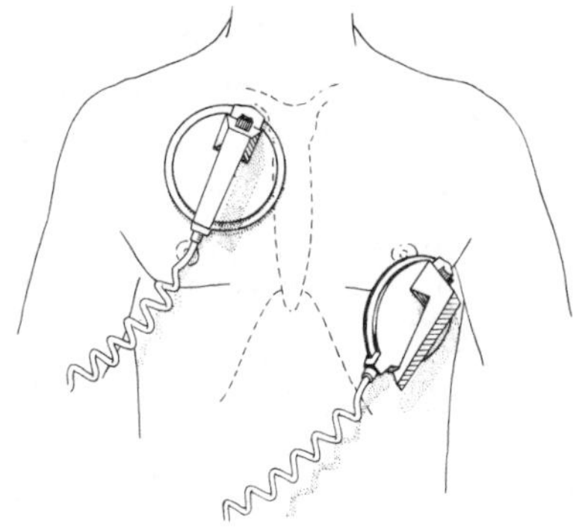

FIG. 11-3. Anteroapical paddle electrode position.

(Fig. 11-2). The weight of the patient usually keeps the electrode in place just beside the lower left scapula. Abducting the patient's left elbow at 45 degrees will move the left scapula away from the posterior electrode and reduce the tissue impedance to the flow of cardioverting current through the chest. Such positioning has been shown to yield a high rate of reversion at lower energies, presumably due to the development of greater current density through the heart.[8] If the other type of cardioverter is used, the 8- to 8.5-cm paddle electrodes should be applied as for ventricular defibrillation (Figs. 11-3 and 12-1). Paddle electrode number one is positioned below the right clavicle just lateral to the upper sternum, and paddle electrode number two is placed just lateral and below the left nipple in the anterior axillary line. Firm pressure (25 pounds; 11.25 kg) should be applied to each electrode during delivery of the shock. In the anteroposterior electrode position, it will only be necessary to press firmly on the anterior electrode.

8. Select the desired energy level. The choice will depend on the type of arrhythmia, urgency of the clinical situation, and whether or not the patient is taking digitalis. Low-energy shocks should be tried first because they elicit less ventricular irritability, less bradycardia, minimize chest wall injury, lessen the risk of myocardial damage, and are less uncomfortable to the patient. Atrial flutter and rapid ventricular tachycardia often require only 5 to 20 joules (watt-seconds), whereas cardioversion of atrial fibrillation usually requires 50 joules or more.

9. Ascertain that there is no contact between the operator or the assistants and the patient or conductive material touching the patient (metal bed frame, side rails, ventilating equipment, etc).
10. Administer the shock when the patient is adequately sedated, using firm (25 pounds; 11.25 kg) pressure on the electrodes.
11. Check the patient's pulse, ECG, and airway immediately after the shock. The immediate cardiac response to transthoracic electric shock appears vagal with significant bradycardia. This initial slow rate response is usually succeeded by tachycardia within 30 seconds, presumably of sympathetic origin. Higher levels of current and energy tend to depress or injure the sinoatrial node and impair subsidiary pacemakers. Ventricular arrhythmias and significant S-T and T wave abnormalities also may reflect cardiac damage from the shock or drug interaction with the shock.
12. If the shock fails, increase the energy dose in a stepwise fashion (10, 25, 50, 100, 200, 300, 360 joules) until the arrhythmia is converted or until 360 joules have failed. Allow 2 minutes between shocks for supraventricular tachycardias, since they frequently may convert late after the shock.

■ POSTPROCEDURE CARE

1. Perform a brief examination, looking for immediate complications such as hypotension, systemic embolization, pulmonary edema, and aspiration.
2. Obtain a 12-lead ECG and monitor the patient's rhythm for at least several hours.

■ COMPLICATIONS

1. Skin burns. Inadequate electrode contact with the skin causes the current to arc between the paddle and the skin, and first- and second-degree burns result. A first-degree burn also may occur if repeated shocks are needed, even with good electrode contact.
2. Arrhythmias. Atrial and junctional ectopic beats, atrioventricular junctional rhythms, ventricular premature beats, ventricular tachycardia, and ventricular fibrillation may appear after direct current shocks. The frequency of ventricular fibrillation is 1.1%,[13] and it occurs predominantly when the shock is administered during the ventricular vulnerable period on the T wave or in the S-T segment. Patients with digitalis intoxication also have a greater risk of ventricular fibrillation with synchronized direct current shock. Slow atrioventricular junctional, His bundle, or ventricular escape rhythms may occur if the sinoatrial node is sluggish, damaged by the shock, or under the influence of drugs like digitalis, beta-adrenergic blockers, or calcium antagonists.
3. Cardiac muscle damage. S-T and T wave changes occur in approximately 1% and significant elevation in serum creatine kinase in 9%[13] of the patients. The significance of these abnormalities is not clear, but no serious residual myocardial damage has been reported.
4. Cardiac enlargement.[13]
5. Pulmonary edema. There are at least 27 reported cases[2] of pulmonary edema, and the cause is believed to be left atrial paralysis. Even though sinus rhythm may be seen, left atrial contraction may be uncoupled.
6. Systemic embolization. The frequency of systemic embolization is approximately 0.8%[13] but may be higher in a patient with a large left atrium, mitral stenosis, congestive heart failure, or a previous embolism. It is due to dislodgment of an intracardiac thrombus.
7. Hypotension. In most patients, hypotension is brief, ends in a few hours, and does not require any therapy.[13]
8. Aspiration pneumonitis.

REFERENCES

1. Bjerkelund, C.J., and Orning, O.M.: The efficacy of anticoagulant therapy in preventing embolism related to DC electrical conversion of atrial fibrillation, Am. J. Cardiol. **23:**208-216, 1969.
2. Dorney, E.R.: The use of cardioversion and pacemakers in the management of arrhythmias. In Hurst, J.W., editor: New York, 1978, The Heart, McGraw-Hill, Inc.
3. Dreifus, L.S.: Use of DC shock in the treatment of cardiac arrhythmias. in Fowler, N.O.: Treatment of cardiac arrhythmias, New York, 1970, Harper & Row, Publishers, Inc.
4. Haft, J.I.: Treatment of arrhythmias by intracardiac electrical stimulation, Prog. Cardiovasc. Dis. **16:**539-568, 1974.
5. Henry, W.L., et al.: Relation between echocardiographically determined left atrial size and atrial fibrillation, Circulation **53:**273-279, 1976.
6. Jenzer, H., and Lown, B.: Cardioversion of atrial fibrillation after value replacement, Am. Heart J. **84:**840-842, 1972.
7. Kleiger, R.E., and Lown, B.: Cardioversion and digitalis. II. Clinical studies, Circulation **33:**878-887, 1966.
8. Kleiger, R.E., and Wolff, G.: Indications and contraindications for cardioversion of arrhythmias, Heart Lung **2:**552-560, 1973.
9. Lister, J.W., et al.: Treatment of supraventricular arrhythmias by rapid atrial stimulation, Circulation **38:**1044-1060, 1968.
10. Lown, B., Kleiger, R., and Wolff, G.: The technique of cardioversion, Am. Heart J. **67:**282-284, 1964.
11. Martin, R.H.: Elective conversion of cardiac arrhythmias with precordial shock. In Stephenson, H.E., editor: ed. 4, St. Louis, 1974, The C.V. Mosby Co.
12. Resnekov, L.: Drug therapy before and after the electroversion of cardiac dysrhythmias, Prog. Cardiovasc. Dis. **16:**531-538, 1974.
13. Resnekov, L., and McDonald, L.: Complications in 220 patients with cardiac dysrhythmias treated by direct current shock and indications for electroconversion, Br. Heart J. **29:**926-936, 1967.

CHAPTER 12

Ventricular defibrillation: unsynchronized transthoracic direct current shock

■ Robert S. Gibson
Richard S. Crampton

■ GENERAL CONSIDERATIONS

Countershock is the application of direct current electric shock to the chest to terminate ventricular fibrillation or ventricular tachycardia that results in life-threatening hemodynamic compromise. It is an emergency procedure involving delivery of an *unsynchronized* electric shock. In contrast, cardioversion is an elective procedure for converting supraventricular or ventricular arrhythmias with an electric shock synchronized to fall at a safe point in the cardiac cycle (R wave of the QRS) (Chapter 11).

■ INDICATIONS

1. Ventricular fibrillation.
2. Ventricular tachycardia without a detectable peripheral arterial pulse or that fails to provide adequate circulation (such as in apnea or collapse).
3. Sudden collapse with loss of pulse. It can be assumed that at least 75% of these patients have ventricular fibrillation.[6] Blind defibrillation[6,9] (without rhythm confirmation) can be satisfactorily accomplished in a few patients

even before cardiopulmonary resuscitation (CPR) is undertaken if the electric shock is applied within 30 seconds of the arrest. However, CPR should be started promptly unless one can immediately apply a shock to defibrillate the heart. If the patient is in cardiac arrest due to ventricular fibrillation before arriving at the hospital, CPR should be initiated within 4 minutes and defibrillation attempted within 8 minutes; half the patients are long-term survivors.[4,10]

■ CONTRAINDICATIONS

There are no absolute contraindications, since persistent ventricular fibrillation always leads to death, and ventricular defibrillation rarely occurs spontaneously.[1,2] The following are contraindications to ventricular defibrillation:

1. The decision to permit the patient to die (those with hopeless, terminal illness).
2. Conscious patients with palpable spontaneous arterial pulse. Regardless of what the oscilloscope or ECG show, these patients do not require *unsynchronized* electric shock. Artifacts on the oscilloscope or ECG strip chart may masquerade as ventricular tachycardia or fibrillation and should not be treated with electric shock or antiarrhythmic drugs. Loose electrodes, muscle tremors, and defective recording equipment are common causes of false ventricular arrhythmias. After exclusion of ECG artifacts in a conscious patient, if electroversion is necessary, the protocol for synchronized direct current shock should be followed.
3. Unkempt or malfunctioning defibrillators with visible hazards, such as broken insulation, frayed wires, broken dials, bent paddle electrodes, cracked electrode handles, etc. In this situation, CPR should be continued until equipment that is safe for the user and patient arrives.

■ EQUIPMENT NEEDED

1. Cardiac defibrillator.
2. Electrically conductive material, such as electrode paste or jelly.

3. Rhythm monitoring equipment (ECG recorder, paddle electrode, and oscilloscope monitor).

TECHNIQUE

1. While another member of the resuscitation team is administering CPR, the operator should proceed as follows:
   a. Turn the off/on switch or push button to the *on* position.
   b. Turn the switch or push button to charge the capacitor.
   c. Adjust the energy level setting to 150 to 200 joules (watt-seconds) for adult patients with ventricular fibrillation of a 2-minute duration or more or of unknown duration.[1] If ventricular fibrillation occurs in a closely monitored situation and the defibrillator is immediately at hand, shocks of 50 to 100 joules may be delivered.[2] Such patients typically have identified themselves by previous episodes of ventricular tachycardia or fibrillation out of the hospital, in the intensive care unit, or in the electrophysiologic laboratory during electroprovocative stimulation tests.[1,2,4,10]
2. Spread conductive jelly on the electrode paddles.
3. Position the paddle electrodes on the patient (Fig. 12-1).
   a. Press firmly (25 pounds; 11.25 kg) one paddle elec-

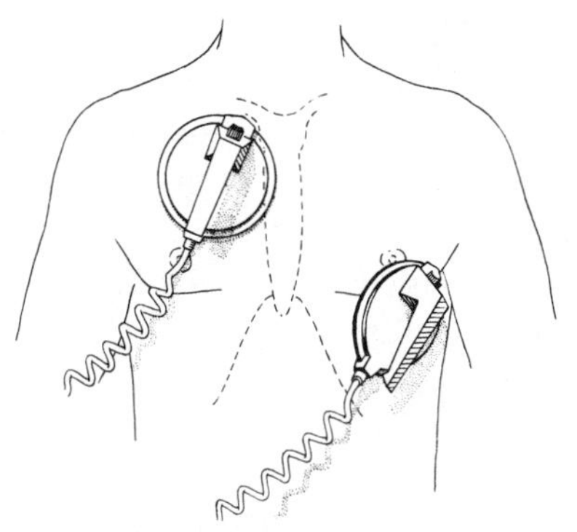

FIG. 12-1. Position paddles on patient's chest.

trode just to the right of the upper sternum, below the right clavicle.

b. Press firmly (25 pounds; 11.25 kg) the other electrode to the left of the cardiac apex, usually left of and below the nipple.

4. Be sure that no personnel contact the patient, metal bed frame, or other conductive material in contact with the patient.
5. Press the buttons on the paddle electrodes simultaneously to discharge the electric shock through the patient's chest and heart.
6. Immediately after the shock, a member of the resuscitation team should palpate for an arterial pulse and obtain an ECG rhythm strip. If no pulse is detected, resume CPR regardless of the rhythm.
7. If the patient's heart defibrillates and then refibrillates, the same energy, or lower energy, shock should be delivered promptly within 5 to 15 seconds.[1,2]
8. Additional countershocks are administered if necessary, while other supportive and therapeutic measures are being carried out simultaneously.[1,2] The shock energy sequence should be 150 to 200, 200, 300, and 360 joules.[1] If one is unable to defibrillate, proceed as follows:
   a. Continue CPR between shocks.
   b. Correct acidosis or alkalosis and abnormal ion ratios (potassium, calcium, magnesium, etc.).
   c. Make sure that pulmonary ventilation is adequate; when possible, serial arterial blood gases should be obtained.
   d. Administer intravenous epinephrine (0.5 mg) and/or calcium chloride (5 ml of 10% solution) (1 gm/10 ml), if there is fine ventricular fibrillation (Fig. 12-2) or asystole on the ECG recording. Magnesium sulfate also may expedite ventricular defibrillation.[2] Not infrequently, these maneuvers will coarsen the ventricular fibrillation (Fig. 12-2) and allow effective defibrillation.
   e. Check the function of the defibrillator. Failure of direct current defibrillator output is higher than sus-

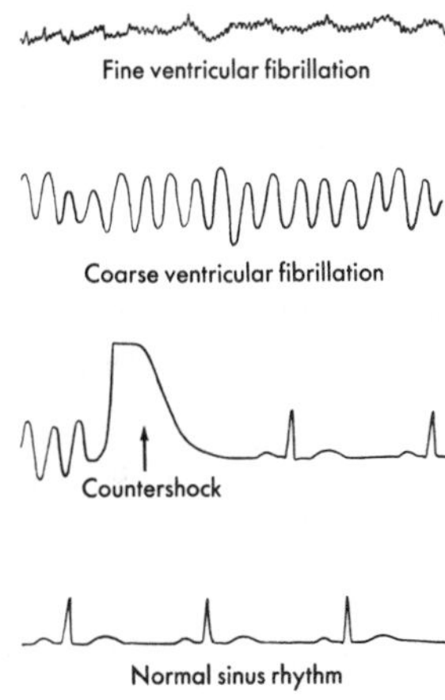

FIG. 12-2. Ventricular fibrillation converting to sinus rhythm with countershock.

pected, and muscular jerks at the time of defibrillator discharge do not indicate adequate flow of electric current through the chest wall and heart.[3] Consider using another defibrillating device while continuing CPR.

f. Consider administration of antiarrhythmic drugs, such as lidocaine (50- to 100-mg bolus injection followed by a 2- to 4-mg/min infusion), procainamide (100 to 500 mg IV over 1 to 5 minutes) and bretylium tosylate (5 mg/kg/IV bolus).[5,7]

■ POSTPROCEDURE PATIENT CARE

Patients who survive ventricular fibrillation require careful ECG monitoring, measures to control arrhythmias and prevent recurrence of ventricular fibrillation, and general management of underlying diseases and pathophysiologic conditions.[1]

1. Transfer the patient to the intensive care unit.
2. Perform a physical examination, looking particularly for complications of resuscitation, such as rib fractures, pneumothorax, or rupture of the liver or spleen. (See Chapter 13.)
3. Obtain a chest roentgenogram and ECG.

4. Carefully monitor the following:
   a. Blood pressure and pulse and respiratory rates.
   b. Cardiac rhythm, especially frequency (5 or more beats/min) and type (couplets, multifocal, bigeminy, R or T phenomenon) of ventricular premature beats, bursts of unsustained ventricular tachycardia, and sustained ventricular tachycardia. Prompt antiarrhythmic therapy is essential to prevent recurrence of ventricular fibrillation.
   c. Cerebral (higher integrative) function.[8]
   d. Arterial blood gases. Acidosis and alkalosis predispose to refibrillation.
   e. Electrolytes and renal function.
   f. Occasionally it will be desirable to monitor hemodynamics precisely, such as measuring PCW pressure and cardiac output (Chapter 8).

■ COMPLICATIONS

The sequellae of CPR (Chapter 13) and defibrillation are numerous and result from mechanical and electrical injury. With medical personnel well trained in basic and advanced life support tactics, the frequency of the following complications should be negligible[1]:

1. Rib fracture(s).
2. Flail chest.
3. Pneumothorax, hemothorax, or pneumomediastinum.
4. Pericardial tamponade (especially following intracardiac injections).
5. Myocardial contusion or burns.
6. Aspiration pneumonitis.
7. Pulmonary edema.

REFERENCES

1. American Heart Association and National Academy of Science—National Research Council: Standards for cardiopulmonary resuscitation and emergency cardiac care, J.A.M.A. **244**:453-509, 1980.
2. Crampton, R.: Accepted, controversial and speculative aspects of ventricular defibrillation, Prog. Cardiovasc. Dis. **23**:167-186, 1980.
3. Edmark, K.W. et al.: DC defibrillator failure, J. Thorac. Cardiovasc. Surg. **55**:741-745, 1968.

4. Eisenberg, M., Bergner, L., and Hallstrom, A.: Paramedic programs and out-of-hospital cardiac arrest. I. Factors associated with successful resuscitation, Am. J. Publ. Health **69:**30-38, 1979.
5. Geddes, J.S. et al.: Prognosis after recovery from ventricular fibrillation complicating ischemic heart disease, Lancet **2:**273-275, 1967.
6. Grace, W.J. et al.: Blind defibrillation, Am. J. Cardiol. **34:**115-116, 1974.
7. Holder, D.A. et al.: Experience with bretylium tosylate by a hospital cardiac arrest team, Circulation **55:**541-544, 1977.
8. Snyder, B.D., Ramirez-Lassepas, M., and Lippert, D.M.: Neurologic status and prognosis after cardiopulmonary arrest, Neurology **27:**807-811, 1977.
9. Stephenson, H.E: Cardiac arrest and resuscitation, ed. 4, St. Louis, 1974, The C.V. Mosby Co.
10. Thompson, R.G., Hallstrom, A.P., and Cobb, L.A.: Bystander initiated cardiopulmonary resuscitation in the management of ventricular fibrillation, Ann. Int. Med. **91:**737-740, 1979.

CHAPTER 13

Cardiopulmonary resuscitation: basic and advanced cardiac life support

Douglas L. Mayers
Robert S. Gibson
Richard S. Crampton

GENERAL CONSIDERATIONS

Cardiopulmonary resuscitation (CPR) is an emergency procedure designed to maintain circulation of oxygenated blood to the brain and other vital organs after sudden, unexpected respiratory or cardiac arrest.[8,10] Effective CPR requires both bystander-initiated basic cardiac life support (BCLS) and application of more definitive techniques of advanced cardiac life support (ACLS).[1] The techniques of BCLS are summarized by the letters A, B, and C, which stand for *a*irway, *b*reathing, and *c*irculation. The first and perhaps most important maneuver during CPR is establishing a patent airway (Chapter 35). If the patient is apneic and has a patent airway, mouth-to-mouth rescue breathing should be started. If a pulse cannot be palpated, rescue breathing is combined with external cardiac compressions. The purpose of BCLS is to restore breathing and circulation by the quickest, simplest means until advanced cardiac life support maneuvers can be administered or until the patient can maintain basic life functions alone.

Advanced cardiac life support (ACLS), as defined by the American Heart Association[1] includes six elements: (1) BCLS, (2) the use of adjunctive equipment and special techniques for ventilation and artificial circulation, (3) cardiac monitoring of arrhythmias, (4) establishment of an intravenous access line, (5) definitive therapy to treat acidosis, hypotension, and arrhythmias, including defibrillation, and (6) ancillary resuscitation care. The combination of bystander-initiated BCLS with prompt application of ACLS techniques has resulted in the successful resuscitation of 40% to 80% of victims with documented cardiac arrest.

INDICATIONS

1. Respiratory arrest.
2. Cardiac arrest.

CONTRAINDICATIONS

1. A patient with a terminal, hopeless illness when the decision to allow death to proceed from natural causes has already been made.
2. An obviously dead victim (with decapitation or when rigor mortis has begun).

EQUIPMENT AND PERSONNEL

Basic cardiac life support

1. One or two individuals trained in BCLS.
2. No equipment is needed.

Advanced cardiac life support

1. Medical or paramedical personnel trained in ACLS. Such individuals should be able to diagnose and treat the following arrhythmias[1,9]: sinus tachycardia, sinus bradycardia, premature atrial contractions, supraventricular tachycardia, atrial flutter, atrial fibrillation, atrioventricular block of all degrees, premature ventricular contractions, ventricular tachycardia, ventricular fibrillation, asystole, and electromechanical dissociation.
2. Adjunctive equipment.
   a. Airway management: a low-flow oxygen source (2 to 15 L/min), oropharyngeal airways, nasopharyngeal airways, lubricating jelly, tongue blades, a suction

device and tonsil tip suction catheter, clean anatomic face masks, Venturi masks, a T piece, and a bag-valve device.

b. Intubation: an esophageal obturator airway with a 30-cc cuff syringe (Chapter 34), a laryngoscope and appropriate endotracheal tube (Chapter 33), a tracheotomy tray (Chapter 35), and blood gas syringes with 1000 units/ml heparin solution.

c. Circulatory assist: a compression board, a manual or automatic chest compressor, a sterile cardiac pacing wire and pacemaker pulse generator, an intraaortic balloon counterpulsation device, MAST suit (Medical Anti-Shock Trousers).

3. Cardiac monitoring: ECG recorder with electrodes and electrode paste.

4. Intravenous access: tourniquets, a skin preparation solution, peripheral intravenous catheters (18 gauge or larger), infusion solution (normal saline, 5% dextrose in water), central venous catheter and catheter introducer kit, a cutdown tray, sterile gloves, suture material, and an antibiotic ointment.

5. Definitive drug therapy.

a. General: oxygen, morphine sulfate, meperidine, sodium bicarbonate, 5% dextrose in water, insulin, and corticosteroids.

b. Airway management: naloxone, succinylcholine, and a short-acting barbiturate, such as methohexital (Brevital).

c. Antiarrhythmic agents: lidocaine, atropine, procainamide, bretylium tosylate, phenytoin, propranolol, digitalis, and verapamil.

d. Cardiotonic agents: calcium chloride, epinephrine, isoproterenol, dopamine, dobutamine, phenylephrine, norepinephrine, metaraminol, sodium nitroprusside, nitroglycerin, and magnesium sulfate.

e. Diuretics: furosemide and ethacrynic acid.

6. Defibrillation: a direct current defibrillator and electrode gel (Chapter 12).

■ TECHNIQUE FOR BASIC CARDIAC LIFE SUPPORT

1. Establish unresponsiveness. Shout "Are you OK?" and shake the victim by the arm or shoulder. If the victim cannot be aroused, call for help.
2. Position the victim. To perform adequate CPR, the victim must be supine on a firm surface. If face down, turn the victim over as a unit, taking care to not twist the head, neck or torso.
3. Open the airway (Fig. 13-1) and assess for spontaneous respiration. Place your ear over the victim's mouth and listen for air movement, feel for airflow on your face, and

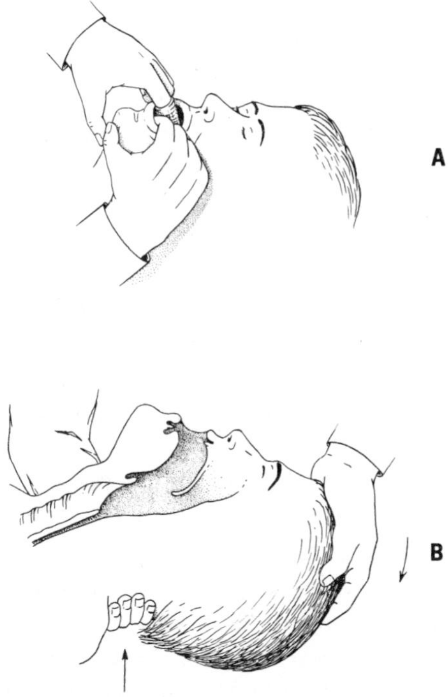

FIG. 13-1. A, Clear the pharynx with a finger wrapped with gauze to remove vomitus, particles of food, or dentures. **B,** Hyperextend head. This maneuver opens the pharynx by lifting the tongue.

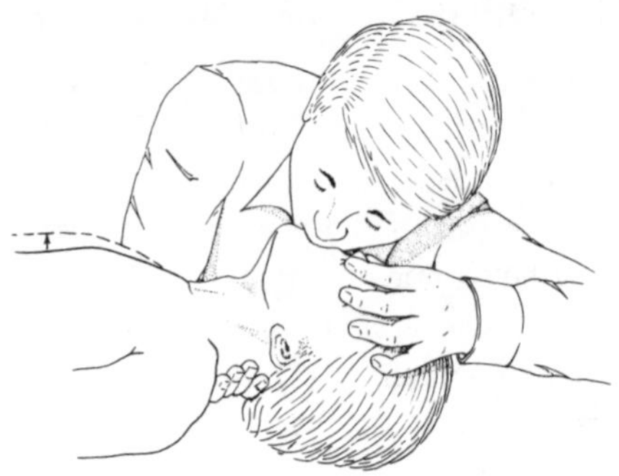

FIG. 13-2. Perform rescue breathing, using mouth-to-mouth technique.

watch for chest movement. If these signs are not present, begin rescue breathing.

4. Perform rescue breathing (Fig. 13-2). Inflate the lungs with four breaths using the mouth-to-mouth technique, while maintaining the victim's neck in the hyperextended position and pinching the nostrils closed. Make sure the chest is expanding by observing the motion out of the corner of the eyes. If adequate ventilation is not obtained, the airway must be cleared promptly (Chapter 35).
5. Check for pulse. While maintaining the victim's airway, palpate the carotid artery. If a pulse is present, continue rescue breathing at a rate of one ventilation every 5 seconds and recheck the pulse each minute. If no pulse is felt, begin external chest compressions.
6. External chest compression (cardiac massage) (Fig. 13-3). The patient must be on a backboard or on the floor for external chest compression to be effective. Place the heel of one hand two finger breadths above the xiphoid process. The other hand is placed on top with the fingers held off the chest wall. With elbows locked, depress the lower sternum 1½ to 2 inches (3.8 to 5 cm). The time of compression should equal the time of expansion.
7. Single-rescuer CPR. After establishing pulselessness, the single rescuer should perform 15 chest compres-

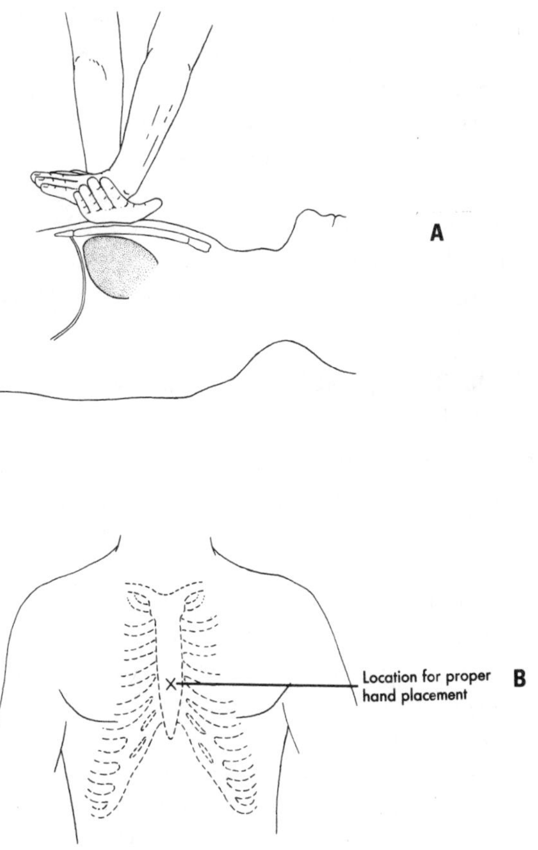

FIG. 13-3. A, External chest cardiac compression. **B,** Location for proper hand placement is indicated by X.

sions followed by two ventilations every 15 seconds (one cycle). After completing four cycles of 15 compressions and two ventilations, check for the return of pulse and spontaneous breathing. If the victim remains pulseless, resume the compression-ventilation cycles. Subsequently, the victim is checked for return of pulse every 4 or 5 minutes. If the pulse returns without spontaneous respirations, continue rescue breathing with one ventilation every 5 seconds.

8. Two-rescuer CPR. After establishing pulselessness, one rescuer should begin chest compressions at a rate of 60 per minute. The second rescuer maintains the victim's airway and interposes a breath on the *upstroke* of every fifth compression. Spontaneous return of the victim's pulse and respiration should be sought after 1 minute, and every 4 or 5 minutes thereafter. The two rescuers should be on opposite sides of the victim. This will allow frequent switches from ventilation to chest compression without rescuer fatigue.

■ TECHNIQUE FOR ADVANCED CARDIAC LIFE SUPPORT

1. Basic life support measures should be continued without interruption, and steps 2 through 8 should be carried out simultaneously by members of the ACLS team.
2. Administer supplemental 100% oxygen to the unresponsive victim through an oropharyngeal airway and bag-valve-mask until either an esophageal obturator airway (Chapter 34) or endotracheal tube (Chapter 33) can be inserted.
3. Begin electrocardiographic monitoring by using either the defibrillator electrode paddles or an attachable lead system. Monitoring of the rhythm should be maintained during a resuscitative effort.
4. Insert a large-bore needle (18 gauge or greater) attached to the intravenous line and begin infusion of 5% dextrose in water for delivery of intravenous medications. An antecubital vein, femoral vein, or central vein may be used. In an unwitnessed arrest, 1 mEq/kg of sodium bicarbonate (one or two ampules) may be given once the line is inserted. Obtain blood samples for arterial blood gas analysis and determination of electrolyte, glucose, calcium, and magnesium status. Before proceeding to definitive therapy, quickly determine the patient's antecedent cardiopulmonary status and the circumstances surrounding the arrest.

Definitive treatment for arrhythmias

1. Ventricular fibrillation.[1,5] Countershock with 200 joules (watt-seconds) and, if necessary, repeat shock with 300 and 360 joules. If ventricular fibrillation continues, administer sodium bicarbonate (1 mg/kg IV bolus), epinephrine (0.5 mg IV bolus), lidocaine (50 to 100 mg IV bolus), followed by a lidocaine drip (2 to 4 mg/min), and repeat the countershock (360 joules). If ventricular fibrillation persists, consider administering either procainamide (100 to 500 mg IV over 1 to 5 minutes) or bretylium tosylate (5 mg/kg IV bolus) prior to repeating the countershock. Once effective rhythm has been reestablished, lidocaine should be continued for the next 24 hours. (More details are given in Chapter 12.)
2. Ventricular tachycardia.[1,5] Treatment depends on the gravity of the clinical setting. Ventricular tachycardia that does not have a detectable peripheral arterial pulse or that fails to provide adequate circulation should be immediately terminated with electric countershock (200 to 360 joules) (Chapter 12), followed by administration of antiarrhythmic therapy (generally IV lidocaine). If the patient is awake and tolerating the arrhythmia, a brief trial of intravenous lidocaine may be used as a first approach (50 to 100 mg bolus, followed by a 2 to 4 mg/min drip). If the arrhythmia persists, countershock may be required (Chapters 11 and 12).
3. Asystole.[4] Administer sodium bicarbonate (1 mg/kg IV bolus), epinephrine (0.5 mg IV bolus), and calcium chloride (5 ml of 10% solution IV bolus). If ventricular fibrillation develops, countershock with 200 to 360 joules. If asystole persists, give atropine (1 mg IV bolus, may be repeated one time). If atropine followed by isoproterenol (2 to 20 μg/min IV) fails to produce a rhythm, insert a pacemaker.
4. Rapid supraventricular arrhythmias with evidence of decreased systemic perfusion. The therapy of choice is rapid synchronized direct current cardioversion with the

following delivered energy levels (Chapter 11):

a. Atrial fibrillation (50 joules).

b. Atrial flutter (25 joules).

c. Paroxysmal atrial tachycardia (25 joules).

If this therapy is unsuccessful, the delivered energy should be doubled sequentially (25, 50, 100, and 200 joules) and cardioversion repeated until a sinus rhythm or slower rate with an adequate cardiac output is obtained.

5. Bradyarrhythmias with evidence of decreased perfusion. Initial therapy is atropine sulfate (0.5 mg IV) administered every 5 minutes until the desired heart rate (more than 60 to 70 beats/min) is obtained. Generally, a total dose of 2 mg should not be exceeded. If atropine is not successful, intravenous isoproterenol (2 μg/min) can be started and gradually increased until a heart rate of 60 to 70 beats/min is obtained. Not exceeding a maximum dose of 20 μg/min is recommended. This measure often allows time for insertion of a temporary pacing electrode (Chapter 10).

6. Atrioventricular block. Initial therapy for atrioventricular block is identical to that for bradyarrhythmias just described. First-degree atrioventricular block and Mobitz type I (Wenckebach) second-degree atrioventricular block generally require no further therapy. Mobitz type II second-degree atrioventricular block and complete heart block require insertion of a temporary transvenous pacing electrode. (More details are given in Chapter 10.)

7. Electromechanical dissociation. Electromechanical dissociation refers to a phenomenon in which adequate electrocardiographic complexes are recorded without perceptible mechanical cardiac function and output.[6] Three kinds of hemodynamic alterations can produce it: inadequate preload (e.g., exsanguinating hemorrhage, inflow-obstructing left atrial masses, and pericardial tamponade), excessive afterload (e.g., pulmonary embolism), and severe pump failure (e.g., extensive ventricular asynergy and rupture of a papillary muscle, interventricular septum, or free wall of the heart). Since electromechanical dissociation carries an extremely grave prognosis, it must be treated aggressively. If tamponade is suspected, immediate pericardiocentesis should be performed (Chapter 9). With exsanguinating hemorrhage, massive and rapid volume replacement is undertaken with saline, plasmanate, and whole blood. Pump failure is treated by administering epinephrine (0.5 to 1 mg IV bolus, may be repeated), sodium bicarbonate (1 mg/kg IV bolus), and calcium chloride (5 ml of 10% solution, may be repeated). Isoproterenol (2 to 20 μg/min IV) may also be given.

8. Premature ventricular contractions (PVCs). Initial therapy includes lidocaine given as a 1 mg/kg IV bolus followed by a 2- to 4-mg/min infusion. If unsuccessful, administer procainamide, 100 mg IV, slowly every 5 minutes until the PVCs are abolished, a total dose of 1000 mg has been given, or signs of toxicity are noted (e.g., hypotension or QRS prolongation $\geq$50% of its original width). If the PVCs are suppressed, a maintenance infusion of 1 or 2 mg/min procainamide can be added along with the lidocaine.

Definitive treatment for acidosis*

1. Respiratory acidosis. Respiratory acidosis is managed by hyperventilation. Failure to correct respiratory acidosis may be due to airway obstruction (e.g., mucous plug, misplaced esophageal obturator airway or endotracheal tube [Chapter 35], pneumothorax, hemothorax, pulmonary edema, or atelectasis).
2. Metabolic acidosis. Metabolic acidosis is managed by administering intravenous sodium bicarbonate according to the following formula: bicarbonate deficit = body weight in kg $\times$ 0.4 $\times$ (desired serum HCO_3 − measured serum HCO_3). The use of intravenous sodium bicarbo-

*The acid-base status of the victim must be assessed by serial arterial blood gas determinations.

nate requires concurrent hyperventilation to prevent respiratory acidosis. Overzealous use of sodium bicarbonate can lead to hypernatremia, volume overload with pulmonary edema, intracellular acidosis, and lethal levels of hyperosmolarity.[3]

Definitive treatment for hypotension*

1. Hypotension due to hypovolemia (e.g., massive hemorrhage or diarrhea). Rapidly replenish the intravascular volume with normal saline, plasmanate, or whole blood as appropriate. A subclavian or internal jugular line (Chapters 5 and 6) should be used if possible for volume replacement. An antishock garment (MAST suit) is helpful until volume can be restored.
2. Hypotension due to depressed myocardial function. Infuse dopamine 2 to 20 μg/kg/min and/or dobutamine 2 to 10 μg/kg/min. Use of the intraaortic balloon pump may be beneficial in certain patients with acute myocardial infarction.
3. Hypotension associated with low peripheral vascular resistance (e.g., bacteremic shock). Volume replacement with normal saline is used to maintain an adequate cardiac preload. A norepinephrine infusion (8 to 32 μg/ml) is then begun to increase peripheral vascular resistance and systolic blood pressure. Specific antimicrobial therapy is imperative.
4. Hypotension due to bradycardia should be treated with atropine, isoproterenol or cardiac pacing. (See definitive treatment for bradyarrhythmias.)
5. Defibrillation (Chapter 12).
6. Ancillary resuscitation care.
   a. Monitoring the progress of resuscitation. The adequacy of CPR can be assessed by the following clinical parameters:
      1. A palpable carotid or femoral pulse during external chest compressions.

*Frequently, a Swan-Ganz catheter and arterial line will be necessary to determine the cause of hypotension and to monitor therapy. A Foley catheter should be inserted to measure urine output.

2. Pupillary responsiveness to light, unless atropine has been administered.
3. Improved color of the patient's skin and nail beds. The oral mucous membranes should be evaluated in black patients.
4. Purposeful spontaneous movement by the victim.
5. Return of spontaneous pulse or respiratory effort by the victim.

b. Termination of resuscitation. The American Heart Association[1] recommends that resuscitative efforts be withdrawn only after "cardiovascular unresponsiveness" has been demonstrated. Examples of this include refractory ventricular fibrillation, asystole, or electromechanical dissociation. Lack of neurologic responsiveness is not an adequate criterion for termination of CPR. In cases of hypothermia, efforts should not be discontinued until the patient has been rewarmed and adequate cardiovascular function fails to return.

c. Postresuscitation care. After restoration of basic life function, the victim should be transferred to an intensive care facility. This should occur only under the following circumstances:
1. The patient's respiratory status and cardiac rhythm are stabilized.
2. There is a functioning intravenous line.
3. A portable monitor and defibrillator are available.
4. Adequate support personnel are available: one person to monitor the patient's pulse and continue (or reinitiate) chest compression, a second person to support ventilation manually if necessary, and a third person to administer drugs and defibrillate the patient. Ideally, one of these individuals should be a physician.

■ COMPLICATIONS OF CPR

The most frequent complications of CPR[2] relate to mechanical trauma during external chest compression. Although the exact incidence of these complications varies, their frequency can be minimized by proper placement of the hands and frequent practice on a mannequin. Following are some of the complications:

1. Fractured sternum or ribs. The incidence of sternal and rib fracture varies from 2% to 6% and 25% to 40% respectively. Signs of this complication are crepitation and bony instability during CPR, but a chest roentgenogram should be used for confirmation. Usually, analgesia is adequate therapy, but a flail chest requires special attention with endotracheal intubation and mechanical ventilation.
2. Pneumothorax and hemothorax due to laceration of the lung are said to be "common" complications, but the actual incidence is probably less than 2%. A pneumothorax should be suspected when absent breath sounds and hyperresonance to percussion are noted over one hemithorax. A hemothorax is suggested when the patient develops dullness to percussion over one hemithorax and signs of shock. A chest roentgenogram will confirm the diagosis. Therapy consists of chest tube placement (Chapter 41). A hemothorax will require volume replacement with whole blood.
3. Pericardial tamponade is suggested when arterial pulsus paradoxus, distended neck veins, and hypotension are seen. The diagnosis may be confirmed by echocardiography, and the treatment is pericardiocentesis (Chapter 9).
4. Rupture of the right ventricular papillary muscle.[7] This appears to be associated with preexistent right ventricular dilation. It can cause severe tricuspid regurgitation.
5. Laceration of the liver or spleen should be suspected in the victim with lower thoracic rib fractures who develop hypotension with a normal ECG rhythm and chest examination. The diagnosis is confirmed by abdominal paracentesis (Chapter 22). Treatment consists of volume replacement and surgical consultation.
6. Fat emboli occur in 33% to 50% of patients. Fat emboli are frequently subclinical. There is no specific therapy.

7. Gastric distention is a common complication. It is detected by abdominal distension with hyperresonance during BCLS. It is usually due to high ventilatory pressures and can be decreased by proper positioning of the head and decreased airway pressures. A nasogastric tube can be inserted to decompress the stomach. If the stomach is not decompressed, the victim may develop decreased tidal volume, regurgitation and aspiration of gastric contents, or perforation of the stomach.

8. Rarely, a patient will have a return of cardiovascular function, but suffer anoxic brain damage with neurologic sequelae.[11]

9. Specific complications of airway insertion, intravenous access, defibrillation, and pericardiocentesis are discussed in other chapters.

REFERENCES

1. American Heart Association: Standards and guidelines for cardiopulmonary resuscitation (CPR) and emergency cardiac care (ECC), J.A.M.A. **244:**453-509, 1980.
2. Atcheson, G., and Fred, H.L.: Letter: Complications of cardiac resuscitation, Am. Heart J. **80:**263-265, 1975.
3. Bishop, P.L., and Weisfeldt, M.D.: Sodium bicarbonate administration during cardiac arrest, J.A.M.A. **235:**506-609, 1976.
4. Brown, D.C., Lewis, A.J., and Criley, J.M.: Asystole and its treatment: the possible role of the parasympathetic nervous system in cardiac arrest, J. Am. Coll. Emerg. Phys. **8:**448-450, 1979.
5. Crampton, R.S.: Accepted, controversial and speculative aspects of ventricular defibrillation, Prog. Cardiovasc. Dis. **28:**167-186, 1980.
6. Friedman, H.S.: Editorial: Diagnostic considerations in electromechanical dissociation, Am. J. Cardiol. **38:**268-269, 1976.
7. Gerry, J.L., Bulkley, B.H., and Hutchins, G.M.: Rupture of the papillary muscle of the tricuspid valve, Am. J. Cardiol. **40:**825-828, 1977.
8. Jude, J.R., Kouwenhoven, W.B., and Knickerbocker, G.G.: External cardiac massage, Monogr. Surg. Sci. **1:**59-117, 1964.
9. Schamroth, L.: How to approach an arrhythmia, Circulation **47:**420-426, 1973.
10. Stephenson, H.E.: Cardiac arrest and resuscitation, ed. 4, St. Louis, 1974, The C.V. Mosby Co.
11. Snyder, B.D., Ramierez-Lassepas, M., and Lippet, D.M.: Neurologic status and prognosis after cardiopulmonary arrest, Neurology **27:**807-811, 1977.

PART THREE

DERMATOLOGIC PROCEDURES

CHAPTER 14

Removal of cutaneous cysts

■ Barbara L. Braunstein
Kenneth E. Greer

■ GENERAL CONSIDERATIONS

A cyst is a sac that contains fluid or semisolid material. The most common type is the epidermal, or keratinous, cyst that frequently occurs on the face, scalp, neck, and trunk. Malignant degeneration of epidermal cysts is quite rare; when it does occur the tumor is usually a low-grade squamous cell carcinoma that does not metastasize.[3] Although cysts may be incised and their contents expressed, only complete removal of the cyst wall is likely to prevent recurrence.

■ INDICATIONS

1. An inflamed and painful cyst.
2. A cyst that discharges foul-smelling cheesy material.
3. A cyst that is cosmetically unacceptable.

■ CONTRAINDICATIONS

The only contraindication is when the resultant scar is likely to be more cosmetically objectionable than the cyst.

■ PATIENT PREPARATION AND EVALUATION

Explain the procedure to the patient.

■ PERSONNEL AND EQUIPMENT

1. A physician or paramedical person trained in cutaneous cyst removal.
2. Principal implements: a scalpel with a number 15 blade, curved hemostat, iris scissors, fine-toothed forceps, suturing material (6-0 nylon for the face, 4-0 nylon for other sites, and absorbable sutures).

3. Alcohol (70% solution), sterile gloves, 4 × 4 inch gauze pads, and sterile towels.
4. Lidocaine, 1%, 2 or 5 ml (with or without epinephrine, 1:100,000), a 5-ml syringe, and 26-gauge needle.
5. A labeled specimen bottle containing 10% buffered formalin for light microscopic studies.

■ TECHNIQUE[1,2]

1. Carefully palpate the cyst to determine its size.
2. Cleanse the area with 70% alcohol.
3. Draw the anticipated incision lines with a skin marking pen. The long axis of the ellipse should be parallel to the skin wrinkle lines to give the best cosmetic results (Fig. 14-1). The width of the ellipse should be approximately half the diameter of the cyst. The length of the ellipse should be approximately three times the width of the ellipse.
4. Inject the local anesthetic into the skin overlying the cyst and into the connective tissue surrounding the cyst wall. Avoid injecting into the cyst to prevent leakage of the cyst contents.
5. Using the needle that was used for the lidocaine injection, scratch the skin along the marked lines. By doing this the ellipse will still be visible after the marking ink is removed by alcohol.
6. Cleanse the skin again with 70% alcohol.
7. Put on sterile gloves and prepare a sterile field with towels.
8. Incise the skin down to the subcutaneous fat along the scratched lines with the number 15 blade held perpendicular to the skin surface. Do not penetrate the cyst wall; if the cyst wall is accidentally entered, wipe away the extruded material and proceed with the dissection.
9. Undermine the skin edges with iris scissors (Fig. 14-2).
10. Hold one end of the ellipse of skin with the fine-toothed forceps and carefully dissect the cyst wall from the surrounding connective tissue with iris scissors. (Fig. 14-3). Alternatively, a curved hemostat may be used for

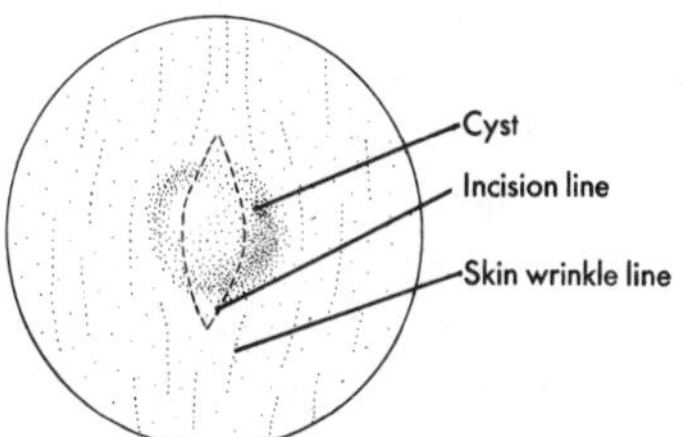

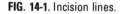

FIG. 14-1. Incision lines.

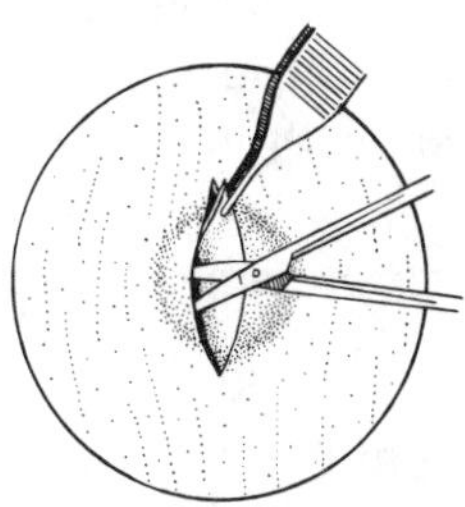

FIG. 14-2. After incising the skin, undermine skin edges.

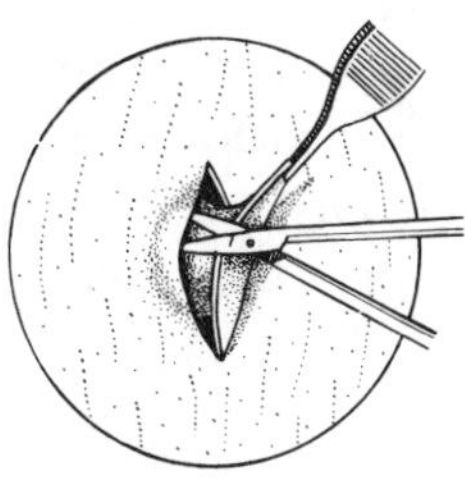

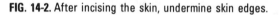

FIG. 14-3. Dissect cyst wall from surrounding tissue.

blunt dissection. NOTE: If the cyst occurs on the lateral face, extreme care should be taken not to traumatize the facial nerve.

11. Obtain hemostasis by applying pressure with a 4 × 4 inch gauze pad. If necessary, bleeding vessels may be tied off with absorbable sutures.

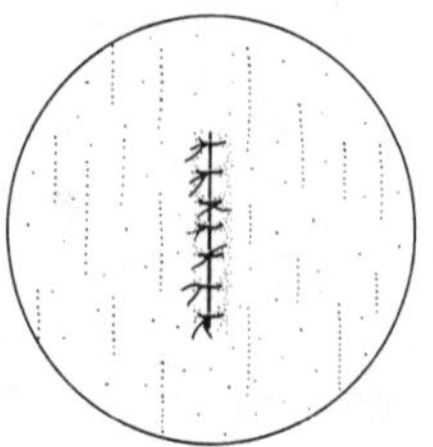

FIG. 14-4. Closure with interrupted sutures.

12. If the cyst is large it may be necessary to close the dead space with subcutaneous absorbable sutures.
13. Close the wound with interrupted nylon sutures (Fig. 14-4).
14. Apply a dry gauze dressing. A pressure dressing may be applied.

■ POSTPROCEDURE CARE

1. Keep water off the excision site for 2 or 3 days.
2. Remove the dressing in 2 days.
3. Cleanse the excision site daily with 70% alcohol until the sutures are removed.
4. Sutures on the face may be removed in 4 or 5 days and skin tapes applied to the wound. Sutures on the trunk and extremities should be removed in 10 to 14 days, at which time no further adhesive materials are required.

■ COMPLICATIONS

1. Hemorrhage. If lidocaine containing epinephrine has been used on a large cyst that requires a moderate amount of dissection, bleeding may occur when the vasoconstrictive effect of the epinephrine wears off. This can usually be controlled with pressure applied with a 4 × 4 inch gauze pad.
2. Infection. The frequency of infection will decrease if the dead space is obliterated with subcutaneous absorbable sutures.

REFERENCES

1. Albom, M.J.: Surgical gems, J. Dermatol. Surg. **1**:73-74, 1975.
2. Epstein, E., and Epstein, E., Jr.: Techniques in skin surgery, Philadelphia, 1979, Lea & Febiger.
3. Fitzpatrick, T.B.: Fundamentals of dermatologic diagnosis. In Fitzpatrick, T.B. editor: Dermatology in general medicine. New York, 1979, McGraw-Hill, Inc.

CHAPTER 15

Removal of nevus cell nevi (moles)

■ Barbara L. Braunstein
Kenneth E. Greer

■ GENERAL CONSIDERATIONS

Nevus cell nevi are benign pigmented lesions that are histologically divided into three types: junctional, compound, and intradermal. These lesions can be removed by either surgical excision with closure by sutures or by shave excision. With surgical excision all of the nevus is removed, whereas with a shave excision only the portion of the nevus elevated above the plane of the surrounding skin is removed. Shave excision is, however, quick and simple, and, because of the superficiality of the cut, yields excellent cosmetic results. Any lesion that may be malignant should be removed by total excision rather than shave excision.

■ INDICATIONS

1. Lesions that are cosmetically unacceptable.
2. Lesions that are repeatedly traumatized.
3. Lesions that are suspected of being malignant.

■ CONTRAINDICATIONS

There are no absolute contraindications.

■ PATIENT EVALUATION AND PREPARATION

Explain the procedure to the patient.

■ PERSONNEL AND EQUIPMENT

1. A physician or paramedical person trained in removal of nevi.
2. Principal implements: a fine-toothed forceps, a scalpel

with a number 15 blade, and iris scissors. For surgical excision: suture material, (6-0 nylon may be used on the face, 4-0 nylon at other sites). For shave excision: aluminum chloride (35% in a 50% isopropyl alcohol solution) and cotton-tipped applicators.

3. Alcohol (70% solution), sterile 4 × 4 inch gauze pads, sterile gloves, and sterile towels.
4. Lidocaine, 1%, (with or without epinephrine, 1:100,000), 1 to 3 ml, a 3-ml syringe, and 26-gauge needle.
5. A labeled specimen bottle containing 10% buffered formalin for light microscopic studies.

■ TECHNIQUE[1,2]

Excision

1. Cleanse the excision site with 70% alcohol.
2. Draw the anticipated elliptic excision lines with a skin marking pen. The long axis of the ellipse should be parallel to the skin wrinkle lines for the best cosmetic result (Fig. 15-1).
3. Inject the local anesthetic (lidocaine with epinephrine should not be used on the digits) so as to raise a wheal at the incision site.
4. Using the needle that was used for the lidocaine injection, scratch the skin along the marked lines. By doing this the ellipse will still be visible after the marking ink is removed by alcohol.
5. Cleanse the skin again with 70% alcohol.

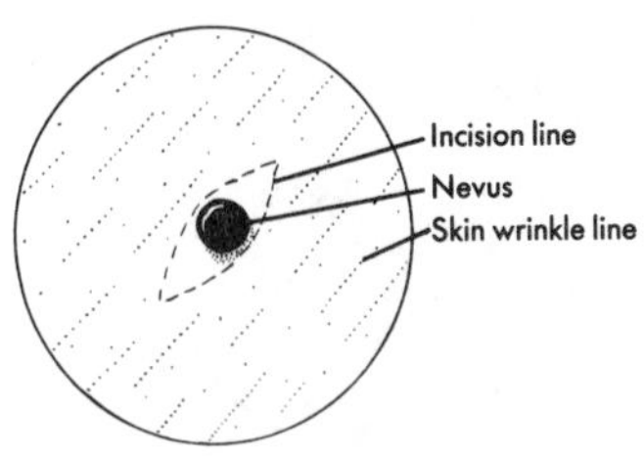

FIG. 15-1. Incision lines.

6. Put on sterile gloves and prepare a sterile field with towels.
7. Incise the skin down to the subcutaneous fat, while holding the number 15 blade perpendicular to the skin surface.
8. Pick up one end of the ellipse with the fine-toothed forceps and exert gentle upward pressure, while freeing the base of the specimen with the iris scissors (Fig. 15-2).
9. Place the specimen into the labeled specimen container.
10. Obtain hemostasis by exerting pressure with a 4 × 4 inch gauze pad.
11. Close the wound with interrupted nylon sutures (Fig. 15-3). To make the wound edges meet evenly, the needle should be inserted perpendicular to the skin surface and passed through the full thickness of the skin.
12. Apply a dry gauze dressing.

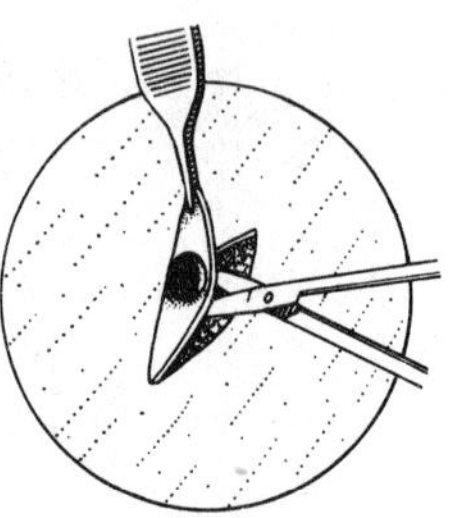

FIG. 15-2. After incising skin, lift ellipse and cut nevus free.

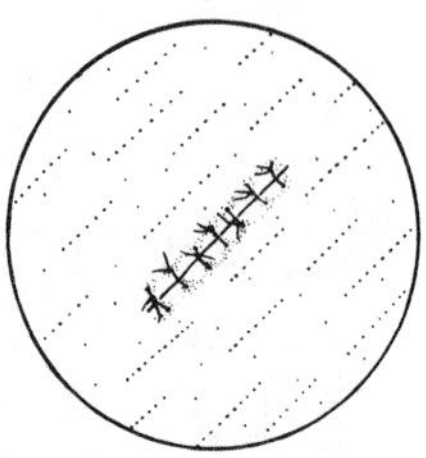

FIG. 15-3. Closure with interrupted sutures.

Shave excision[3]

1. Cleanse the excision site with 70% alcohol. Inject the local anesthetic under the nevus, raising it slightly above the level of the surrounding normal skin (Fig. 15-4).
2. Allow a few minutes for the swelling to subside.
3. Put on sterile gloves and prepare a sterile field with towels.
4. Immobilize the skin by holding it taut between the index finger and thumb.
5. Hold the number 15 blade nearly horizontal to the skin surface. Use a sawing motion and slice off the lesion flush with the surrounding skin (Fig. 15-5). It may be necessary to smooth the edges with the iris scissors.

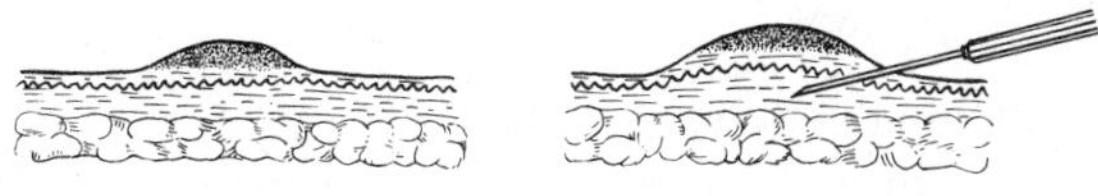

FIG. 15-4. Anesthetic injection for shave excision.

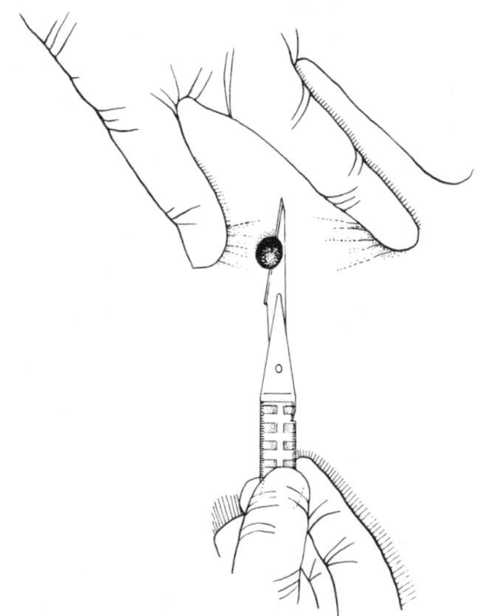

FIG. 15-5. Shave excision.

6. Apply aluminum chloride solution with a cotton-tipped applicator to obtain hemostasis.
7. Place the specimen into the labeled specimen container.
8. No dressing is needed.

■ POSTPROCEDURE CARE

Excision

1. Keep water off the excision site for 2 or 3 days.
2. Remove the dressing the following day.
3. Cleanse the excision site daily with 70% alcohol until the sutures are removed.
4. Sutures may be removed as early as 3 days from the face or as late as 14 days from areas subjected to stress or trauma, such as the back, chest, or over joints.

■ COMPLICATIONS

1. Infection. Infection is extremely rare with shave excision because of the superficiality of the excision.
2. Hemorrhage. Hemorrhage is rare with a shave biopsy. This can usually be controlled by applying pressure with a 4 × 4 inch gauze pad.
3. Repigmentation may occur with shave excisions, but the lesions rarely recur with any appreciable elevation.

REFERENCES

1. Arndt, K.: Manual of dermatologic therapeutics, ed. 2, Boston, 1978, Little, Brown & Co.
2. Beerman, H.: The biopsy. In Epstein, E., editor: Skin surgery, Springfield, Ill., 1970, Charles C Thomas, Publisher.
3. Kopf, A.W., and Popkin, G.L.: Letter: Shave biopsies for cutaneous lesions, Arch. Dermatol. **110**:637, 1974.

CHAPTER 16

Skin biopsy

Barbara L. Braunstein
Kenneth E. Greer

GENERAL CONSIDERATIONS

Skin biopsies are performed to obtain specimens for light microscopic examination, cultures, immunofluorescent studies, or electron microscopic studies. Biopsies may be excisional, incisional, or punch. With an excisional biopsy the entire lesion is removed. All suspected malignancies should be excised unless the lesion is too large to allow primary wound closure or an acceptable cosmetic result. Excisional biopsies may be curative as well as diagnostic. With an incisional biopsy only a portion of the lesion is removed. This is the most commonly used biopsy technique and is done when only a portion of a large lesion or of an extensive dermatosis is needed for diagnostic purposes. With a punch biopsy a small cylinder of skin is removed with a skin punch. This method is quick, simple, and generally does not require sutures. Disadvantages, however, include slower healing, and an oval, rather than linear, scar.

INDICATIONS

1. A skin lesion that may be malignant.
2. Dermatoses that have been unresponsive to therapy.
3. Other skin lesions or eruptions for which the diagnosis is unknown.

CONTRAINDICATIONS

There are no contraindications when a biopsy is needed to make or confirm a diagnosis.

PATIENT EVALUATION AND PREPARATION

Explain the procedure to the patient.

PERSONNEL AND EQUIPMENT

1. A physician or paramedical person to perform the skin biopsy.
2. Principal implements: a fine-toothed forceps and an iris scissors. For excisional and incisional biopsy: a scalpel with a number 15 blade and nylon sutures (6-0 nylon suture should be used on the face, 4-0 nylon sutures may be used at other sites). For punch biopsies: a 3- or 4-mm skin punch.
3. Alcohol (70% solution), sterile gloves, sterile 4 × 4 inch gauze pads, and sterile towels.
4. Lidocaine, 1%, 3 ml (with or without epinephrine, 1:100,000), a 3-ml syringe, and a 26-gauge needle.
5. A labeled specimen bottle containing 10% buffered formalin for light microscopic studies. When special stains or other studies are requested, different fixatives may be required.

TECHNIQUE[2,4,6]

For all three types of biopsies the following steps apply:

1. When more than one lesion is present, choose the best site for the biopsy.[7]
   a. Select a lesion that is well developed and representative of the eruption. When doing a biopsy on a patient with a vesiculobullous disease, however, choose a very early lesion. This may be an edematous papule rather than a vesicle.[1]
   b. Select a lesion from a location that is commonly involved in the disease process being considered.
   c. Avoid lesions that are excoriated, secondarily infected, or "burnt out."
   d. Avoid cosmetically important areas if possible.
   e. Avoid the lower legs of persons over 40 because these areas heal slowly.
2. Cleanse the biopsy site with 70% alcohol.

Excisional biopsy and incisional biopsy

1. Use a skin marking pen to draw the proposed incision lines around the area to be excised. Draw an ellipse

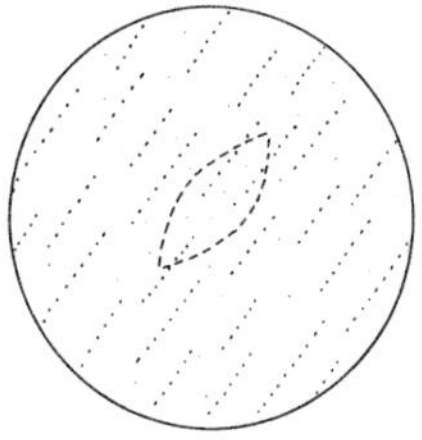

FIG. 16-1. Incision lines.

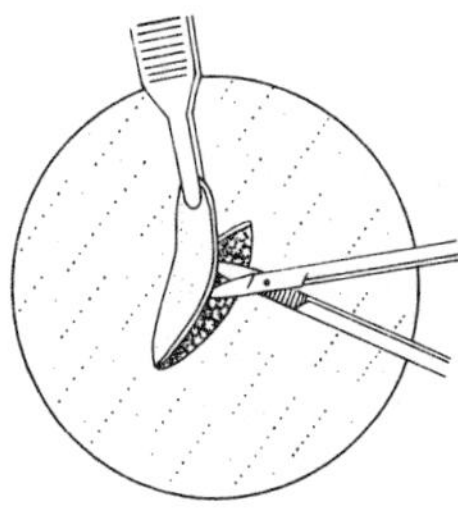

FIG. 16-2. After incising skin, lift ellipse and cut specimen free.

with the long axes parallel to the skin wrinkle lines to improve the cosmetic results (Fig. 16-1).

2. Inject the local anesthetic (lidocaine with epinephrine should not be used on the digits). The injection should be superficial enough to raise a wheal at the biopsy site.
3. Using the needle that was used to inject the lidocaine, scratch the skin along the marked lines. By doing this the ellipse will remain visible after the marking ink is removed by alcohol.
4. Cleanse the area again with 70% alcohol.
5. Put on sterile gloves and prepare a sterile field with towels.
6. Incise the skin down to the subcutaneous fat with a number 15 blade held perpendicular to the skin surface.
7. Pick up one end of the ellipse with a fine-toothed forceps and exert gentle upward pressure on the specimen while cutting the base with iris scissors (Fig. 16-2).

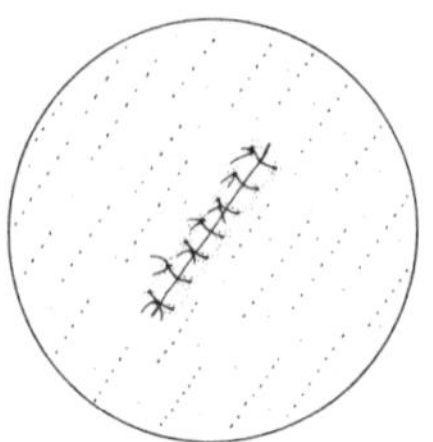

FIG. 16-3. Closure with interrupted sutures.

8. Place the specimen into the labeled specimen container.
9. Obtain hemostasis by exerting pressure with a 4 × 4 inch gauze pad.
10. Close the wound with interrupted nylon sutures (Fig. 16-3). To made the wound edges meet evenly the needle should be inserted perpendicular to the skin surface and passed through the full thickness of the skin.
11. Apply a dry gauze dressing.

Punch biopsy[3]

1. Inject the local anesthetic (lidocaine with epinephrine should not be used on the digits). The injection should be superficial enough to raise a wheal at the biopsy site.
2. Put on sterile gloves and prepare a sterile field with towels.
3. Hold the skin punch perpendicular to the skin surface.
4. Stretch the skin taut in a plane perpendicular to the skin wrinkle lines (Fig. 16-4). This will result in an oval, rather than a round, defect, which will yield a better cosmetic result.[5,8]
5. Simultaneously press and twist the skin punch into the tissue (Fig. 16-4). A give will be felt as the punch reaches subcutaneous fat. To avoid traumatizing the specimen, twist the skin punch in only a single direction, either clockwise or counterclockwise.
6. Grasp the edge of the specimen with a fine-toothed forceps. Apply gentle upward pressure and cut the base

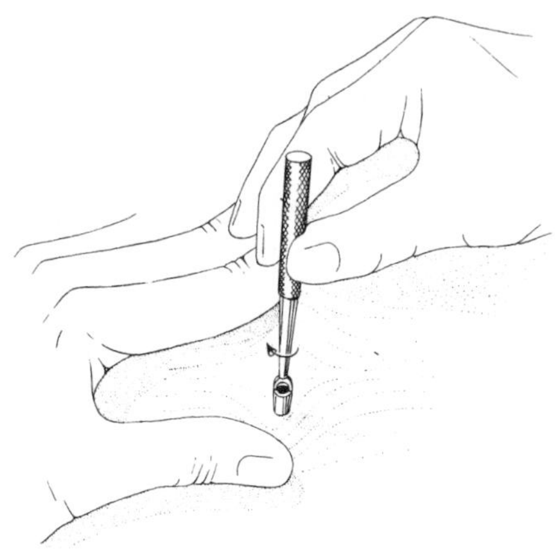

FIG. 16-4. Hold skin taut in a plane perpendicular to skin lines. Press and twist skin punch into tissue.

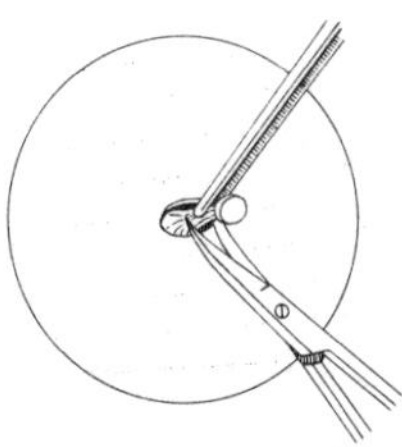

FIG. 16-5. Lift specimen up and cut it free with scissors.

of the specimen with iris scissors (Fig. 16-5). Be sure to include fat in the specimen. An oval defect will be left in the skin (Fig. 16-6).

7. Place the specimen in the labeled specimen container.
8. Obtain hemostasis by applying pressure with a 4 × 4 inch gauze pad.
9. Sutures are usually not used except for hemostasis or to obtain a linear scar rather than an oval defect. If indicated, close the wound with interrupted nylon sutures (Fig. 16-7).
10. Apply a dry gauze dressing.

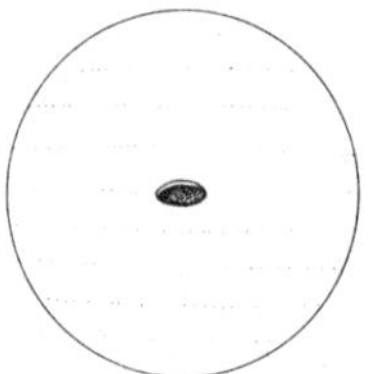

FIG. 16-6. Oval defect left after removal of punch.

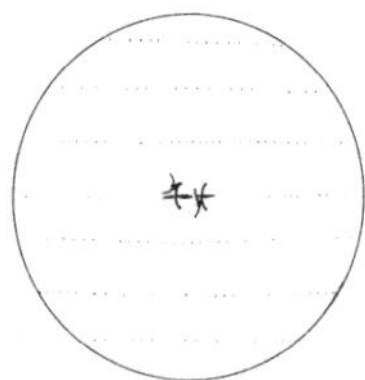

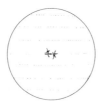

FIG. 16-7. Closure with interrupted sutures when linear, rather than oval, scar is desired.

POSTPROCEDURE CARE

1. Keep water off the biopsy site for 2 or 3 days.
2. Remove the dressing the following day.
3. Cleanse the biopsy site daily with 70% alcohol until the sutures are removed.
4. Sutures may be removed as early as 3 days from the face or as late as 10 days from areas subjected to stress and trauma, such as the back, chest, or over joints.

COMPLICATIONS

1. Infection. Inflammation around sutures may occur, but significant infection is unusual.
2. Hemorrhage. Hemorrhage can usually be controlled by the application of pressure with a 4 × 4 inch gauze pad.
3. Keloids or hypertrophic scars may develop wherever surgery has been performed. It is important to anticipate this complication in anyone who has a history of keloid formation.

REFERENCES

1. Ackerman, B.A.: Biopsy: why, where, when, how, J. Dermatol. Surg. **1**:21-23, 1975.
2. Anderson, P.C.: Skin biopsy, J.A.M.A. **201**:762-764, 1967.
3. Arndt, K.: Manual of dermatologic therapeutics, ed. 2, Boston, 1978, Little, Brown & Co.
4. Beerman, H.: The biopsy. In Epstein, E., editor: Skin surgery, Springfield, Ill., 1970, Charles C Thomas, Publisher.
5. Caro, M.: Skin biopsy technique, Arch. Dermatol. **76**:9-12, 1957.
6. Epstein, E., and Epstein, E., Jr.: Techniques in skin surgery, Philadelphia, 1979, Lea & Febiger.
7. Krull, E.A., and Babel, D.E.: Diagnostic procedures of the skin. Part 2: Skin biopsy and other tests, J. Family Prac. **3**:427-431, 1976.
8. Whyte, H.J. et al.: A simple method to minimize scarring following large punch biopsies, Arch. Dermatol. **81**:520-521, 1960.

PART FOUR

EARS, NOSE, AND THROAT PROCEDURES

CHAPTER 17

Epistaxis control

■ Michael E. Johns

■ GENERAL CONSIDERATIONS

The treatment of epistaxis is not always the solution to the problem. It is most important to look for and consider the etiology of the nosebleed.[2,4,5]

If the patient has failed to control the nosebleed at home using external pressure or cotton placed in the anterior nares, there are several techniques that should be considered, such as external pressure, silver nitrate cautery, anterior nasal packing, and posterior nasal packing. If none of these maneuvers controls the epistaxis, consult an otolaryngologist to consider surgical ligation of the appropriate blood vessels.

■ INDICATIONS: PERSISTENT EPISTAXIS

1. Anterior septal bleeding. Anterior septal bleeding will usually be controlled by pressure or silver nitrate cautery.
2. Other anterior nasal bleeding sites. These may respond to silver nitrate cautery or require anterior nasal packing.
3. Posterior nasal bleeding. Posterior nasal bleeding will require posterior and anterior nasal packs.

■ CONTRAINDICATIONS

1. Clotting abnormalities. When coagulation studies are abnormal, aggressive nasal packing may cause further bleeding. This is particularly true for posterior packs. Nevertheless, clotting abnormalities are a relative contraindication. Prior to removing the nasal packs, clotting mechanisms should be normalized as much as possible.

Light anterior packing with oxidized cellulose (Surgicel) soaked in phenylephrine (Neo-Synephrine) is preferable to aggressive packing with petrolatum gauze whenever possible.

2. Patients with severe chronic obstructive pulmonary disease may have a significant drop in their pO_2 if a posterior nasal pack is placed. These patients should be closely monitored and given supplemental oxygen.

■ PATIENT EVALUATION AND PREPARATION

1. Obtain hemoglobin and hematocrit values, blood type and cross match, prothrombin time, partial thromboplastin time, and platelet count.
2. Arterial blood gases should be checked if a posterior pack might be placed.
3. Insert an intravenous line if the patient is hypotensive or has lost a significant amount of blood.

■ PERSONNEL AND EQUIPMENT

1. A physician who understands nasal anatomy and can use a headlight and an assistant who is familiar with the equipment.
2. Principal implements.
   a. For the patient: a chair with a headrest, a gown, and a basin.
   b. For the physician: a headlight (or head mirror and light source), suction pump, nasal suction tips, bayonet forceps, tongue depressor, 16 French rubber catheter, scissors, and gown.
3. Principal supplies: absorbent cotton, 1-inch continuous petrolatum gauze, 4 × 4 inch gauze pads, silver nitrate sticks, oxidized cellulose, one silk suture (heavy fishline will do), ½-inch adhesive tape, a Foley catheter with 15-ml balloon, a number 16 French rubber catheter, and umbilical clamps.
4. Drugs: cocaine, 4%, 5 ml, (or 3% ephedrine with 1% tetracaine), morphine, and an antibiotic ointment (such as bacitracin ointment).

■ TECHNIQUE

Examination and cauterization[7]

1. Position the patient sitting straight and leaning forward so that blood drips from the front of the nose into the basin.
2. Examine the nose for the source of the bleeding (Figs. 17-1 and 17-2) using a strong headlight, the nasal speculum, and suction to remove any clots from the nose. Go to step 3 if the bleeding point is on the anterior septum or anterior end of the inferior turbinate; if not, skip to step 6.

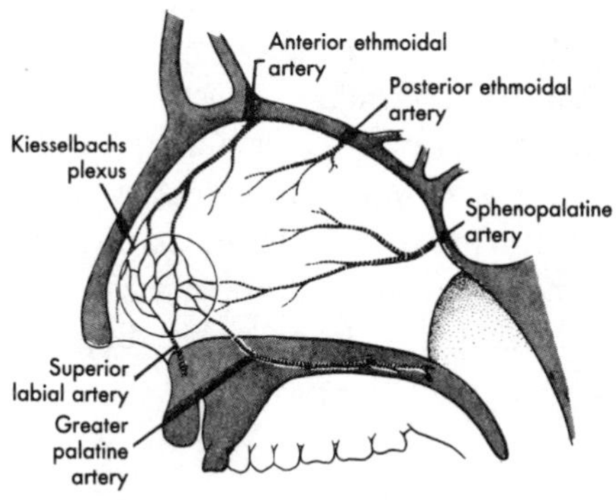

FIG. 17-1. Blood supply of nasal septum.

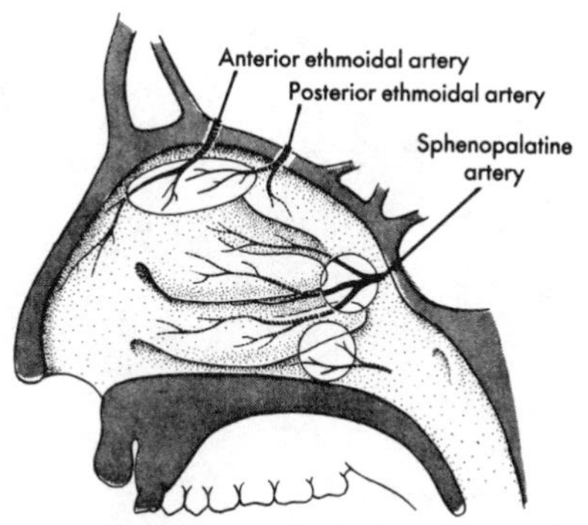

FIG. 17-2. Blood supply of lateral nasal wall.

3. Soak a piece of cotton with 4% cocaine, squeeze out the excess, and, using a bayonet forceps, insert it into the nasal chamber against the bleeding point. Have the patient pinch the nostrils together for 5 to 10 minutes.
4. Remove the cotton. The bleeding should have slowed to a trickle or stopped, and the nasal mucosa should be anesthetized and constricted. Using a silver nitrate stick, cauterize the mucosa in a circle surrounding the bleeding point and then cauterize the bleeding point itself (Fig. 17-3). Remove the silver nitrate stick, then take a cotton swab and hold pressure against the bleeding point and cauterized area for 3 minutes. This serves to hold the silver nitrate in contact against the bleeding point and completes the cauterization. This is especially important when bleeding persists after vasoconstriction, since the blood tends to wash away the silver nitrate.
5. Apply bacitracin ointment into the nasal chamber to keep the mucosa lubricated. No packing is necessary. A pledget of cotton placed in the nasal vestibule keeps the patients fingers away from the bleeding point and can be removed several hours later.

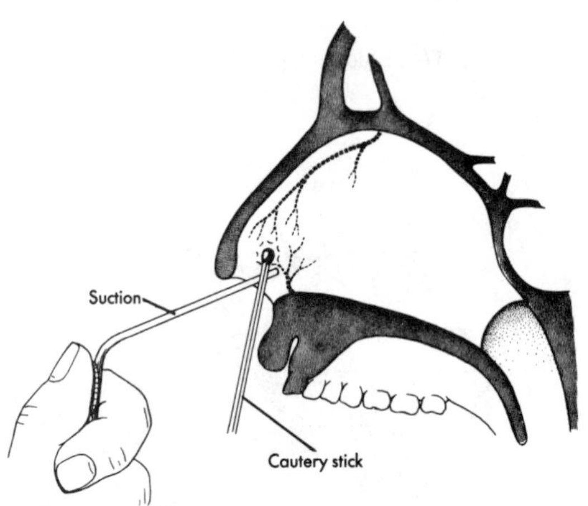

FIG. 17-3. Most epistaxes (80% to 85%) originate from anterior nasal septum and can be managed by visualization and silver nitrate stick cautery.

6. If the bleeding is not visualized anteriorly, suction blood from the nostril working from the anterior to the posterior end until the bleeding is anterior to the suction. At this point you have gone past the bleeding point. Back the suction tip up a short distance until the suction tip fills readily with blood. If the bleeding is from the posterior portion of the nasal chamber, posterior packing will most likely be necessary. A posterior pack requires an anterior pack along with it, but the posterior pack must be placed *first*. The posterior pack rarely applies pressures against the bleeding point but serves as a posterior wall against which a tight posteriorly placed anterior pack can be placed. For a posterior pack, proceed to pp. 156 to 158 and then place an anterior pack. Anterior bleeding can be controlled by a carefully placed anterior pack.

Anterior packing

1. Insert one or two cotton pledgets moistened with 4% cocaine along the length of the nasal chamber to obtain anesthesia. Consider the administration of a sedative or narcotic (intramuscular or intravenous). Anterior, and especially posterior, packing is painful!!
2. Pack the nose using 1-inch wide petrolatum gauze. Use a bayonet forceps to place the packing in the desired areas (Fig. 17-4). Begin packing the gauze tightly against the roof of the nose, folding it back and forth in layers and pushing each layer up tightly against the previous one. This should be carried out to the level of the middle turbinate and down to the floor of the nose. If the bleeding occurs under the inferior turbinate, begin the nasal packing in the posteroinferior portion of the nose, forcing layers of gauze under the inferior turbinate to bring pressure against the bleeding point, then layer the gauze from the floor of the nose up to the roof. Always start at the bleeding point area and pack tightly against that area and then proceed up, down, or out as the situation dictates.

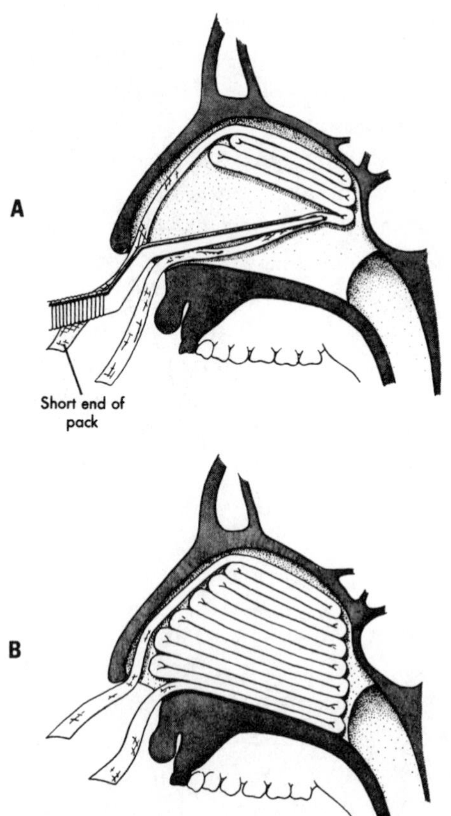

FIG. 17-4. Anterior nasal packing. A, Anterior nasal packing begins high in nasal vault and proceeds inferiorly. Note that at beginning of inserting packing, short end of pack is left outside nose. **B,** Anterior pack completed.

Posterior packing

Posterior nasal packing can be accomplished with a Foley catheter or a gauze pack.

Foley catheter

Insert a deflated 30-ml number 12 French Foley catheter along the floor of the nose until it reaches behind the palate. The tip of the catheter may be cut off to decrease pharyngeal irritation. Inflate the balloon with 10 ml of water and pull the catheter toward you until it fits snugly in the posterior choana. The tube should then be held firmly in position by the assistant while the nose is packed as described in steps 1 and 2 of anterior packing. The Foley catheter is then secured anteriorly by securing it to a gauze roll with an umbilical clamp so it does not cause pressure on the nasal ala.

Gauze pack

1. Fold a 4 × 4 inch gauze in half and then roll it into a cylinder. (Some physicians prefer cut vaginal tampons.) Tie a heavy silk suture around the midpoint of the rolled gauze, leaving the two ends of the suture at least 12 inches (30 cm) long. These will serve to pull the pack into the nasopharynx (Fig. 17-5, *B*). A second suture is tied around the midpoint of the rolled gauze, but this time the knot is tied on the opposite side of the pack. One end is left long to serve as a trailer and to be used for removal of the pack.
2. Insert the 16 French rubber catheter through the nasal chamber on the side of the nosebleed until it appears in the posterior pharynx. Grab it with a hemostat or bayonet forceps and bring the tip out the mouth (Fig. 17-5, *A*).
3. Secure the two leading sutures to the tip of the catheter and make sure the trailing suture is secure.
4. Pull the rubber catheter and, using your finger, guide the posterior pack up behind the soft palate until it is firmly seated in the posterior choana (Fig. 17-5, *C*).
5. Tape the trailing suture to the cheek. It will be used to remove the pack!
6. Detach the two sutures from the catheter, and while the assistant maintains continuous tension, place the anterior nasal packing as previously described on both sides of the nasal septum.
7. Separate the two sutures holding the posterior pack, place a narrow roll of gauze or dental roll between them, and tie the two sutures around the dental roll.

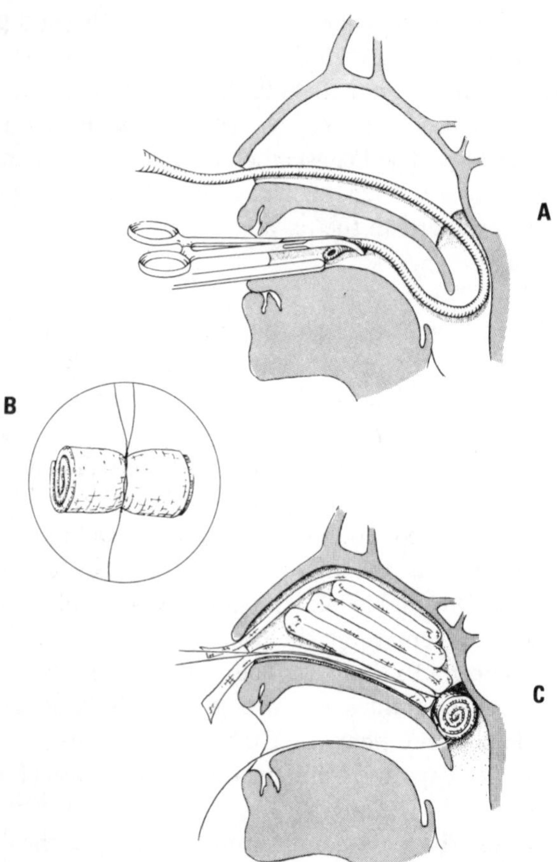

FIG. 17-5. Posterior nasal pack. A, Rubber catheter passed and retrieved from nasopharynx. **B,** Sutures on posterior pack that will be tied to rubber catheter tip coming from mouth. **C,** Posterior pack is then pulled through mouth and firmly seated in nasopharynx, and nasal cavity is packed anteriorly.

This will maintain an anterior pull on the posterior nasal pack, keeping it in position.

8. Begin antibiotic coverage to prevent stasis sinusitis while the packs are in place.
9. Sedation and pain medication are helpful in controlling the epistaxis and discomfort of the packs.
10. Hospitalize all patients requiring nasal packing.

Pack removal

1. Leave anterior packing in place for 3 full days. Remove it by slowly wiggling the packing from the nasal chamber with a bayonet forceps until it is completely removed.
2. Leave posterior nasal packing in place for 3 or 4 days. Remove the anterior pack first, then free the single suture from the cheek and cut the double sutures free from the dental roll. Deliver the posterior pack through the mouth by pulling on the single suture.
3. The patient should be observed for 24 hours in the hospital for signs of recurrent bleeding.

■ COMPLICATIONS

1. Pressure necrosis of the nasal ala. Pressure necrosis is always preventable if care is taken to place the Foley catheter or sutures of the posterior pack in the proper position.
2. Sinusitis can result from obstruction of the natural sinus ostia with resulting secondary infection. This is usually controlled by prophylactic antibiotics during the interval of nasal packing and coating the nasal packing with antibiotic ointment.
3. Severe hypoxia has been observed in young and particularly older patients who have posterior or anterior nasal packs in place.[1,6] Agitation in patients such as these may represent cerebral hypoxia and must be treated with oxygen, *not* sedatives! Administering oxygen through a face mask and monitoring blood gases are recommended in these patients.
4. Blood in the middle ear or in the eye is the result of retrograde blood flow through the eustachian tube or lacrimal duct system and is frequently seen when the nose is packed tightly until the nosebleed stops. The hemotympanum will resolve spontaneously with removal of the packing.
5. Otitis media is a potential complication secondary to blockage of the eustachian tube with secondary bacterial overgrowth. I have never seen this problem.

6. Cocaine reactions are a potential complication in the patient who is sensitive or who is overdosed. This is manifested by signs of central nervous system stimulation, seizures, and respiratory failure. The dose used should be less than 250 mg in an adult, and this much is rarely needed. To treat this complication the patient should be intubated and given respiratory and cardiovascular support until the cocaine is metabolized.[3]

REFERENCES

1. Cassisi, N.J., Biller, H.F., and Ogura, J.H.: Changes in arterial oxygen tension and pulmonary mechanics with the use of posterior packing in epistaxis, Laryngoscope **81**:1261-1266, 1971.
2. El Bitar, H.: The etiology and management of epistaxis: a review of 300 cases, Practitioner **207**:800-804, 1971.
3. Henderson, R., and Johns, M.E.: Cocaine use by the otolaryngologist: a survey, Ann. Otol. Rhinol. Laryngol. **84**:969-973, 1977.
4. Juselius, H.: Epistaxis. A clinical study of 1724 patients, J. Laryngol. Otol. **88**:317-327, 1974.
5. Sessions, R.B.: Nasal hemorrhage, Otol. Clin. North Am. **6**:727-744, 1973.
6. Slocum, C.W., Maisel, R.H., and Cantrell, R.W.: Arterial blood gas determination in patients with anterior packing, Laryngoscope **86**:869-873, 1976.
7. Smith, R.O.: Managing epistaxis, Postgrad. Med. **55**:143-149, 1974.

CHAPTER 18

Indirect laryngoscopy

■ **Michael E. Johns**

■ GENERAL CONSIDERATIONS

Hoarseness and other laryngeal symptoms may be an early sign of malignancy. Any hoarseness persisting for 2 weeks mandates laryngeal examination. In many cases indirect laryngoscopy coupled with the history will lead to the diagnosis.[1] Those patients in whom the larynx cannot be adequately visualized and determined to be normal should be referred to an otolaryngologist for further evaluation. Some patients are impossible to indirectly examine even by the expert laryngologist.

■ INDICATIONS

1. Persistent hoarseness.
2. Upper airway obstruction.
3. Stridor, particularly inspiratory stridor.
4. Hemoptysis.
5. Dysphagia.

■ CONTRAINDICATIONS

Suspected acute epiglottiditis contraindicates indirect laryngoscopy. Instrumentation of the oropharynx or larynx may precipitate acute airway obstruction.

■ PATIENT PREPARATION

Careful counseling as to how the examination is done should help the patient relax. A relaxed, cooperative patient is a prerequisite to adequate visualization of the larynx.

■ PERSONNEL AND EQUIPMENT

1. A physician who knows the laryngeal anatomy and can use a headlight or head mirror.

2. Principal implements.
   a. For the patient: a straight-back chair with headrest.
   b. For the physician: headlight, numbers 4 and 5 laryngeal mirrors, 4 × 4 inch gauze sponges, and an alcohol lamp or bowl of hot water.
   c. Drugs: a topical anesthetic.

TECHNIQUES[2]

1. Remove dentures.
2. Position the patient sitting with the body straight, upright, and leaning slightly forward. The head and jaw should be jutting forward as if to sniff a flower (Fig. 18-1).
3. Select the largest laryngeal mirror that will comfortably fit in the back of the mouth.
4. Warm the mirror in the flame of the alcohol lamp or in hot water. Check the temperature of the mirror on the back of the hand.
5. Have the patient protrude the tongue; then the examiner should cover it with the gauze square and grasp the tongue with the thumb and middle finger (Fig. 18-2). The index finger is used to lift the upper lip. The

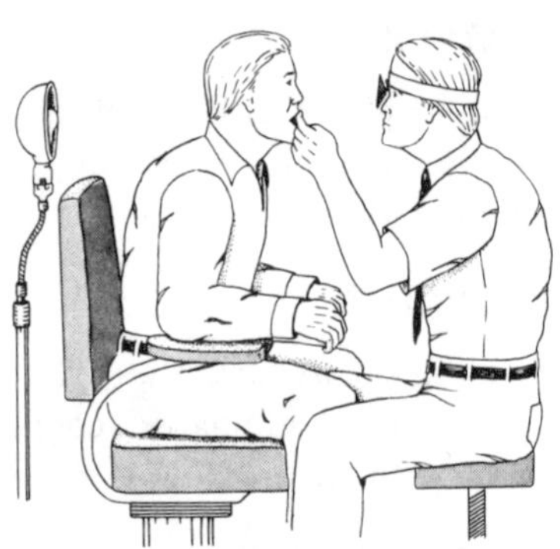

FIG. 18-1. Proper positioning of patient is essential if successful visualization of larynx is to be accomplished. Patient is sitting straight up with neck flexed and head extended as if "sniffing a rose."

tongue should be firmly held but not pulled so hard as to cause discomfort.

6. Ask the patient to breathe in and out through the mouth or to "pant like a puppy." This will form a space between the soft palate and the tongue to allow placement of the mirror.
7. Pass the mirror face side down over the tongue to the level of the uvula (Fig. 18-2). Turn the mirror to face outward, pushing the uvula and soft palate upward out of the way. Take care to avoid the posterior pharyngeal wall.

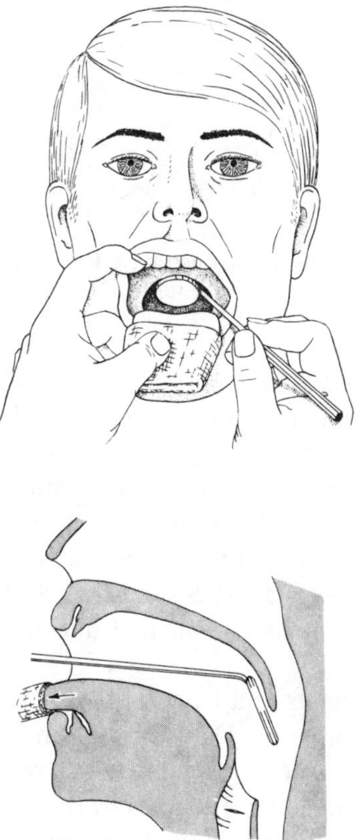

FIG. 18-2. Laryngeal mirror is inserted into pharynx, lifting uvula but avoiding contact with posterior pharyngeal wall. Tongue is pulled forward with gauze.

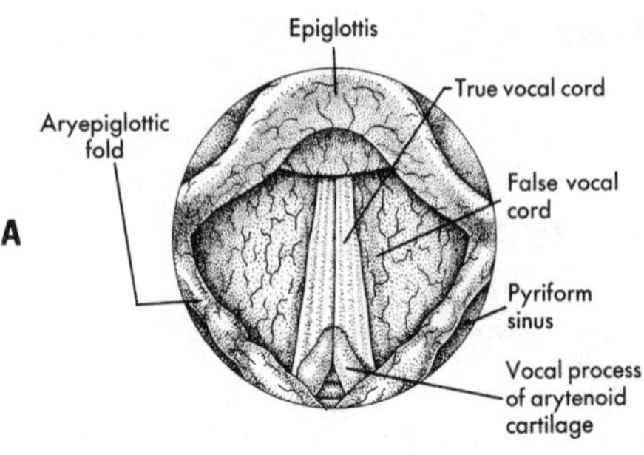

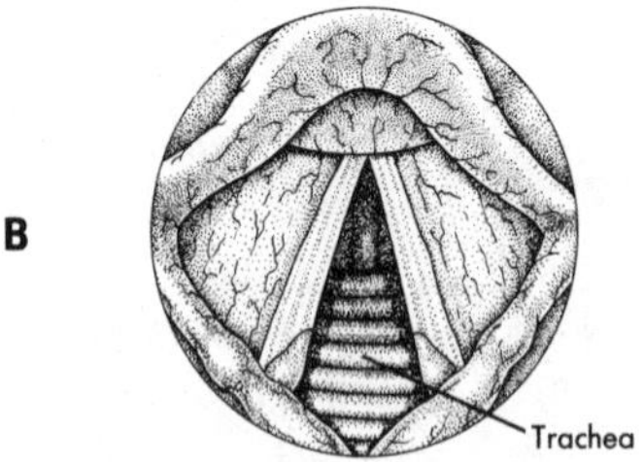

FIG. 18-3. View of larynx through mirror. **A,** Normal vocal cord positioning during phonation. **B,** Normal vocal cord positioning during inspiration.

8. Focus the headlight on the mirror and tilt the mirror in different directions to visualize the different anatomic parts of the larynx, hypopharynx, and tongue base (Fig. 18-3). All these anatomic areas cannot be visualized at one time with the mirror held in one position, but by tilting the mirror the various images can be pieced together to form a composite in the viewer's mind. Vocal cord movement is evaluated during phonation of the vowel "e."
9. Some patients will have an overactive gag reflex and may require topical anesthesia of the posterior pharynx and soft palate to visualize the larynx. A few patients' larynx will not be visualized by this technique and may require a direct examination with a flexible laryngoscope or even a general anesthetic.
10. Practice is the only way to improve one's technique.

▪ COMPLICATIONS

Laceration of the undersurface of the tongue may occur from stretching the tongue firmly over the teeth.

REFERENCES

1. Benign lesions of the larynx. In English, G.M., editor: Otolaryngology, Hagerstown, Md., 1976, Harper & Row, Publishers, Inc.
2. Methods of examining the larynx and tracheobronchial tree. In Ballantyne, J., and Groves, J., editors: Scott-Brown's diseases of the ear, nose and throat, vol. 4, Philadelphia, 1971, J.B. Lippincott Co.

PART FIVE

GASTROINTESTINAL PROCEDURES

CHAPTER 19

Gastric intubation

Michael J. Oblinger
Byrd S. Leavell, Jr.

GENERAL CONSIDERATIONS

Gastric intubation is used to remove gastric contents for diagnostic or therapeutic purposes or to instill various substances into the upper gastrointestinal tract.

DIAGNOSTIC INDICATIONS

1. Determining the presence of upper gastrointestinal tract bleeding.
2. Determining gastric acid content.
3. Assaying for intrinsic factor.
4. Measurement of gastric volume.
5. Drug analysis in suspected overdose cases.
6. *Mycobacterium tuberculosis* cultures.

THERAPEUTIC INDICATIONS

1. Decompression of the stomach and proximal small bowel by suction for a paralytic ileus, postoperative states, and mechanical obstruction.
2. Removal of stomach contents in drug overdose or toxin exposure (usually done with large-bore tubes).
3. Removal of blood from the stomach prior to diagnostic endoscopy or in hepatic encephalopathy.
4. Lavage of the stomach, usually with iced saline, in upper gastrointestinal tract hemorrhage.
5. As a component of treatment in selected cases of peptic ulcer disease, postoperative states, pancreatitis, severe vomiting, and gastric atony.
6. Instillation of fluids, electrolytes, and nutritional supplements.

ABSOLUTE CONTRAINDICATIONS

1. Nasal fractures or head and neck injuries that prevent the passage of tube through the nose or mouth.
2. Esophageal obstruction that prevents passage of tube.

RELATIVE CONTRAINDICATIONS

1. Facial or cranial trauma with potential skull fracture. Special precautions are necessary in these circumstances to prevent intracranial insertion of the nasogastric tube.[2,3]
2. Inability of the patient to protect the airway from aspiration. A comatose patient may require special precautions, such as endotracheal intubation, to prevent aspiration.

PATIENT EVALUATION AND PREPARATION

1. Explain the procedure and enlist the patient's cooperation.
2. Examine the nose and nasal passage to exclude anatomic abnormalities that would prevent passage of the tube.
3. Endotracheal intubation should be performed to protect the airway of the comatose patient prior to gastric intubation.

PERSONNEL AND EQUIPMENT

1. A physician or nurse trained in gastric intubation.
2. Gastric tube. For routine suctioning the preferred tube is a double-lumen (Levine) flexible nasogastric catheter. For most purposes a tube 14 to 18 mm in circumference (14 to 18 French) is used. For aspiration of pill fragments or blood clots, the larger Edlich or Ewald tube (30 to 34 French) is recommended. This tube must be passed through the mouth.
3. A water-soluble lubricant, a stethoscope, nonallergic tape, benzoin, a towel, an emesis basin, and a syringe that will fit the tube selected.
4. A suction machine and ice water for lavage as indicated.
5. Specimen containers.

6. For nasogastric insertion of standard size tubes, a glass of water with a straw may be useful.

■ TECHNIQUE

Nasogastric tube insertion

1. Place the patient, if possible, sitting up in a comfortable position. Otherwise place the patient in the left lateral decubitus position with the head turned to the side to prevent aspiration.
2. Measure the approximate length of tube needed by extending the tube from the end of the nose, along the side of the face past the ear to the xiphoid process. Mark this length with a piece of tape or by noting the mark on the tube just beyond this point.
3. Assess the patency of both nostrils by occluding the opposite side and having the patient sniff. Choose the more patent nostril.
4. Check the tube to be sure it is patent and free of ruptures and lubricate the first 5 cm.
5. Insert the end of tube into the chosen nostril and pass it along the the floor of the nose toward the ear (*not up* the nose) until it passes around the corner of the nasopharyngeal junction (Fig. 19-1). If difficulty in passing the tube is encountered, the tube should be withdrawn and the other nostril tried. At times it may be helpful to

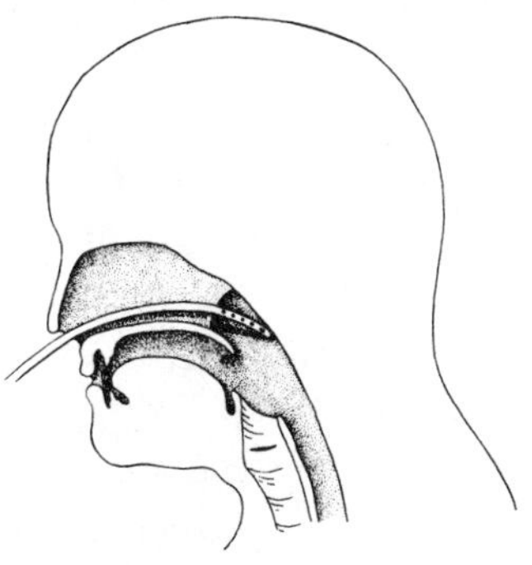

FIG. 19-1. Pass tube along floor of nose to nasopharynx.

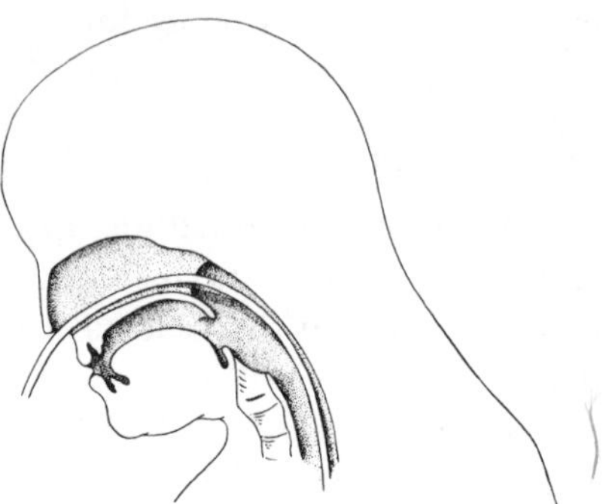

FIG. 19-2. Have patient flex head and gently advance tube while asking patient to swallow.

cool the tube in ice water to add stiffness and curve the distal 5 to 6 inches (12.5 to 15 cm) by coiling it tightly around your hand. The tube is passed with the curve pointing first inferiorly and then with a slight medial rotation of approximately 45 degrees as it is advanced.

6. When the tube is in the pharynx, have the patient bend the head forward toward the chest and gently advance the tube while asking the patient to swallow (Fig. 19-2). In the alert, cooperative patient this can be facilitated by having the patient sip a few mouthfuls of water through a straw. Check the pharynx to be sure the tube is passing down the esophagus and not coiling in the throat.
7. Gently advance the tube to the previously measured mark.
8. Check the position of the tube by gently aspirating with the syringe. If stomach contents are obtained, the tube is in the stomach. If not, advance the tube 2 or 3 inches (5 to 7.5 cm) and aspirate again. Placing the patient in the left lateral decubitus position may also facilitate aspiration of contents.[5] Another way to confirm the proper location is to listen over the epigastrium or left upper quadrant with the stethoscope for the characteristic "whoosh" heard when air is introduced through the tube (Fig. 19-3). *If any doubt exists as to position, check*

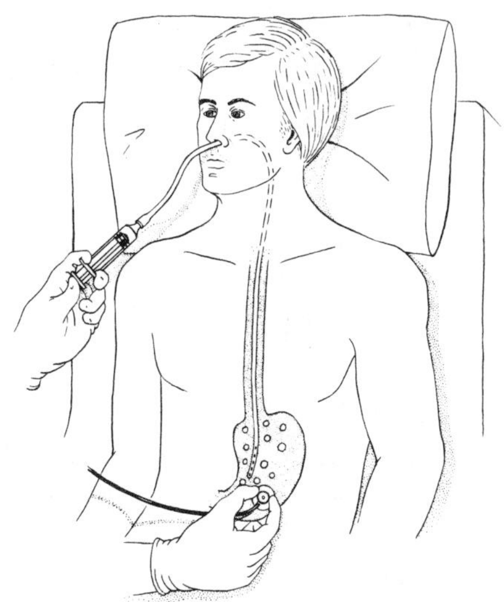

FIG. 19-3. Checking tube positioning in stomach by pushing air through tube and listening for "whoosh" sound.

it with an x-ray examination prior to instilling any material. Holding the end of the tube under water and observing for bubbles does not completely exclude the possibility of tracheal intubation and may lead to aspiration. Hence, it is not recommended.

Large-bore tube placement (oral)

1. Position and prepare the patient as just described.
2. Mark the tube as explained in step 2. Note that Edlich tubes are generally not premarked.
3. Because of the large size of the tube it should be passed orally.
4. If the patient is not alert or has an inadequate gag reflex an endotracheal tube should be passed first.
5. Spray the throat lightly with a short-acting topical anesthetic (such as benzocaine) or use a small amount of viscous lidocaine. Do not completely anesthetize the throat unless the airway is mechanically protected.

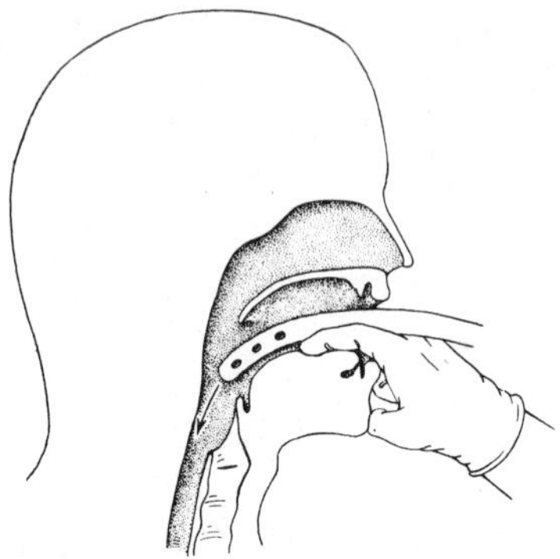

FIG. 19-4. Inserting large-bore tube. Hold tube between your index and middle finger and guide it over base of tongue toward esophagus.

6. In an agitated patient 2 to 10 mg of IV diazepam may be given cautiously in 2-mg increments to increase cooperation. The patient should be calm but not asleep.
7. Lubricate the tip of the tube with a water-soluble lubricant.
8. Have the patient bend the head forward as far as possible and insert your index and middle fingers over the base of the patient's tongue. Holding the tube in your other hand, use your index and middle fingers to guide the tube over the base of the tongue and toward the esophageal opening (Fig. 19-4).
9. Instruct the patient to breathe through the nose and make the motion of swallowing while gently pushing the tube forward. Excessive gagging may require more topical anesthetic. With mild gagging the tube can usually be advanced immediately after the patient gags, since this opens the cricopharyngeal musculature. Once in the esophagus, advance the tube gently to the previously made mark.
10. Check the position as explained in step 8 of nasogastric tube insertion. A large-bore tube should not be inserted, secured, and left. A nurse or physician should be in attendance at all times.

POSTPROCEDURE CARE

1. Secure the nasogastric tube in place by looping tape around the tube and applying it to the nose so that it hangs enough to allow movement with swallowing. Place a rubber band around the tube in a slip-knot fashion and attach it to the patient's gown with a safety pin, being sure to leave enough slack to allow full movement of the head.
2. Failure to drain properly may be related to plugging of the lumen or malposition. Follow step 8 of nasogastric tube insertion to assure position and irrigate gently. If no return is obtained, the tube may be clogged and require replacement.

COMPLICATIONS

1. Pulmonary aspiration is most likely to occur with a comatose or uncooperative patient. This risk can be minimized by protecting the airway if necessary during insertion and keeping the patient in an upright position once the t be is in place.
2. Intracranial insertion of the tube may occur when the nasogastric tube is passed in a patient with a fracture of the cribriform plate.[3] This can be prevented by first passing a precurved nasopharyngeal airway and inserting the nasogastric tube through it. Positioning the tube in patients with head or neck trauma should be checked fluoroscopically.
3. Esophageal perforation is an unusual complication that occurs with overforceful insertion of the tube, usually through an obstructing lesion.
4. Esophageal stricture may occur with prolonged use of the nasogastric tube.[1]
5. Significant fluid and electrolyte imbalance may occur with nasogastric suction. Volume and electrolyte content of gastric aspirate must be replaced on a daily basis.
6. Irritation occurs when the tube is secured in such a position that undue pressure is applied on the nose. Necrosis may occur if not corrected.

7. Trauma in nasal structures on insertion can be prevented by careful adherence to correct procedure and identification of structural abnormalities prior to insertion.
8. Gastric mucosal irritation with suction is minimized with a double-lumen tube, and, although significant gastric ulceration has been described,[4,6] this is an unusual phenomenon. Minor blood loss as detected by chemical testing is not unusual, but significant bleeding is rare.

REFERENCES

1. Benfield, W.J., and Hurwitz, A.L.: Esophageal stricture associated with nasogastric intubation, Arch. Intern. Med. **74:**1083-1086, 1974.
2. Bouzarth, W.F.: Nasogastric intubation, Ann. Emerg. Med. **9:**73, 1980.
3. Galloway, D.C., and Crudis, J.: Inadvertent intracranial placement of a nasogastric tube through a basal skull fracture, South. Med. J. **72:**240-241, 1979.
4. Green, J.F., Jr., Sawicki, J.E., and Doyle, W.F.: Gastric ulceration: a complication of double lumen nasogastric tubes, J.A.M.A. **224:**338-339, 1973.
5. Hector, R.M.: Improved technique of gastric aspiration, Lancet **1:**15-16, 1968.
6. Schmerl, E.F., and Steiner, P.: Porthole ulcers associated with gastric intubation, West. J. Med. **124:**172-173, 1976.

CHAPTER 20

Specialized gastric and intestinal feeding tubes

■ Byrd S. Leavell, Jr.
Michael J. Oblinger

■ GENERAL CONSIDERATIONS

Specialized gastric and intestinal feeding tubes are used to administer enteral hyperalimentation to patients who cannot eat but who have gastrointestinal tracts that will absorb nutrients. These tubes, unlike conventional nasogastric tubes, are small in diameter (1 or 2 mm), will not stiffen after 4 days of use, and can be inserted into the small bowel. Enteral hyperalimentation should be tried before intravenous hyperalimentation, since the latter may cause sepsis and is more expensive than enteral hyperalimentation.[6] Discussion of enteral formulas is beyond the scope of this chapter, but several excellent reviews of this subject are available.[3,5]

■ INDICATIONS

1. Malnourished patients, those who have lost 10% of their usual weight and are unable to eat enough food to correct their malnutrition.
2. Patients who are unable to eat and are likely to remain this way for at least a week, such as neurologically impaired or postoperative patients.

■ ABSOLUTE CONTRAINDICATIONS

1. Nasal fractures or head and neck injuries preventing passage of the tube through the nose or mouth.
2. Esophageal obstruction preventing passage of the tube.

■ RELATIVE CONTRAINDICATIONS

The inability of the patient to protect the airway from aspiration is a relative contraindication. A comatose patient may require special precautions, such as endotracheal intubation, to prevent aspiration or selection of a tube designed to prevent aspiration (Dobbhoff tube).

■ PATIENT EVALUATION AND PREPARATION

1. Explain the procedure and enlist the patient's cooperation.
2. Examine the nose and nasal passage to exclude anatomic abnormalities that would prevent passage of the tube.
3. Endotracheal intubation should be considered to protect the airway of the comatose patient prior to gastric intubation.

■ PERSONNEL AND EQUIPMENT

1. A physician or nurse trained in gastric intubation.
2. An appropriate tube (Table 20-1).
3. A water-soluble lubricant, stethoscope, nonallergic tape, benzoin, a towel, an emesis basin, and a large syringe (30 to 50 ml).
4. For comatose patients, a gelatin capsule for passing the nasogastric tube.

TABLE 20-1. ENTERAL ALIMENTATION TUBES

Trade names	Materials	Circumferences (French)	Lengths (inches/cm)	Feedings	Duration of use
Keofed	Silicone	5, 7.3, 9.6	43 (107.5)	Gastric or intestinal	Up to 6 weeks
Dobbhoff	Polyurethane	8	43 (107.5)	Gastric or intestinal	Up to 6 weeks
Duo-Tube	Silicone	5, 6, 8	40 (100)	Gastric or intestinal	Up to 6 weeks
Entriflex	Polyurethane	8	36, 43, (90, 107.5)	Gastric or intestinal	Up to 6 weeks

■ TECHNIQUE

1. Place the patient in a sitting or semirecumbent position with the head flexed to the chest. If this is not possible, then place the patient in the left lateral decubitus position with the head turned to the side to prevent aspiration.
2. Measure the approximate length of the tube needed. For gastric feeding 50 cm of tube is required, and for small bowel feedings 75 cm of tube must be passed.
3. Assess the patency of both nostrils by occluding the opposite side and having the patient sniff. Choose the more patent nostril; occasionally preparatory shrinkage of the nasal mucous membranes with a decongestant is helpful.
4. Lubricate the distal 5 cm of the tube.
5. Insert the end of the tube into the chosen nostril and pass it along the floor of the nose toward the ear until it passes around the corner of the nasopharyngeal junction (Fig. 20-1, *A*). If difficulty in passing the tube is

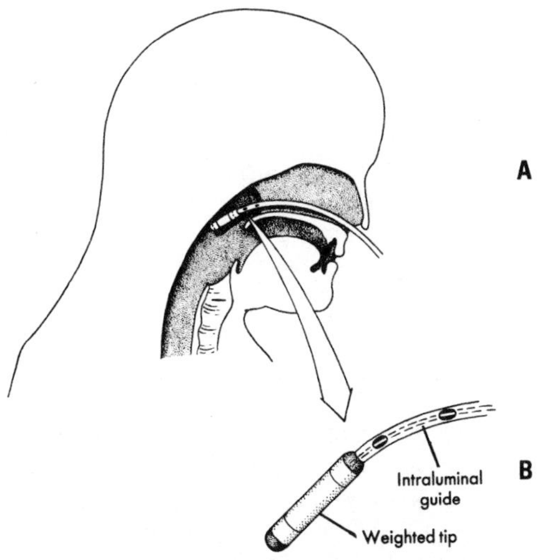

FIG. 20-1. A, Pass tube along floor of nose and beyond nasopharyngeal junction. **B,** Keofed tube with intraluminal guide in place.

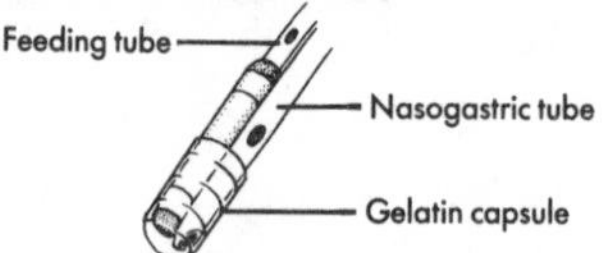

FIG. 20-2. "Piggybacking" feeding tube to stiffer plastic nasogastric tube with gelatin capsule.

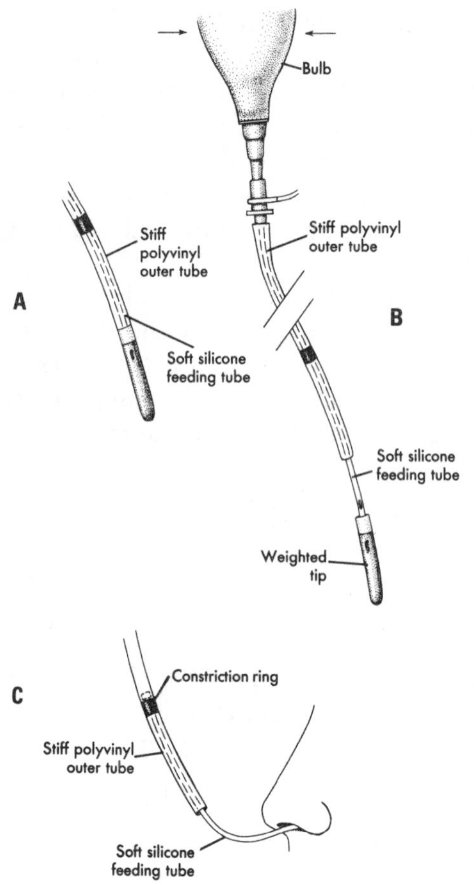

FIG. 20-3. Duo-Tube. **A,** Tube is placed in stomach in this configuration. **B,** When tube is in stomach, bulb is attached and squeezed, ejecting 2 inches (5 cm) of feeding tube into stomach. Bulb is detached, filled with water, and squeezed again to fully express feeding tube out of polyvinyl outer tube. **C,** Withdraw polyvinyl tube until about 3 inches (7.5 cm) of silicone tube emerge from nose; tape silicone tube to face.

encountered, the tube should be withdrawn and the other nostril tried. If this does not work, an intraluminal guide, if supplied, should be used to give more rigidity to the tube (Fig. 20-1, *B*).

6. When the tube is in the pharynx, have the patient bend the head forward toward the chest and gently advance the tube, asking the patient to swallow. This may be facilitated with a few mouthfuls of water thrugh a straw. In comatose patients, a guide may be needed, or the feeding tube may be "piggybacked" into the stomach using a stiff plastic nasogastric tube by impinging the distal ends of both tubes into the base of a suitably sized gelatin capsule (Fig. 20-2).
7. Check the pharynx to be sure the tube is passing down the esophagus and not coiling in the throat.
8. When passage of a flexible feeding tube is difficult, one may succeed with the Duo-Tube, which is a soft silicone tube inside a stiffer outer polyvinyl tube (Fig. 20-3).
9. Gently advance the tube to the 50-cm mark.
10. Confirm the intragastric location by injecting a small amount of air (20 to 40 cc), while auscultating over the left upper quadrant with the stethoscope for the characteristic "whoosh" of air entering the stomach. If any doubt exists as to the position, check it with an abdominal radiograph prior to instilling any material.
11. If small bowel feeding is desired, the patient should lie on the right side and have the tube advanced 10 cm every 2 to 4 hours until the 75-cm mark is passed.
12. Verify the small bowel location by a flat-plate abdominal roentgenograph. If passing the tube beyond the pylorus is a problem, endoscopic guidance may be necessary.

■ POSTPROCEDURAL CARE

1. Secure the nasogastric tube in place by looping tape around the tube and applying it to the nose so that it hangs enough to allow movement with swallowing. Place a rubber band around the tube in a slip-knot fash-

ion and attach it to the patient's gown with a safety pin, being sure to leave enough slack to allow full movement of the head.

2. Extubation is a problem with some disoriented patients and special anchoring maneuvers have been described.[1,4]
3. In the smaller gauge tubes, continuous infusion of nutrients is required to maintain patency of the tube and achieve the maximum caloric intake with the least amount of side effects.[2]
4. Transpyloric placement of the feeding tube decreases the risk of reflux gastritis and aspiration.

COMPLICATIONS

Problems with the tube itself are infrequent, with the exception of occlusion of the tube lumen with the nutrient solution. Following are common problems associated with administration of the solutions[5]:

1. Tube lumen clogged by solution. Clogging of the tube lumen is said to occur in less than 10% of intubations and can usually be eliminated by flushing the tube with water.
2. Aspiration of stomach contents occurs in less than 1% of patients and is unlikely if the head of the bed is elevated.
3. Erosion of the esophagus has occurred with conventional nasogastric tubes but must be very rare with the specialized tubes.

REFERENCES

1. Carr, G.C., and Heimlich, H.J.: Circle tie to prevent removal of nasogastric tube by patient, Surg. Gynecol. Obstet. **134**:317-318, 1972.
2. Dobbie, R.I., and Hoffmeister, J.A.: Continuous pump-tube enteric hyperalimentation, Surg. Gynecol. Obstet. **143**:273-276, 1976.
3. Malt, R. et al.: Nutritional support of hospitalized patients, N. Engl. J. Med. **304**:1147-1152, 1981.
4. McGuire, W.F., and Strout, J.J.: Securing of intermediate duration feeding tubes, Laryngoscope **90**:2046-2048, 1980.
5. Rudman, D. et al.: Enteral hyperalimentation: an alternative to central venous hyperalimentation, Ann. Intern. Med. **90**:63-71, 1979.
6. Rudman, D. et al.: Nasogastric hyperalimentation through a polythylene catheter: an alternative to central venous hyperalimentation, Am. J. Clin. Nut. **32**:1112-1120, 1979.

CHAPTER 21

Intestinal intubation

■ **Matthew J. Lambert III**

■ GENERAL CONSIDERATIONS

Intestinal intubation with a "long tube" is a method of decompressing small intestine that has become distended because of mechanical obstruction or paralytic ileus.[1]

■ INDICATIONS

Mechanical intestinal obstruction

Complete intestinal obstruction is a surgical condition, and intestinal intubation is no substitute for operative correction of the obstruction.[1] Intestinal intubation should be considered in individuals with the following conditions:

1. Acute or recurrent partial intestinal obstruction.
2. Obstruction due to disseminated carcinoma.
3. Obstruction due to inflammatory bowel disease.
4. Enterocutaneous fistulae in which evacuation of proximal small intestinal content is desirable.

Paralytic ileus

Paralytic ileus is common after most abdominal operations but usually resolves in 48 to 72 hours spontaneously or with the use of a nasogastric tube. Paralytic ileus may also occur after spinal fractures, retroperitoneal hemorrhage, trauma, electrolyte disturbances, or the use of certain medications (e.g., narcotic analgesics and atropine-like drugs).[2] In cases where such an ileus is prolonged or associated with significant abdominal distention, a "long tube" may facilitate intestinal decompression.[1-3]

■ CONTRAINDICATIONS

1. Nasal fractures or head and neck injuries that prevent passage of the tube through the nose or mouth.

2. Esophageal obstruction that prevents tube passage.
3. Need for urgent surgical correction of the obstruction.
4. Inability of the patient to protect the airway from aspiration. A comatose patient may require special precautions, such as endotracheal intubation, to prevent aspiration.

■ PATIENT EVALUATION AND PREPARATION

1. Explain the procedure to the patient.
2. Examine the nose and nasal passages to exclude abnormalities that would prevent successful tube passage.
3. Protect the comatose patient from aspiration by performing endotracheal intubation prior to inserting the "long tube."

■ PERSONNEL AND EQUIPMENT

1. A physician familiar with the technique of intestinal intubation and one assistant to aid in the proper positioning of the patient.
2. Principal implements: a tube, lubricant, syringe (10 to 20 ml), needle (21 gauge), mercury, cotton-tip applicators, suction apparatus, a cup filled with water, and a straw.

■ TECHNIQUE

I prefer to use the Cantor tube for intestinal intubation. It is radiopaque and siliconized. A 16 French tube is employed in adults.

1. Aspirate mercury into the syringe with a 21-gauge needle. Use 5 ml in patients with active peristalsis and 7 to 9 ml in patients with paralytic ileus and absent bowel sounds.
2. Expel all remaining air from the syringe.
3. Insert the needle into the middle of the bag, inject the mercury, and then aspirate all air from the bag prior to needle withdrawal.
4. Lubricate the bag with a small amount of water-soluble lubricant.

5. Place the patient in a sitting or semirecumbent position with the head hyperextended.
6. Grasp the bag at the tip and let the mercury fall back toward the tube (Fig. 21-1).
7. Insert the bag into the nostril (Fig. 21-2) and then squeeze the mercury toward the tip of the bag. The bag should then fall easily into the nasopharynx. A cotton-tip applicator may be used to propel the tube if necessary.
8. Ask the patient to sip water and swallow the tube (Fig. 21-3) until the letter S on the tube is at the external

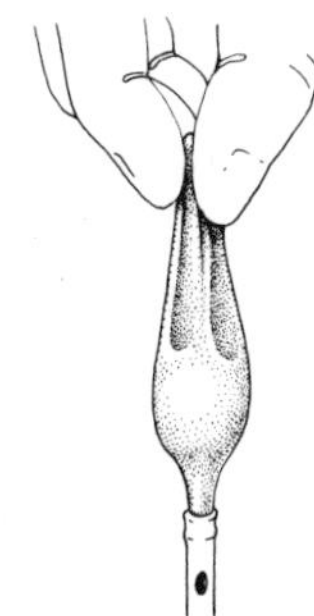

FIG. 21-1. Grasp bag at tip and let mercury fall back toward tube.

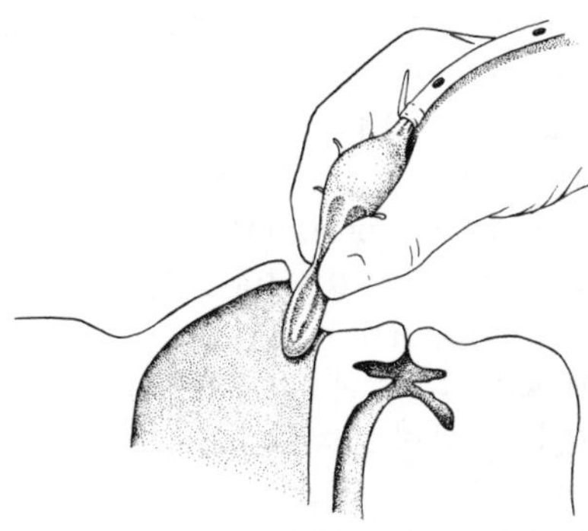

FIG. 21-2. Insert bag into nostril.

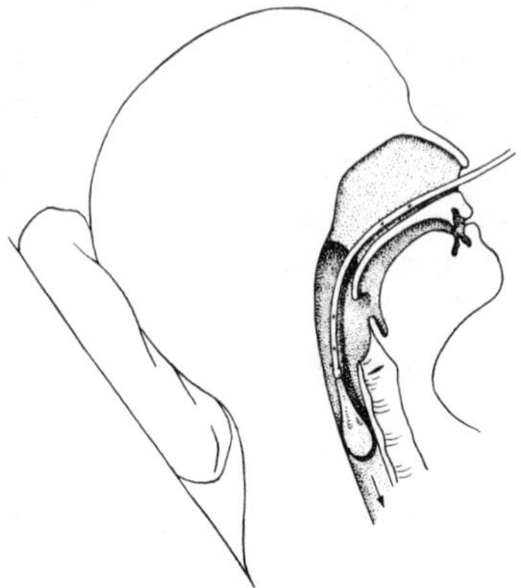

FIG. 21-3. Ask patient to swallow bag. Do not push tube down.

nares. This indicates the tube is in the stomach. Confirmation can be obtained by injecting a small amount of air into the tube and auscultating the left upper quadrant.

9. Connect the tube to intermittent suction.
10. Do not allow the tube to advance more rapidly than 4 inches (10 cm) every 2 hours. A quicker rate of insertion may cause the tube to curl in the stomach.
11. After the tube has reached the stomach, the patient should lie on the right side with the foot of the bed elevated 12 inches (30 cm). Sufficient tube should be allowed to pass to bring the letter P to the nostril. The tube should then be at the pylorus. This position should be maintained for 2 hours.
12. Place the patient on the back with the foot of the bed lowered (Fowler's position) for 2 hours. The tube should then pass into the duodenum bringing the letter D to the external nares.
13. Turn the patient to the left side, lying flat in bed. Allow 4 inches (10 cm) of tube to pass. Maintain this position for 2 hours.
14. Allowing the patient to move about encourages tube passage. The tube should not be secured with tape.

15. Determine tube position in 6 hours with an abdominal roentgenograph.

■ TUBE REMOVAL

1. Change the tube if it is in place longer than 2 weeks or if stiffening of the tube occurs.
2. Remove the tube with gentle but firm traction. If resistance is encountered, wait until the peristaltic wave has released the balloon and resume traction.

■ COMPLICATIONS

1. Pulmonary aspiration is most likely to occur with a comatose or uncooperative patient. This risk can be minimized by protecting the airway during insertion (endotracheal intubation) and keeping the patient in an upright position once the tube is in place.
2. Fluid and electrolyte abnormalities may occur with prolonged enteral suction. The volume and electrolyte content of aspirated fluid should be replaced daily.
3. Loss of mercury from the balloon into the gastrointestinal tract will not lead to toxicity because it is unabsorbable.

REFERENCES

1. Jones, R.S.: Intestinal obstruction. In Sabiston, D.C., editor: Davis-Christopher textbook of surgery, Philadelphia, 1977, W.B. Saunders Co.
2. Schwartz, S.I., and Storer, E.H.: Manifestations of gastrointestinal disease. In Schwartz, S.I., editor: Principles of Surgery, New York, 1974, McGraw-Hill, Inc.
3. Welch, C.E., and Hedberg, S.E.: Complications in surgry of the colon and rectum. In Artz, C.P., and Hardy, J.D., editors: Management of surgical complications, Philadelphia, 1975, W.B. Saunders Co.

CHAPTER 22

Proctosigmoidoscopy

■ William Cunningham
Paul M. Suratt

■ GENERAL CONSIDERATIONS

Proctosigmoidoscopy is a method of visually examining the rectum and distal sigmoid colon with a rigid tube. Biopsies can also be obtained through the scope. Approximately 60% of colorectal tumors can be seen with and examined through this instrument. The procedure is relatively safe and is frequently used as a screening procedure for cancer in patients over 50 years of age.[9,14]

■ INDICATIONS

1. Hematochezia (red blood in stool).
2. Symptoms suggesting colorectal disease, such as unexplained diarrhea, tenesmus, and rectal pain.
3. A barium enema suggestive of cancer, polyps, or inflammatory bowel disease.
4. Screening for colorectal cancer in patients over 50 years of age or in patients with diseases predisposing them to colorectal cancer.[2,9]
5. Sigmoid volvulus.[1]
6. Staging of pelvic tumors.
7. Suspected systemic disease that may be diagnosed by proctoscopic biopsy such as amyloidosis, cerebrosidosis, and schistosomiasis.[8,9]
8. Polypectomy.

■ CONTRAINDICATIONS

There are no absolute contraindications to protosigmoidoscopy,[13] although bleeding diathesis contraindicates a proctoscopic biopsy, LeFrock et al.[11] have noted an unconfirmed[5] 10% frequency of bacteremia, mostly enterococcal, with proctoscopy. This should be considered when performing the study in subjects with immunodeficiency or abnormal or prosthetic heart valves. The necessity for antibiotic prophylaxis is unsettled.

PATIENT EVALUATION AND PREPARATION

1. Routine bowel preparation is not required and is undesirable in patients with diarrhea.
2. A saline or phosphate enema may be given if formed stool obscures the examination.
3. Coagulation studies should be performed prior to the biopsy.
4. The bowel should be evacuated if electrocautery is to be performed. This can be achieved by giving the patient clear liquids only for 48 hours, followed by magnesium citrate, 240 ml, 24 hours prior to the procedure. Then tap water enemas can be given 12 hours before and just prior to the procedure.
5. The biopsy must be coordinated with barium enema studies, since there is a risk of barium extravasation during the first few days after the biopsy and barium obscures amebae.
6. Explain the procedure and its potential complications to the patient and obtain written informed consent, particularly if a biopsy or polypectomy is planned.

PERSONNEL AND EQUIPMENT

1. A physician trained in proctoscopy and one assistant.
2. Principal implements: a proctosigmoidoscope with a light source, obturator, suction source and catheter, insufflation bag, biopsy forceps, silver nitrate lubricant, cotton swabs, cautery sticks, and gloves.
3. Specimen containers: 10% formalin solution in a jar for material excised, glass slides, and culture plates or a holding media.

TECHNIQUE[12,13]

1. Inform the subject of all the effects of the examination, including cramps and the urge to defecate.

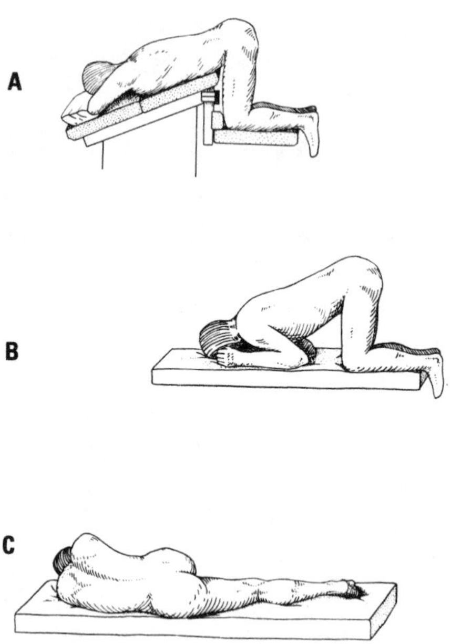

FIG. 22-1. Positioning patient. A, Position using proctoscopy table. **B,** Position using flat examination table. **C,** Position for patient who is unable to assume knee-chest position illustrated in **A** and **B.**

2. Position the patient, if possible, in the knee-chest position; otherwise position the patient in the left decubitus position (Fig. 22-1).
3. Inspect the perineal area and perform a digital rectal examination to lubricate and dilate the anal canal and to assure a patent pathway.
4. Introduce the proctoscope with the obturator in place 3 or 4 cm into the anus, with the tip directed toward the umbilicus. Direct the tip posteriorly and advance it another 2 or 3 cm and remove the obturator (Fig. 22-2). Advance the instrument *only* when the lumen can be visualized! The rectosigmoid junction at 13 cm is negotiated by directing the proctoscope tip anteriorly and occasionally to the right where the lumen will reappear (Fig. 22-3). Insert the scope to 25 cm if possible.

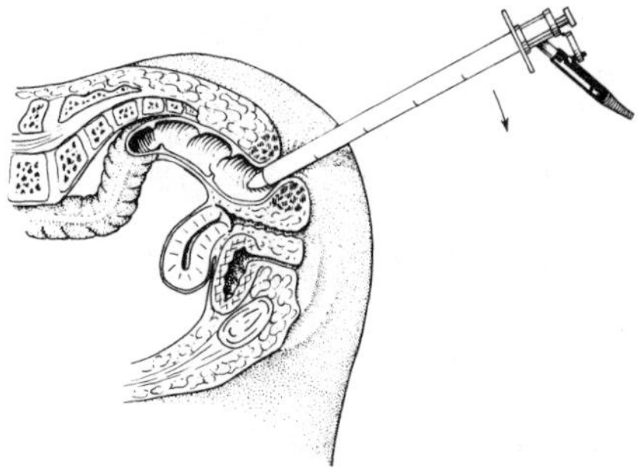

FIG. 22-2. Proctoscope with obturator in place, inserted 3 or 4 cm into anus. Note that tip is pointed toward umbilicus. Next point tip posteriorly by moving proctoscope in direction of arrow, advance it another 2 or 3 cm, and remove obturator.

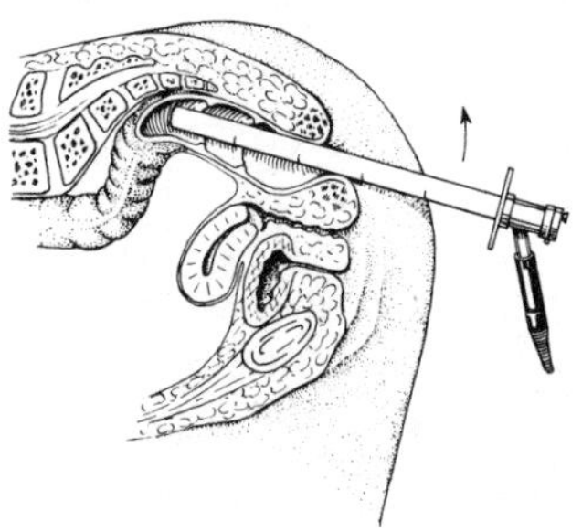

FIG. 22-3. Negotiate rectosigmoid junction by moving proctoscope in direction of arrow so that tip will move anteriorly.

5. After maximal insertion, withdraw the instrument slowly and scan the entire mucosal surface. The proximal surface of the rectal valves should be examined by flattening the valves with the instrument tip.
6. Mucosal features to evaluate include the presence or absence of submucosal vessels, friability to swabbing, and granularity. The location of all discrete lesions should be recorded in their distance from the anal verge and in anterior, posterior, right-left orientation with reference to the subject. The size and appearance of the lesions should be recorded. Collection of mucus for wet

preparation, methylene blue stain, Gram-stain examination, or culture may be appropriate, using the nonabsorbent end of a swab.

7. Biopsies are performed only by a trained physician on the posterior wall in the distal 10 cm of the rectum.

■ INTERPRETATION OF FINDINGS

Rectosigmoid appearance[12]

Diffuse abnormalities

1. Disappearance of submucosal vessels: submucosal edema or infiltration.
2. Granularity: subepithelial edema or infiltration.
3. Contact friability: mucosal inflammation.

These changes are nonspecific and may be seen in inflammatory bowel disease, bacterial infections (shigella, invasive *Escherischia coli*, gonococcus, etc.), amebiasis, radiation, antibiotics, and lymphogranuloma venereum.

4. Pigmentation: melanosis coli (anthracene cathartics).

Discrete abnormalities

1. Ulcer: amebiasis, Crohn's disease, radiation, stercoraceous, nonspecific.
2. Cobblestoning: Crohn's disease.
3. Dull yellow-gray adherent plaques: pseudomembranous colitis.
4. Stricture: carcinoma, radiation, inflammatory bowel diseases, lymphogranuloma venereum, extrinsic compression (endometriosis, carcinoma, abscess).
5. Blue collapsible cysts: pneumatosis cystoides intestinalis.
6. Minute gray blebs: colitis cystica superficialis.
7. Telangiectasis: radiation.
8. Polyp: neoplasm, hyperplasia, hematoma, inflammatory bowel disease, schistosomiasis, amebiasis.

Anal appearance[12]

1. Polyp: hemorrhoid, papilla, skin tag, neoplasm.
2. Fissure: nonspecific, syphilitic, inflammatory bowel disease.

3. Fistula: inflammatory bowel disease, radiation, lymphogranuloma venereum, crypt abscess drainage site, tuberculosis, carcinoma, traumatic.
4. Stricture: surgical, lymphogranuloma venereum, inflammatory bowel disease, carcinoma.

Rectal mucus

1. Methylene blue stain[10]: neutophils indicate inflammatory bowel disease, pseudomembranous colitis, invasive bacterial infection (*Escherischia coli*, shigella, salmonella, gonococcus, etc.)
2. Gram stain: detects staphylococcal and *Candida* overgrowth, and invasive candidiasis (mycelia).[6]
3. Saline wet preparation: amebic trophozoites.[4]
4. Iodine preparation: parasitic cysts, eggs.[4]

Stool

Stool samples may be examined for muscle fibers, fat (Sudan stain), pH level, reducing substances, eggs, larvae (*Strongyloides stercoralis*). Many other analyses beyond the scope of this summary are possible.

■ COMPLICATIONS

1. Bowel perforation, 0.002% to 0.7% frequency,[7] results in retroperitoneal abscess, peritonitis, and sepsis.
2. Bacteremia, 0% to 9.5% frequency.
3. Hemorrhage following the biopsy or other operative techniques.
4. Intestinal gas explosion following electrocautery.[3]

REFERENCES

1. Arnold, G., and Nance, F.: Volvulus of the sigmoid colon, Ann. Surg. **177:**527-531, 1973.
2. Bolt, R.: Sigmoidoscopy in detection and diagnosis in the asymptomatic individual, Cancer **28:**121-122, 1971.
3. Bond, J., Levy, M., and Levitt, M.: Explosion of hydrogen gas in the colon during proctosigmoidoscopy, Gastrointest. Endosc. **23:**41-42, 1976.
4. Brown, H.: Basic clinical parasitology, ed. 4, New York, 1975, Appleton-Century-Crofts.
5. Engeling, E. et al.: Letter: Bacteremia after sigmoidoscopy: another view, Ann. Int. Med. **85:**77-78, 1976.

6. Eras, P., Goldstein, M., and Sherlock, P.: *Candida* infection of the gastrointestinal tract, Medicine **51**:367-379, 1972.
7. Fielding, J. et al.: Large bowel perforation in patients undergoing sigmoidoscopy and barium enema, Br. Med. J. **1**:471-473, 1973.
8. Gear, E., and Dobbins, W.: Rectal biopsy: a review of its diagnostic usefulness, Gastroenterology **55**:522-544, 1968.
9. Gilbertsen, V.: Proctosigmoidoscopy and polypectomy in reducing the incidence of rectal cancer, Cancer **34**(Suppl.):936-939, 1974.
10. Harris, J., DuPont, H., and Hornick, R.: Fecal leukocytes in diarrheal illness, Ann. Int. Med. **76**:697-703, 1972.
11. LeFrock, J. et al.: Transient bacteremia associated with sigmoidoscopy, N. Engl. J. Med. **289**:467-469, 1973.
12. Sleisenger, M., and Fordtran, J.: Gastrointestinal disease, ed. 2, Philadelphia, 1978, W.B. Saunders Co.
13. Thompson, W.G.: Sigmoidoscopy, Can. Med. Assoc. J. **110**:683-685, 1974.
14. Winawer, S. et al.: Screening for colon cancer, Gastroenterology **70**:783-789, 1976.

CHAPTER 23

Abdominal paracentesis and lavage

■ Robert S. Gibson

■ GENERAL CONSIDERATIONS

Abdominal paracentesis and lavage is a method of removing fluid from or introducing therapeutic agents into the abdominal cavity.[2-6] The procedure is easy to perform and safe if one avoids adhesions, solid viscera or masses, distended bowel loops, and the bladder.

■ DIAGNOSTIC INDICATIONS

1. When intraperitoneal bleeding, hollow viscus perforation, or bacterial peritonitis is suspected.
2. Ascites of unknown etiology.

■ THERAPEUTIC INDICATIONS

1. Ascites causing abdominal discomfort, impaired respirations, or when contributing to high portal pressures.[1]
2. Treatment of hemorrhagic pancreatitis.
3. Instillation of antineoplastic agents for carcinomatous peritonitis.

■ CONTRAINDICATIONS

1. Multiple previous abdominal operations.
2. Significant bowel distention.
3. Hemorrhagic dyscrasia that cannot be corrected.
4. Disease of the abdominal skin, such as cellulitis or furunculosis.
5. During pregnancy midline paracentesis should be avoided.
6. Uncooperative patient.

■ PATIENT EVALUATION AND PREPARATION

1. Examine the patient's abdomen for surgical scars, dermatitis, distention, masses, and hepatosplenomegaly.
2. Obtain the prothrombin time, partial thromboplastin time, and platelet count.
3. Obtain the necessary abdominal roentgenograms, particularly if a distended or perforated bowel is suspected.
4. Before aspiration or lavage, the bladder must be emptied, either voluntarily or by catheterization.
5. Explain the procedure to the patient, including its potential complications, and obtain written informed consent.

■ PERSONNEL AND EQUIPMENT

1. A physician skilled in abdominal paracentesis.
2. Principal implements: a peritoneal dialysis catheter (Trocath); an intravenous administration set, Ringer's lactate solution (1 L), a 35-ml syringe, and a number 15 scalpel blade and handle. Optional equipment (for simple needle aspiration) includes an 18-gauge intracatheter (IV Cath, Becton-Dickinson) and a 20-ml syringe.
3. Asepsis and sterile field: antiseptic solution; sterile sponges; a mask, hair cap, gown, and gloves; draping towels, and towel clips.
4. Anesthesia: lidocaine (1%, 10 ml), a 23-gauge needle (1 inch; 2.5 cm), and a 3-ml syringe.
5. Dressing: an adhesive bandage, silk suture (3-0) on a cutting needle, suture scissors, antibiotic ointment, sterile sponges, and adhesive tape (1-inch).

■ TECHNIQUE

Abdominal lavage

1. Place the patient in the supine position.
2. Select one of the following puncture sites (Fig. 23-1): (1) a point in the midline, approximately midway between the umbilicus and symphysis pubis, (2) a point in either lower abdominal flank (pelvic fossae) lateral to

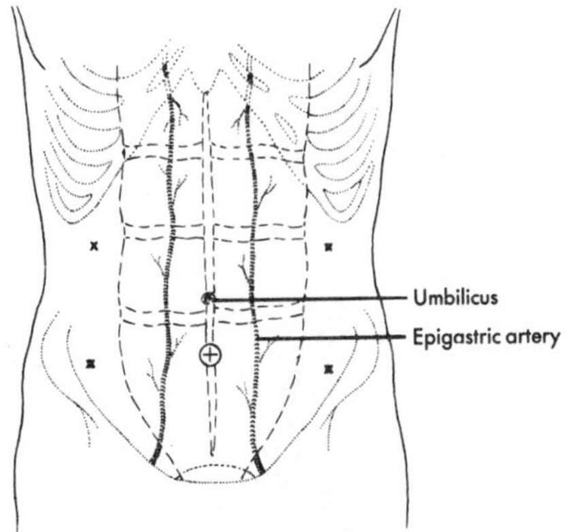

FIG. 23-1. Anatomic landmarks.

the rectus muscle, or (3) all four abdominal quadrants.

3. Put on a hair cap, gown, mask, and gloves.
4. Prepare the skin with an antiseptic solution and drape a sterile field with towels.
5. Anesthetize the skin and tissues down to and including the peritoneum.
6. Make a 3-mm incision in the skin at the needle puncture site with a number 15 scalpel blade.
7. Place the stylet into the Trocath until the pointed tip is exposed.
8. Instruct the patient to lift the head to tense the abdominal wall.
9. Hold the Trocath vertically and insert it into the peritoneal cavity with a twisting motion, using forceful restraint (Fig. 23-2). Entry through the peritoneum is indicated by a "pop" or "give."
10. Withdraw the inner stylet several centimeters so that its sharp point is no longer protruding out of the catheter. Grasp the catheter with your thumb and index finger, and advance it toward the right or left pelvic fossa (whichever side is likely to give a positive tap) while withdrawing the stylet (Fig. 23-3). Remove the stylet from the catheter when the catheter is properly placed.

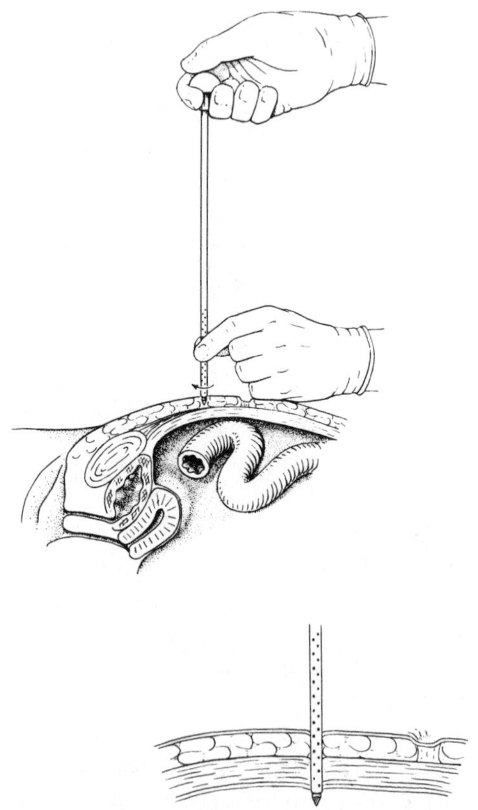

FIG. 23-2. Place stylet into Trocath so that pointed tip is exposed. Hold Trocath vertically and enter peritoneal cavity with twisting forceful motion.

Ascertain that all catheter perforations are in the peritoneal cavity.

11. Aspirate peritoneal fluid with the 35-ml syringe. If sufficient fluid is obtained for diagnostic or therapeutic purposes, remove the catheter and proceed to step 13. If a definitive diagnosis (such as recovery of blood or bowel contents) is not made or the desired therapeutic effect is not achieved, proceed to step 12.
12. Peritoneal lavage. Attach the elbow of the connecting tube to the end of the catheter (Fig. 23-4). Infuse 1 L of

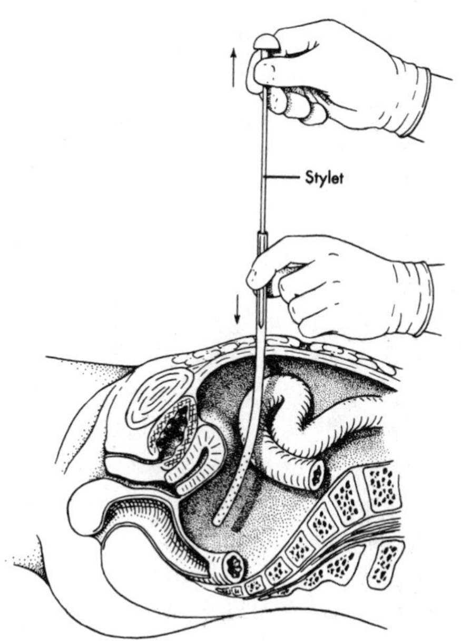

FIG. 23-3. Advance Trocath toward right or left pelvic fossa while withdrawing stylet.

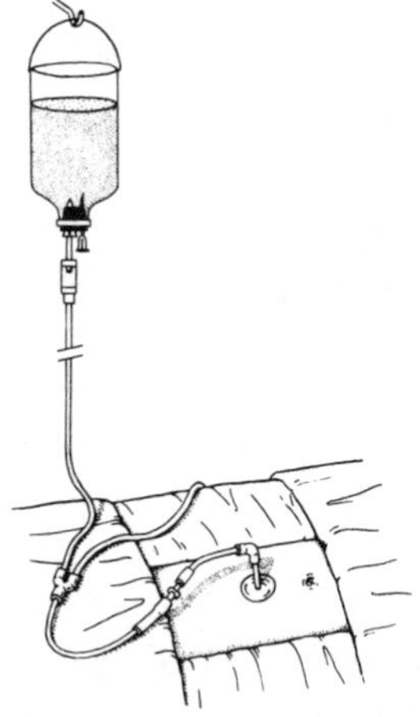

FIG. 23-4. Lavage of peritoneal cavity.

Ringer's lactate solution into the abdomen, clamp the intravenous tubing, and roll the patient from side to side to disperse the fluid. Transfer the intravenous tubing to the vent hole of the intravenous bottle, unclamp the tubing, and lower the intravenous bottle to siphon the fluid. Aspiration through a 35-ml syringe can also be used to evacuate fluid. For therapeutic lavage, the catheter should be secured to the skin with sutures and appropriate fluid infused and allowed to drain; repeat this as often as necessary (Chapter 25).

13. Evaluate fluid. Obtain sufficient fluid for a cell count; Gram stain; culture; protein, glucose, amylase, and cytology examination; and cell block. Greater than 500 white blood cells per cubic millimeter in peritoneal fluid indicates peritonitis. Intraperitoneal hemorrhage is present when the red blood cell count (obtained by a hemacytometer) is greater than 100,000 per cubic millimeter or the hematocrit value is greater than 2%.[7]
14. Remove the catheter and apply a sterile absorbent dressing.

Simple needle aspiration

1. Follow steps 1 to 6 of the technique for abdominal lavage.
2. Instruct the patient to lift the head and tense the abdominal wall.
3. Hold the 18-gauge intracatheter needle vertically and insert it into the peritoneal cavity. Entry through the peritoneum is indicated by a "pop" or "give."
4. Advance the cannula into the peritoneal cavity and withdraw the needle back over the cannula. *Do not* withdraw the cannula over the needle.
5. Attach a 20-ml syringe to the cannula and aspirate the peritoneal fluid. Obtain sufficient fluid for a cell count; Gram stain; culture; protein, glucose, amylase, and cytology examination; and cell block.
6. Remove the cannula and apply a sterile absorbent dressing.

POSTPROCEDURE CARE

1. Observe the patient for fever, signs of peritonitis, and other complications. The patient may be mobilized as much as tolerated.
2. If a drainage catheter is left in place, the dressing should be removed, inspected, and replaced daily. Since the risk of infection rises rapidly after 48 hours, the catheter should be removed after this length of time. Prior to removing an indwelling catheter, it is advisable to obtain a specimen for culture.

COMPLICATIONS

1. Bleeding from the puncture site. Bleeding from the puncture site is usually caused by laceration of the epigastric vessels. It almost always stops spontaneously and very rarely requires blood transfusion. It can be avoided by puncturing the abdominal wall in the midline or lateral to the rectus sheath (Fig. 23-1).
2. Bowel perforation. Iatrogenic bowel perforation is most likely to occur in the presence of an ileus or when a loop of bowel adheres to the anterior peritoneum. It should be considered when feculent, malodorous, or cloudy material is recovered from the lavage fluid. When bowel perforation is suspected, obtain a surgical consultation and observe the patient for signs of peritonitis. To lessen the risk of this complication, avoid inserting the catheter through surgical scars and do not advance the stylet once the peritoneal cavity has been entered.
3. Intraabdominal hemorrhage. Intraabdominal hemorrhage is due to laceration of a major omental or mesenteric vessel. It can be serious and require blood transfusion. When suspected, obtain a surgical consultation and observe the patient for signs of hypovolemia. To avoid this complication, the stylet should not be plunged too deeply, nor should it be advanced once the peritoneal cavity has been entered.
4. Peritonitis. Peritonitis may be caused by bowel perforation, intraperitoneal bleeding, or wound contamination

(especially when a drainage catheter is left in the abdominal cavity). It is usually first recognized when the peritoneal fluid becomes cloudy and the white blood cell count exceeds 300 to 500 per cubic millimeter. Typical signs of peritoneal irritation and fever may not occur early in the course. Early recognition and treatment of this problem is imperative to prevent local abscess formation, septicemia, and formation of adhesions. Antibiotic selection should be based on the interpretation of a Gram stain of peritoneal fluid. If no organisms are seen in the Gram stain, the patient should be treated for both *Staphylococcus aureus* and gram-negative bacilli with antibiotics, such as vancomycin or cephalosporin, and an aminoglycoside.

5. Perforation of the bladder. This may occur when the puncture site is too close to the symphysis pubis or the bladder is full at the time of catheter insertion.

6. Pneumoperitoneum. Pneumoperitoneum occurs when air is introduced through the catheter. It causes no complications but makes interpretation of roentgenograms difficult.

REFERENCES

1. Boyer, J.L. et al: Effect of plasma-volume expansion on portal hypertension, N. Engl. J. Med. **275:**750-755, 1966.
2. Ceelen, G.H.: The cytologic diagnosis of ascitic fluid, Acta. Cytol. **8:**175-185, 1974.
3. Engrav, I.H., et al.: Diagnostic peritoneal lavage in blunt abdominal trauma, J. Traumatol. **15:**854-859, 1975.
4. McCay, J., and Wolma, F.J.: Abdominal tap, Am. J. Surg. **122:**693-695, 1971.
5. McPartin, J.F. and McCarthy, W.: An appraisal of diagnostic paracentesis of the abdomen, Br. J. Surg. **58:**498-501, 1971.
6. Sachatello, C.R., and Bivens, B.: Technic for peritoneal dialysis and diagnostic peritoneal lavage, Am. J. Surg. **131:**637-640, 1976.

CHAPTER 24

Liver biopsy

■ William Cunningham
Paul M. Suratt
Robert S. Gibson

■ GENERAL CONSIDERATIONS

Percutaneous liver biopsy is a method of obtaining a small section of liver tissue. Its speed and simplicity allow its use at the bedside in alert patients. Although the procedure is generally performed on hospitalized patients, there is evidence that it might be done safely on ambulatory patients.[5] Since many liver diseases can have a patchy distribution, a blind percutaneous biopsy may miss the diseased area. The yield of diseased tissue is higher in patients who have hepatomegaly, deranged liver function tests, and significant elevation of liver enzymes. Patients who appear at high risk for complications from the procedure may be candidates for other methods, such as laparoscopy, transjugular biopsy, "minilaparotomy," and laparotomy.[2]

■ INDICATIONS[3]

1. Unexplained hepatomegaly, liver dysfunction, or injury.
2. Assessment of liver involvement in certain systemic disorders, including cancer,[4] unexplained fever,[9] and metabolic diseases.
3. Monitoring toxic or beneficial effects of therapy.
4. Clinical research.

■ CONTRAINDICATIONS[3]

1. Uncooperative patient.
2. Inability to percuss hepatic dullness.
3. Bleeding diathesis.
4. Infection lying in the path of needle.

5. Ascites.
6. Severe extrahepatic obstruction.
7. Severe anemia.

The last three are strictly relative.[10] Conn[2] gives thoughtful consideration to this subject.

PATIENT EVALUATION AND PREPARATION

1. Obtain a chest roentgenograph.
2. Obtain hematocrit values, prothrombin time, partial thromboplastin time, and a platelet count.
3. Nothing should be given by mouth 6 hours prior to the procedure.
4. Explain the procedure and its potential complications to the patient and obtain written informed consent.

PERSONNEL AND EQUIPMENT

1. A physician trained in liver biopsy and an assistant familiar with the equipment.
2. Principal implements: a Menghini needle, a number 11 blade with handle, a 30-ml glass syringe, filter paper, and 10 ml of sterile saline.
3. An antiseptic solution and a cup to hold it, sterile gloves, 4 × 4 inch gauze pads, sterile towels, and an adhesive bandage.
4. Lidocaine, 2%, 10 ml, 5-ml glass syringe, and needles (25 gauge, ¾ inch; 21 gauge, 1½ inches).
5. Specimen containers: 10% formalin and culture tubes as appropriate.

TECHNIQUE[3,7]

1. Place the patient in a supine position with the right hand under the head.
2. Mark the site of the biopsy, unless *situs inversus,* right midaxillary line, one to one and a half interspaces below the superior margin of maximum hepatic dullness after a full expiration.
3. Put on sterile gloves, prepare the skin with antiseptic, and form a sterile field with draping towels.

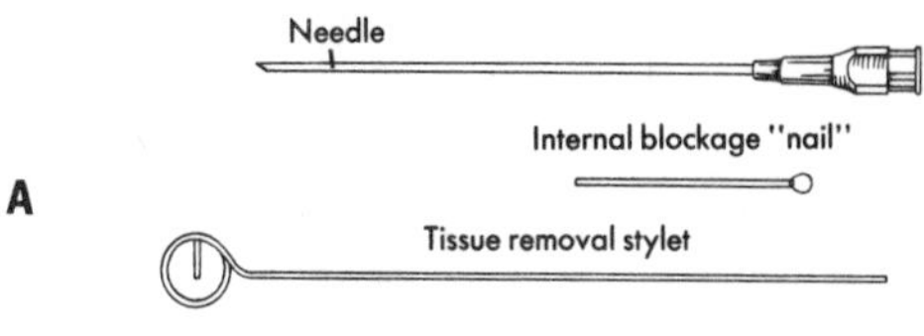

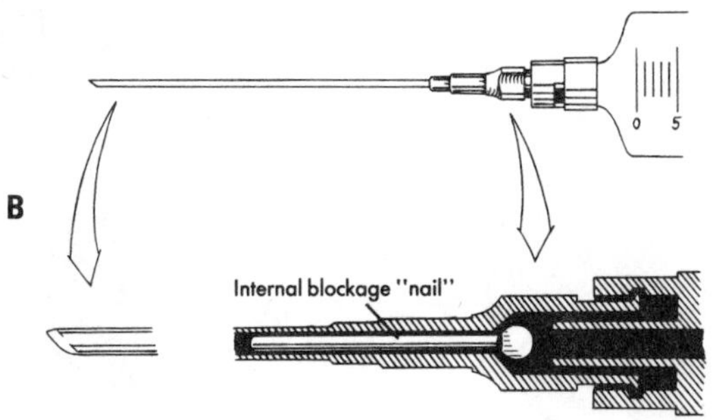

FIG. 24-1. Menghini liver biopsy needle. A, Unassembled, tissue-removal stylet is rarely used. **B,** Assembled and attached to syringe. Internal blockage "nail" prevents tissue specimen from being drawn up into syringe and fragmented.

4. Assemble the needle (Fig. 24-1).
5. Have the patient practice blowing out all air and holding his breath for 10 to 15 seconds.
6. Anesthetize the skin and the anticipated needle track down to Glisson's capsule.
7. Incise the skin 2 or 3 mm to allow needle insertion. Blot the wound every 30 seconds with a gauze pad and time the duration of bleeding. If bleeding continues for more than 6 minutes, the biopsy should probably not be performed.
8. Fill the 30-ml syringe with about 6 ml of sterile saline; then attach the biopsy needle and flush out about 1 ml of saline to check the patency of the needle.
9. Insert the Menghini needle at a right angle to the skin into intercostal tissue to a depth of 4 or 5 mm (Fig.

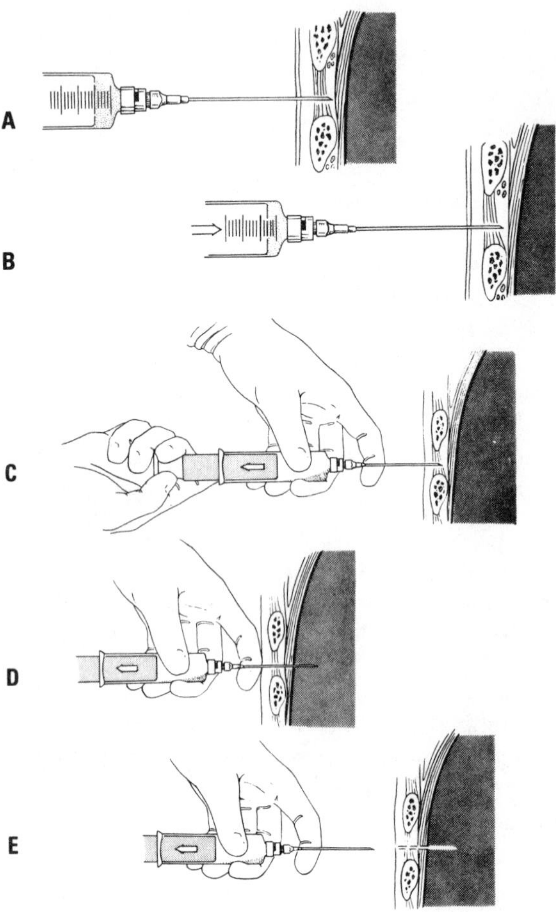

FIG. 24-2. Liver biopsy technique. A, Needle inserted through skin 4 to 5 mm into subcutaneous tissue. **B,** Expel tissue fragments from needle by injecting 2 ml of saline. **C,** Place left index finger against needle as "stop" 4 or 5 cm from the needle tip in normal-sized individual. Pull back on plunger to about 15-ml line to create vacuum. **D,** Quickly but smoothly advance needle into liver to depth of your left index finger and then withdraw it. This entire phase should last only brief fraction of a second. **E,** Needle withdrawn from patient.

24-2, *A*). Clear the needle by injecting 2 ml of saline (Fig. 24-2, *B*).

10. Instruct the patient to exhale all air and hold his breath.
11. Pull back the plunger to about the 15-ml line to create a vacuum in the syringe (Fig. 24-2, *C*) and quickly (about 0.1 second) pass the needle in (Fig. 24-2, *D*) and out (Fig. 24-2, *E*) of the liver.[8] Withdraw the needle.
12. Place the biopsy specimen on a piece of filter paper by pushing on the syringe plunger. If no tissue is expelled, remove the needle from the syringe and insert the tissue-removal stylet into the cutting tip of the needle and gently express the tissue out the other end of the needle. Portions for culture should be cut off with the knife and placed with their underlying filter paper in sterile culture tubes; a few drops of sterile saline are used to prevent desiccation if there is no medium. The remainder is left on a piece of filter paper and placed in 10% formalin for light microscopic studies.

POSTPROCEDURE CARE

1. Position the patient in the right lateral decubitus position for 1 hour.
2. Restrict the patient to bed for 24 hours.
3. Obtain a blood pressure, pulse, and respiratory rate every 15 minutes for 2 hours; if stable, check these signs every 30 minutes for 2 hours. If stable, check the vital signs every hour for 4 hours. Vital signs may then be obtained every 4 hours thereafter if stable.
4. Obtain a hematocrit value the following day.

COMPLICATIONS

1. Pain over the puncture site or in the shoulder is moderate or severe in 5%.[11]
2. Clinically significant hemorrhage, 0.5%[5]; 7% have evidence of intrahepatic hematoma.[14] Significant bleeding is usually intraperitoneal, but may appear as hemobilia.[1]

3. Hypotension, 2%.[5]
4. Arteriovenous fistula of liver, 5.4%[13].
5. Septicemia.[6]
6. Bile peritonitis, 0.1%.[15]
7. Pneumothorax.[3]
8. Penetration and injury to the adjacent organs.[3]
9. Drug reaction.[3]
10. Menghini needle fracture within the liver.[12]
11. Death, 0.2%.[8]

REFERENCES

1. Ball, T.J. et al.: Hemobilia following percutaneous liver biopsy, Gastroenterology **68:**1297-1299, 1975.
2. Conn, H.: Liver biopsy in extrahepatic biliary obstruction and in other contraindicated disorders, Gastroenterology **68:**817-821, 1975.
3. Edmondson, H., and Schiff, L.: Needle biopsy of the liver. In Schiff, L., editor: Diseases of the liver, ed. 4, Philadelphia 1975, J.B. Lippincott Co.
4. Grossman, E. et al.: Cytological examination as an adjunct to liver biopsy in the diagnosis of hepatic metastases, Gastroenterology **62:**56-60, 1972.
5. Knauer, C.M.: Percutaneous biopsy of the liver as a procedure for outpatients, Gastroenterology **74:**101-102, 1978.
6. LoIudice, T. et al.: Septicemia as a complication of percutaneous liver biopsy, Gastroenterology **72:**949-951, 1977.
7. Menghini, G.: One second needle biopsy of the liver, Gastroenterology **35:**190-199, 1958.
8. Menghini, G.: One second biopsy of the liver-problems of its clinical application, N. Engl. J. Med. **283:**582-585, 1970.
9. Mitchell, D.P. et al.: Fever of unknown origin: assessment of the value of percutaneous liver biopsy, Arch. Int. Med. **137:**1001-1004, 1977.
10. Morris, J.S. et al.: Percutaneous liver biopsy in patients with large bile duct obstruction, Gastroenterology **68:**750-754, 1975.
11. Perrault, J. et al.: Liver biopsy: complications in 1000 inpatients and outpatients, Gastroenterology **74:**103-106, 1978.
12. Purow, E., Grosberg, S., and Wapnick, S.: Menghini needle fracture after attempted liver biopsy, Gastroenterology **73:**1404-1405, 1977.
13. Okuda, K. et al.: Frequency of intrahepatic arteriovenous fistula as a sequela to percutaneous needle puncture of the liver, Gastroenterology **74:**1204-1207, 1978.
14. Raines, D., Van Heertum, R., and Johnson, L.: Intrahepatic hematoma: a complication of percutaneous liver biopsy, Gastroenterology **67:**284-289, 1974.
15. Terry, R.: Risks of needle biopsy of the liver, Br. Med. J. **1:**1102-1105, 1952.

PART SIX

GENITOURINARY PROCEDURES

CHAPTER 25

Urethral catheterization

■ Arthur W. Wyker, Jr.

■ GENERAL CONSIDERATIONS

A urethral catheter may be passed into the bladder for diagnostic or therapeutic purposes. For single, in-out catheterization, blunt-nosed catheters are preferred. If the catheter is indwelling, use a self-retaining Foley catheter.

Insertion of a Foley catheter into the bladder is the simplest and most direct way of providing continuous urinary drainage when there is anatomic or physiologic urinary obstruction of the lower urinary tract. By keeping the bladder empty and the intravesical pressure low, catheter drainage may reverse back-pressure effects on the upper urinary tract and allow overdistended bladder muscle to regain its tone and contractile power.

■ INDICATIONS

1. Inability of the patient to empty the bladder or frank urinary retention. This indication should be based on the physical findings of a distended bladder and not on the lack of urine output over a specified period of time. The empty or near-empty bladder is neither palpable nor percussible because of its anatomic location in the pelvis. When it contains about 125 ml of urine, it rises out of the pelvis into the lower abdomen and projects one finger breadth above the pubis. With further filling, it rises progressively toward the umbilicus. When percussing a distended bladder, the normally resonant note is replaced by dullness and the induced rise in intravesicle pressure often causes the patient to experience a desire to void.

2. To provide a dry environment for severely obtunded or comatose patients.
3. To control urinary incontinence.
4. To monitor urine output in patients with shock, major trauma, severe burns, or those undergoing long or complicated operations.
5. Diagnostic purposes: to obtain urine for culture or special laboratory studies, for cystourethrograms, cystometrograms, urodynamic studies, and determination of residual urine after voiding.
6. To facilitate healing following surgery or injury to the lower urinary tract.

▪ ABSOLUTE CONTRAINDICATIONS

An anatomic abnormality of the urethra that prevents passage of a catheter is considered to be an absolute contraindication.

▪ RELATIVE CONTRAINDICATIONS

The risk of passing a urethral catheter must be weighed against the potential benefit achieved via improved urinary drainage or by more accurate information about the status of the urinary tract.

1. Urinary tract infection, especially urethritis in males.
2. An immunocompromised host.
3. Diabetes mellitus.

▪ PATIENT EVALUATION AND PREPARATION

1. Urinalysis and urine culture, if feasible.
2. Explain to the patient the reason for and the nature of the procedure.

▪ PERSONNEL AND EQUIPMENT

1. An individual familiar with the proper technique of urethral catheterization.
2. Principal implements: a fenestrated drape, lots of lubricant, sterile containers, sterile gloves, and the appropriate catheter.

a. For in-out catheterization: a number 14 or 16 French blunt-nose catheter.
b. For indwelling catheterization: a number 18 or 20 French Foley catheter with a 10-ml syringe of sterile water to inflate the balloon and a drainage bag and tubing.

3. An antiseptic solution and cup to hold it, 4 × 4 inch gauze sponges.
4. An antibacterial solution, such as 0.1% neomycin, 30 ml.

■ TECHNIQUE IN MALES

1. The patient should be supine with the legs slightly apart.
2. Saturate the gauze sponges with antiseptic solution and thoroughly wash the penis, especially the glans and urethral meatus. If the patient is uncircumcised, gently retract the foreskin before starting the preparation.
3. Put on sterile gloves and place the fenestrated drape over the genitalia so that the penis is exposed.
4. If a Foley catheter is being inserted, inject sterile water into the balloon to make sure it is functioning properly.
5. Lubricate the catheter liberally from end to end, since this greatly facilitates its passage and reduces frictional irritation of the sensitive urethral mucosa.
6. Hold the penis on stretch at right angles to the body and pass the well-lubricated catheter slowly and gently (Fig. 25-1). Avoid quick and jerky movements.
7. Resistance is usually encountered when the catheter reaches the external urinary sphincter (Fig. 25-1). By applying gentle, steady pressure the sphincter will relax and allow the catheter to pass. Do not repeatedly jab the catheter against the urinary sphincter, since this may cause pain and sphincter spasm. In some men with urinary retention due to benign prostatic hyperplasia (BPH), the entrance into the bladder is displaced anteriorly by an enlarged median lobe so that standard

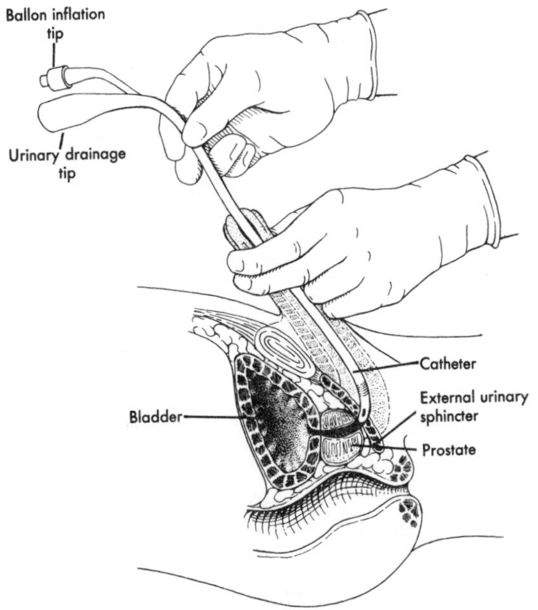

FIG. 25-1. Passing the catheter.

catheters may hang up in the prostatic urethra. If this occurs, do not use a smaller size catheter; use a larger one, such as a number 24 French Foley, or one with an angled tip (Coudé). These catheters will easily ride over the projecting lobe of the prostate into the bladder. If the catheter still cannot be passed, ask for assistance from a urologist.

8. The catheter is in the bladder when urine flows through it. If urine does not flow but 25 to 50 ml of sterile saline flushed through the catheter returns freely, the catheter is in the bladder.

9. If an indwelling Foley catheter has been inserted, fill the balloon with 5 ml of sterile water and connect the catheter to a sterile closed drainage system (Fig. 25-2). Tape it to the anterior thigh, allowing some redundancy so that movement of the legs will not pull on the catheter. If long-term drainage is planned (more than a few

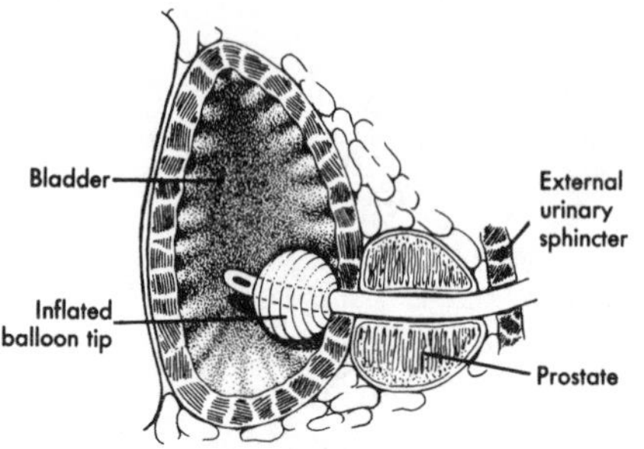

FIG. 25-2. Inflated balloon catheter in bladder.

days), tape the catheter to the abdomen to prevent catheter damage to the knuckled urethra at the penoscrotal junction.

10. After single in-out catheterization, 30 ml of an antibacterial solution, such as 0.1% neomycin solution, may be left in the bladder to prevent infection.
11. Obtain a urine culture just prior to removal of an indwelling catheter.

■ TECHNIQUE IN FEMALES

1. The patient should be supine with the legs slightly apart.
2. Saturate gauze sponges with antiseptic solution and thoroughly wash the vulva, especially the inside of the labia and the area around the urethral meatus.
3. Put on sterile gloves and place the fenestrated drape in such a fashion that the vaginal introitus and urethral meatus are exposed.
4. If a Foley catheter is being inserted, inject sterile water into the balloon to make sure it is functioning properly.
5. Lubricate the tip and distal 3 or 4 inches (7.5 to 10 cm) of the catheter.
6. Separate the labia with the thumb and index finger and pass the well-lubricated catheter gently into the urethral meatus. It usually encounters no significant resistance, entering the bladder easily. If the catheter is inadvertently passed into the vagina, discard it and try again

with a fresh sterile catheter. If you have difficulty locating the urethral meatus, place the patient in the lithotomy position, focus a bright light on the external genitalia, and have an assistant retract one labium while you retract the other.

7. Return of urine through the catheter or free flow of sterile saline washed through the catheter confirms its position in the bladder.
8. If an indwelling Foley catheter has been inserted, fill the balloon with sterile water and connect the catheter to a sterile closed drainage system. Tape it to the anterior thigh, allowing some redundancy so that movement of the legs will not tend to pull on the catheter.

POSTPROCEDURE CARE

Write appropriate orders for catheter management.

COMPLICATIONS

1. Infection is the most common and most significant complication.
   a. After single catheterization, 1% to 2% of normal adults develop a urinary tract infection.[2] The incidence rises with more susceptible groups—diabetics, the elderly, or the debilitated and those with significant residual urine.
   b. Indwelling catheters are associated with a greater frequency of infections than single catheterizations. Of patients on catheter drainage for 2 to 7 days, 8% to 10% had significant bacteriuria when the catheter was removed, but only 0.7% experienced subsequent clinical infections.[1]
   c. The catheter is the leading cause of nosocomial-induced urinary tract infections and the most common predisposing factor in fatal gram-negative sepsis in hospitals.[2]
   d. Longstanding indwelling catheters in males may obstruct the ducts draining into the urethra with resultant urethritis, prostatitis, or epididymitis.

2. Hematuria. Hematuria is infrequent and usually mild and transient.
3. Painful urination. Painful urination is usually present one or two times following single in-out catheterization.
4. Catheterization may precipitate urinary retention in male patients with BPH. Catheters cause edema of the urethral mucosa, and this may aggravate preexisting lower urinary tract obstruction with resultant urinary retention.

REFERENCES

1. Guinan, P.D., Bayley, B.C., Metzger, W.I., Shoemaker, W.C., and Bush, I.M.: The case against "The case against the catheter": initial report, J. Urol. **101**:909-913, 1969.
2. Kunin, C.M.: Care of the urinary catheter. In Detection, prevention, and management of urinary tract infections, ed. 3, Philadelphia, 1979, Lea & Febiger.

CHAPTER 26

Peritoneal dialysis

■ Nuzhet O. Atuk

■ GENERAL CONSIDERATIONS

Peritoneal dialysis is a method of removing specific toxins and fluid from the blood.[1,2] It is accomplished by introducing dialysis fluid into the peritoneal cavity. Substances that can diffuse across the peritoneal membrane will enter the fluid, which can then be removed. The procedure can be performed at the bedside, using simple equipment.

■ GENERAL INDICATIONS FOR DIALYSIS

1. Acute or chronic renal failure.
2. Fluid overload.
3. Endogenous intoxication (hyperkalemia, hypermagnesemia, hyperuricemia, or hypercalcemia) that cannot be corrected by other therapy.
4. Specific exogenous intoxications.[6]

■ INDICATIONS FOR PERITONEAL DIALYSIS

Peritoneal dialysis should be performed when the following conditions and those previously listed are present:

1. Hypotension.
2. Active bleeding.
3. When anticoagulation (required for hemodialysis) would be exceptionally hazardous.
4. Infants or elderly patients.
5. Difficulty in achieving or maintaining vascular access; while awaiting maturation of an atrial or ventricular fistula or healing of a bovine or Gore-tex graft.[4]
6. Peritonitis complicating renal failure and intraperitoneal antibiotic therapy is desired.
7. Possibly in patients with acute pancreatitis.
8. Hemodialysis is not available.

■ CONTRAINDICATIONS

There are no absolute contraindications to peritoneal dialysis. However, hemodialysis is preferred in the following situations:

1. Pregnancy.
2. Severe uremia in patients with a high catabolic rate.
3. Severe electrolyte and acid-base disturbances requiring rapid correction.
4. Poisonings known or presumed to benefit by dialysis, when hemodialysis is preferable.
5. Disorders compromising the efficiency of peritoneal dialysis, such as heat stress, vasculitis, scleroderma, and aortic aneurysm.
6. Respiratory failure in a patient who is not receiving ventilation therapy.[3]

■ PATIENT EVALUATION AND PREPARATION

1. Question and examine the patient regarding previous abdominal surgery, hernia, organomegaly (liver, spleen, bladder, polycystic kidneys), bowel distention, and ileus and bowel tumors. If any of these are present, the catheter should be placed surgically using direct visualization.[4]
2. Explain the procedure and its potential complications to the patient and obtain written permission.
3. Usually sedation is not needed unless the patient is excessively apprehensive or agitated. In that case, 50 mg of meperidine can be given before the procedure.

■ PERSONNEL AND EQUIPMENT

1. A physician trained in peritoneal dialysis and a nurse trained in dialysis procedure and familiar with the equipment and solutions.
2. Principal implements: a catheter (Trocath), a peritoneal dialysis stylet, a catheter with connecting tube, surgical scissors, a small (mosquito) hemostat, and a long 15-gauge spinal needle blade with holder.
3. An antiseptic solution with a cup to hold it, sterile gloves

and gowns, hair caps, 4 × 4 inch gauze pads, and draping towels.

4. Lidocaine, 1% 10 ml, a 10-ml syringe, and needles (25 gauge, ¾ inch; 21 gauge, 1½ inches).
5. Dialysis solutions and an administration set, potassium chloride and acetate as needed, tincture of benzoin, and tape.

TECHNIQUE FOR CATHETER INSERTION

1. Place the patient on his back and empty the bladder with a catheter.
2. Select a puncture site in the midline of the abdomen one third of the distance from the umbilicus to the pubis (Fig. 26-1).
3. Put on a cap, gown, mask, and gloves. The patient should also wear a mask.
4. Disinfect the skin and drape with sterile towels.
5. Anesthetize the skin and tissues down to and including the peritoneum.
6. Make a 3-mm incision in the skin at the needle puncture site with a scalpel tip.
7. Place the stylet into the catheter until the pointed tip is exposed.

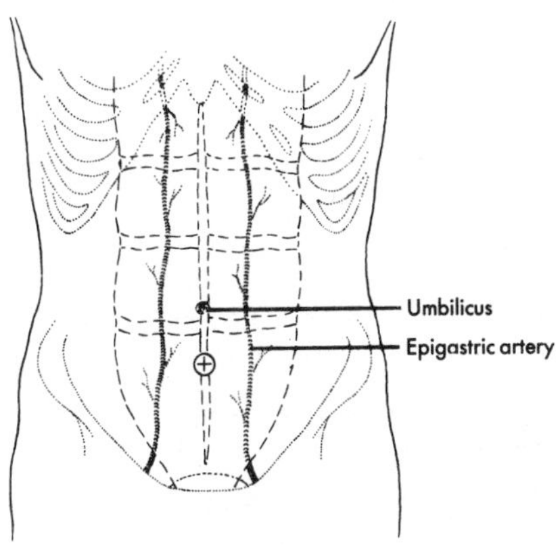

FIG. 26-1. Site of trocar placement.

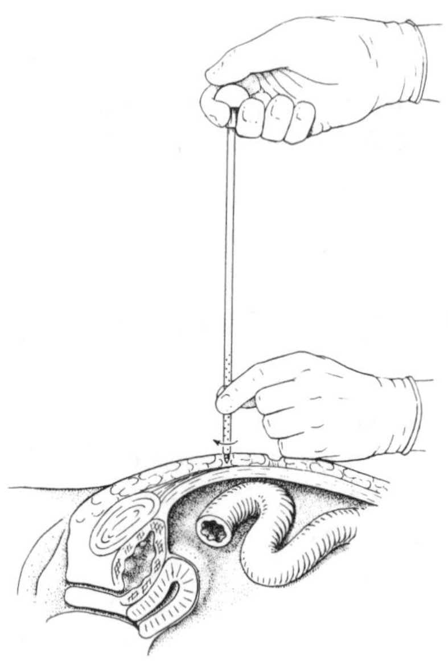

FIG. 26-2. Insert trocar into peritoneum with twisting motion.

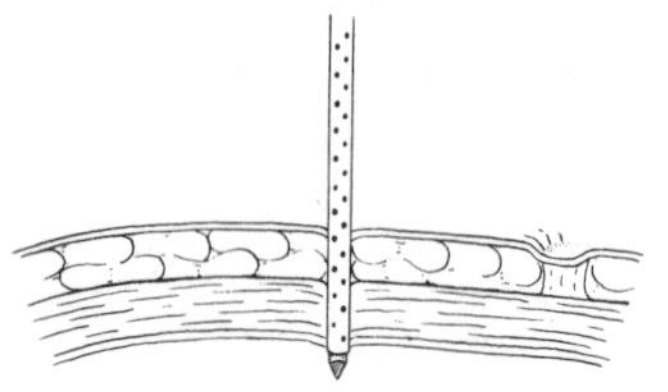

FIG. 26-3. Trocar inserted into peritoneum.

8. Hold the Trocath vertically and insert it into the peritoneal cavity with a twisting motion, using forceful restraint (Figs. 26-2 and 26-3). Entry through the peritoneum is indicated by a "pop."
9. Withdraw the inner stylet several centimeters, so that its sharp point is no longer protruding out of the catheter. Grasp the catheter with your thumb and index finger, advance it toward the right or left pelvic fossa with

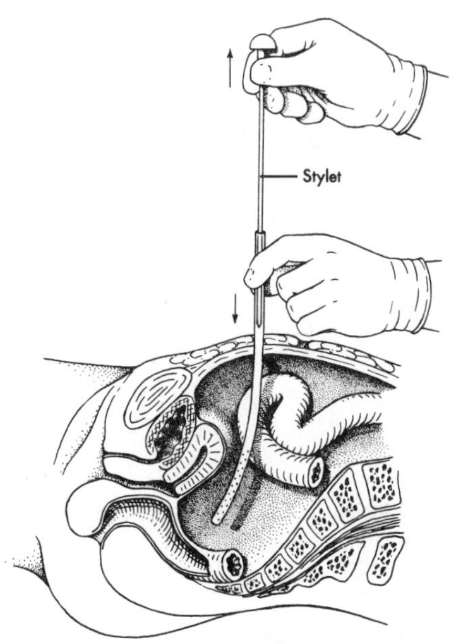

FIG. 26-4. Advance catheter over trocar into iliac fossa.

the curve directed anteriorly (Fig. 26-4). Remove the inner stylet from the catheter when the catheter is properly placed.

10. Attach the elbow of the connecting tube to the proximal end of the catheter and to the administration set. Run 1 L of warmed dialysate into the abdomen rapidly. After establishing that drainage is satisfactory, disconnect the connecting tube from the catheter. Place the catheter clip over the end of the catheter and slide it into place against the skin. Trim the catheter to within 5 cm of the skin (do not cover an excessively long catheter with a paper cup or other device) (Fig. 26-5).

11. Secure the clip with several pieces of paper tape. Attach the catheter to the connecting tube once again and proceed with dialysis. Place 4 × 4 pads around the catheter and tape it securely in place, fixing the connecting tube to the skin with tape to prevent dislodgment.

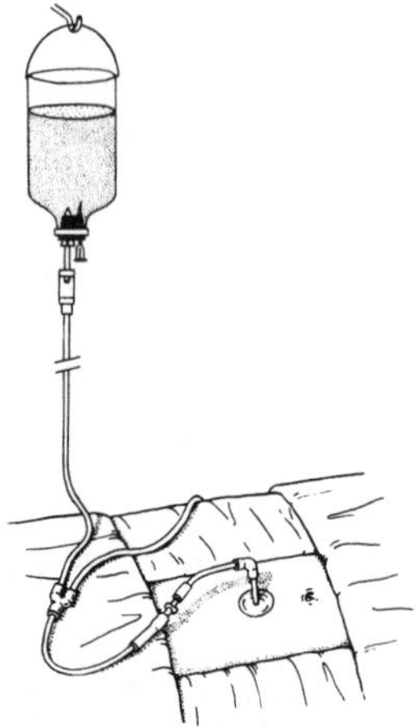

FIG. 26-5. Catheter attached to elbow connector, which is in turn connected to dialysate bottle and drainage catheter.

■ TECHNIQUE FOR DIALYSIS

1. We prefer using the American Medical Products Cycler, since it provides virtually closed circuits, thus reducing the risk of infection and the amount of nursing time. Manual peritoneal dialysis (individual bottles of dialysate for each exchange) offers more opportunity for contamination and requires almost constant nursing attention. Manual dialysis requires simpler equipment and is more widely available though.
2. Standard dialysate contains either 1.5% or 4.25% glucose. The former promotes relatively little, if any, osmotic fluid removal. The more concentrated solution is used when maximum fluid removal is needed. One may blend the two, depending on each patient's needs and responses.[5] A hyperglycemic hyperosmolar syndrome may develop with the repeated use of concentrated solutions. Heparin, 250 units/L, should be added to the dialysis solution. Potassium chloride, 3 or 4 mEq/L, may also be added, depending on the serum potassium concentration. Potassium acetate may be substituted to provide additional bicarbonate in severely acidotic patients.

When the serum potassium is higher than 6 mEq/L or the ECG shows signs of hyperkalemia, no potassium should be added. In patients receiving digitalis who have normal serum potassium levels, dialysis fluid should contain 4 mEq/L of potassium to prevent cardiac arrhythmias.

3. Dialysis effectiveness approaches maximal at a dialysate flow of 4 L per hour. For noncatabolic individuals 2 L per hour often suffices. Most adults will tolerate 2-L exchanges, but some tolerate only 1 L or less.
4. For any desired exchange rate, the greatest efficiency is achieved with brief inflow and outflow times yet long dwell times.
5. Routine daily cultures are an admission of poor technique and are expensive. Daily effluent microscopic examination in the event of abdominal symptoms or fever will guide sound culture policy.
6. Short (15 to 18 hours), frequent (every 2 or 3 days) dialyses are preferable to prolonged (72 hours or more) runs at infrequent intervals.

■ TROCATH CATHETER REMOVAL

At the completion of dialysis, the Trocath is removed from the peritoneal cavity, and the skin opening is closed with butterfly tape. The fluid at the tip of the catheter is cultured for contamination.

■ POSTPROCEDURE CARE

Observe the patient for fever, peritonitis, and complications. The patient may be mobilized as much as tolerated.

■ COMPLICATIONS

1. Bowel perforation. Return of feculent, malodorous or cloudy material in the dialysate suggests bowel perforation. If this occurs, obtain surgical consultation and observe the patient closely for signs of peritonitis. Abdominal exploration and removal of the dialysis catheter are rarely necessary though.

2. Peritonitis. The frequency of this complication varies between 1% and 12%. It is usually first recognized when the dialysate becomes cloudy and the white blood cell count exceeds 300 per cubic millimeter. Typical signs of peritoneal irritation and fever may not occur early in the course of the infection. Early recognition and treatment of this problem are imperative to prevent local abscess formation, septicemia, adhesion formation, and excessive protein losses. To treat preexisting or dialysis-related peritonitis use both intraperitoneal and systemic antibiotics and continue dialysis. Antibiotic selection should be based on the interpretation of a Gram stain of peritoneal fluid. If no organisms are seen in the Gram stain, the patient should be treated for both *Staphylococcus aureus* and gram-negative bacilli with either vancomycin or cephalosporin and an aminoglycoside. If the patient is not seriously ill, a cephalosporin antibiotic alone may suffice.
3. Intraabdominal hemorrhage. Laceration of major abdominal vessels is rare; most bleeding is associated with peritoneal catheter placement in the abdominal wall or skin vessels. The hemorrhage almost invariably stops spontaneously and rarely is severe enough to require blood transfusions.
4. Fluid leakage. Fuid leakage can occur both into and out of the peritoneal cavity and can thus be a source of infection.
5. Inadequate drainage of dialysate. Inadequate drainage of dialysate can lead to abdominal distension and fluid gain.
6. Seizures. Hypoglycemia and severe hypertension may be associated with seizures.
7. Pain.

REFERENCES

1. Boen, S.T.: Peritoneal dialysis in clinical medicine, Springfield, Ill., 1964, Charles C Thomas, Publisher.
2. Boen, S.T.: Overview and history of peritoneal dialysis, Dialysis Transplant. **6:**12-18, 46-48, 1977.

3. Odriozola, J., Bahlmann, J., and Fabel, H.: Effect of peritoneal dialysis on pulmonary function, Klin. Wochenschr. **49:**484-488, 1971.
4. Tenckhoff, H.: Chronic peritoneal dialysis—a manual for patients and dialysis personnel, Seattle, 1974, University of Washington.
5. Vidt, D.G.: Recommendations on choice of peritoneal dialysis solutions, Ann. Intern. Med. **78:**144-146, 1973.
6. Winchester, J.F., Gelfraud, M.C., Knepshield, J.H., and Schreiner, G.E.: Transactions, American Society for Artificial Organs **23:**762-842, 1977.

PART SEVEN

HEMATOLOGIC PROCEDURE

CHAPTER 27

Bone marrow aspiration and biopsy

■ Richard P. Keeling

■ GENERAL CONSIDERATIONS

Bone marrow aspiration is a technique of obtaining semisolid bone marrow tissue for histologic and histochemical examination to assist in diagnosis of disease of the blood-forming system.[5,7] Marrow aspirates can also be cultured for bacteria and fungi and used for chromosome studies. In adults, the preferred site for marrow aspiration is the posterior iliac crest; aspiration of sternal marrow is seldom indicated because of a greater risk of complications. For patients in whom the posterior iliac crest in unsuitable (because of inaccessibility or previous radiotherapy), the anterior iliac crest or greater femoral trochanter may be used. In many cases, marrow aspiration and trephine biopsy[2,3,4,6] are done as a combined procedure. Care should always be taken to obtain good specimens and make slides carefully to ensure useful and reliable results.

■ INDICATIONS FOR ILIAC ASPIRATION[5,7]

1. To define the mechanism of anemia when it is not clear from blood studies or to confirm a suspected cause of anemia.
2. To define the mechanism of thrombocytopenia. Bone marrow examination is critical in determining whether thrombocytopenia results from insufficient platelet production (as in myelosuppression) or accelerated platelet destruction (as in immune purpuras).
3. To define the cause of leukopenia or leukocytosis. Marrow aspiration may be required either as an initial diagnostic evaluation (e.g., suspected chronic myelogenous leukemia in a patient with sustained leukocytosis) or in

the management of a patient with a known bone marrow disease (e.g., progressive leukopenia in a patient with disseminated lymphoma). It is also occasionally necessary to aspirate marrow to evaluate leukopenia in patients taking medications with dose-related or idiosyncratic myelosuppressive effects.

4. To define the etiology of dysproteinemias. Marrow plasmacytosis is required in making a diagnosis of multiple myeloma.
5. To establish or clarify diagnosis of acute or chronic leukemias. Even when the diagnosis seems clear from peripheral blood studies, marrow aspiration may provide additional useful data. In cases of acute leukemia, abundant marrow cells provide excellent material for histochemical and immunologic studies, leading to clarification of a specific cell type. In chronic myelogenous leukemia, aspiration yields material for chromosome analysis, looking for the characteristic Philadelphia chromosome.
6. To evaluate iron metabolism and storage for deficiency, overload, or abnormality. This is of special importance when serum iron, iron-binding capacity, and ferritin studies are contradictory, unreliable, or unrevealing. It is essential when sideroblastic or "refractory" anemias are being considered.
7. To look for histologic evidence of fungal or parasitic infection. In most cases, this will be combined with marrow cultures for possible fungal disease.
8. To obtain culture material for evaluation of possible tuberculosis, atypical infection with *Mycobacterium* organisms, or fungal disease or in the workup of fever of unknown origin.
9. To obtain material for chromosomal analysis, especially in the investigation of leukemias.
10. As part of the staging evaluation of lymphomas or to assess the extent of disease in solid tumors (aspiration generally combined with biopsy).
11. To assess response to therapy and status of disease in leukemia, lymphoma, or myeloma. Repeated bone mar-

row examinations are vital to the proper management of acute leukemia, because peripheral blood findings are often deceptive. Decisions regarding duration and scheduling of treatment courses depend on assessment of bone marrow response (aspiration generally combined with biopsy).

■ INDICATION FOR STERNAL ASPIRATION

When iliac crest aspiration is impossible or unsuccessful and the need for marrow examination is pressing, sternal aspiration is performed.

■ INDICATIONS FOR BONE MARROW BIOPSY[2,3,4,6]

1. To assess marrow cellularity or evaluate pancytopenia. Assessment of cellularity by aspirate alone is unreliable, because aspiration destroys marrow architecture. Marrow biopsy is necessary in differentiating the various etiologies of pancytopenia, such as fibrosis, myeloid hypoplasia-aplasia, marrow infiltration by foreign cells, marrow necrosis, or peripheral cell destruction. When fibrosis is suspected, a reticulin stain of marrow is important.
2. The inability to obtain material by aspiration ("dry tap") when examination of bone marrow is deemed necessary. "Dry taps" commonly occur when marrow is fibrotic and crowded with young cells, as in some patients with acute leukemia. For technical or other reasons, aspiration occasionally results in a dilute sample; in these cases, biopsy may provide more reliable information.
3. To stage Hodgkin and non-Hodgkin lymphomas (generally done bilaterally). Examination of bone marrow is an important early procedure in staging lymphocytic lymphomas, which commonly involve marrow. Involvement is much less common in histiocytic lymphomas and in Hodgkin disease.
4. To evaluate the extent of disease in the workup of solid tumors. This step is particularly important when leukoerythroblastic peripheral blood exists, since this finding suggests marrow invasion by tumor. Marrow infiltration

can also occur in the absence of peripheral leukoerythroblastosis. Marrow biopsy is commonly employed in staging small cell cancer of the lung and breast cancer.

5. To evaluate possible leukemia or the course and status of treated leukemia. Knowledge of marrow cellularity is vital to treatment decisions.
6. To confirm or augment findings on aspiration in the evaluation of anemia, leukopenia, thrombocytopenia, dysproteinemias, fever of unknown origin, granulomatous disease, or leukoerythroblastosis.
7. To evaluate unexplained splenomegaly. Storage diseases, amyloidosis, and lymphomas are often occult in these cases, and marrow is easily accessible tissue for study. When amyloidosis is suspected, Congo red staining is essential.

■ CONTRAINDICATIONS

1. Skin infection or osteomyelitis in the area of proposed marrow aspiration.
2. Previous radiation therapy in the area of proposed marrow aspiration. Aspiration or biopsy in this situation may yield unreliable material.
3. Lack of good patient cooperation, especially in sternal aspirations.
4. Serious coagulation defects. Thrombocytopenia is not an absolute contraindication, but requires special attention to the wound after the procedure.

■ PATIENT EVALUATION AND PREPARATION

1. Obtain a complete blood count, white cell differential count, and platelet count.
2. Carefully evaluate the patient's ability to cooperate.
3. Carefully examine the proposed marrow aspiration site. Identify all relevant anatomic landmarks and inspect the skin for areas of infection.
4. Explain the procedure, including its potential complications, to the patient and obtain written informed consent.

5. Consider premedication for the anxious or apprehensive patient. Moderate doses of analgesics or minor tranquilizers are helpful in some situations.

PERSONNEL AND EQUIPMENT

1. A physician skilled in bone marrow aspiration and biopsy and one assistant.
2. Principal implements:
   a. For marrow aspiration: a bone marrow aspiration needle (4 cm, 18 gauge), a glass or plastic syringe (2 ml); 5 to 10 sterile microscopic slides (1 × 3 inches; 2.5 × 7.5 cm) and several coverslips (1 × 1 inch; 2.5 × 2.5 cm).
   b. For marrow biopsy: a Jamshidi bone marrow biopsy needle, a number 11 scalpel, a blade and a 10% formalin solution.
3. Sterile culture tubes with screw tops, if required.
4. Cell culture medium, if chromosome studies are desired.
5. Asepsis and a sterile field: an antiseptic solution, sterile sponges, gloves, and a draping towel with a window.
6. Anesthesia: lidocaine, 1%, 10 ml, needles (21 gauge, 1½ inches; 23 gauge, ⅝ inch), and a syringe (12 ml).
7. Dressing: an adhesive bandage, sterile sponges, and adhesive tape (1 inch).

TECHNIQUE FOR ILIAC ASPIRATIONS

1. Place the patient comfortably in a prone or lateral decutus position so that the posterior iliac crest is easily accessible.
2. Identify the posterior iliac crest and select a site for aspiration. Mark the site by indenting the skin with a coin or fingernail if desired (Fig. 27-1).
3. Put on gloves while the assistant opens and prepares the bone marrow tray.
4. Prepare the selected aspiration site with antiseptic solution and drape a sterile field.
5. Anesthetize the skin by raising an intradermal wheal with the 23-gauge needle. Infiltrate the subcutaneous

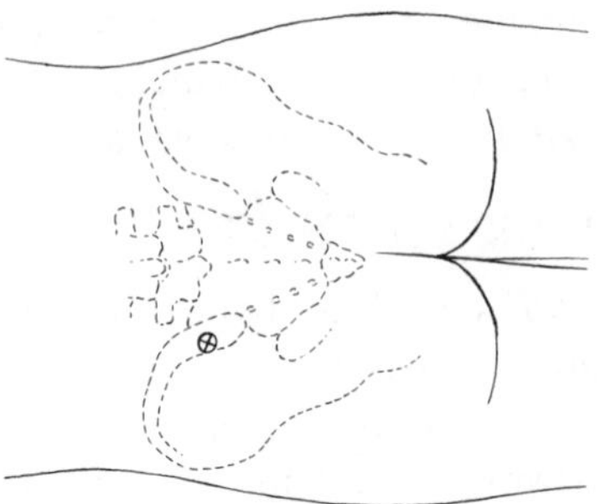

FIG. 27-1. Posterior iliac crest anatomy.

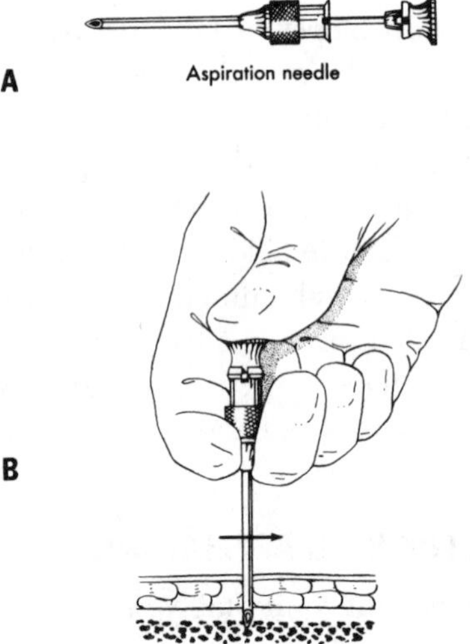

FIG. 27-2. A, Bone marrow aspiration needle. **B,** Insert needle with stylet in place.

tissue and periosteum in four quadrants, using the 21-gauge needle.

6. Insert the bone marrow aspiration needle with stylet in place (Fig. 27-2). Hold the needle perpendicular to the skin. Advance the needle through the skin and subcutaneous tissue to the periosteum. After locating a site on the bone that has been satisfactorily anesthetized, penetrate the periosteum and cortical bone with a steady twisting motion. Entry into the marrow cavity is indicated by a "give."

7. Aspirate the specimen. Remove the stylet from the aspiration needle. Attach a 2-ml syringe to the needle. Gently aspirate not more than 0.2 to 0.4 ml of marrow contents; larger amounts result in dilution of the specimen. If no material is obtained, replace the stylet and advance the aspiration needle carefully another 1 or 2 mm. For repeated failure to obtain material, remove the aspiration needle and try aspiration at a different site. The marrow disruption caused by aspiration will cause a brief, sharp pain; it is advisable to warn the patient of this in advance.
8. Prepare the specimens (Fig. 27-3). Place a single drop of marrow aspirate on each of five or six sterile slides. Make smears by spreading the marrow tissue under the leading edge of another slide and moving this second slide quickly down the longitudinal axis of the underlying slide (Fig. 27-3, *A*). A thin "feather edge" smear should result, and semisolid marrow spicules should be seen distributed in the thin portion of the smear. If few or no spicules are seen, try to isolate them in a larger drop of marrow applied to a slide or coverslip, and smear this material as just directed. A thick smear should be made if iron stain studies are contemplated (Fig. 27-3, *B*). This is done by applying a large drop of spicular marrow aspirate to a slide, dropping a second slide on top of the first (thereby crushing and spreading the aspirate), and then pulling the two slides apart. If chromosome studies are required, the first marrow sample is used, and a second marrow sample is drawn for slides. After slides are made, material for culture can be obtained. Use a fresh sterile syringe. Usually 0.5 to 1 ml of marrow is adequate. Transfer this material immediately to the sterile culture tube(s).
9. Remove the aspiration needle and stylet together with a twisting motion. Apply pressure until bleeding ceases.

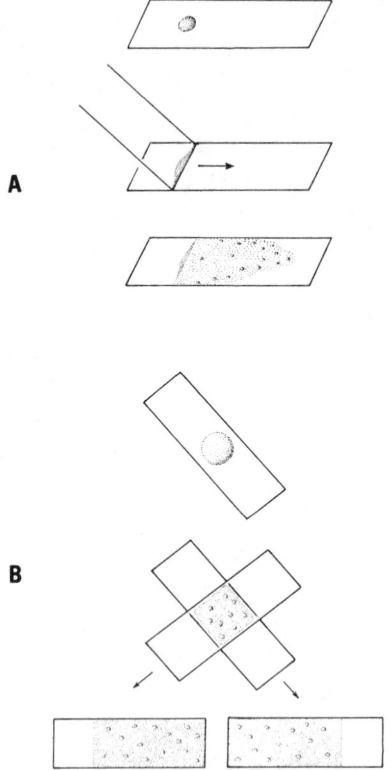

FIG. 27-3. Slide preparation.

10. Apply an adhesive bandage to the puncture site after cleaning off excess antiseptic with an alcohol swab.

■ TECHNIQUE FOR STERNAL ASPIRATION

1. Place the patient comfortably in the supine position.
2. Identify sternal landmarks, including the sternal notch, sternal angle, and intercostal spaces. Select the site for aspiration in the body of the sternum at the level of the second or third intercostal space (never lower) in the midline (Fig. 27-4).
3. Put on gloves, while an assistant opens and prepares the bone marrow tray.
4. Prepare the selected aspiration site with antiseptic solution and drape a sterile field.

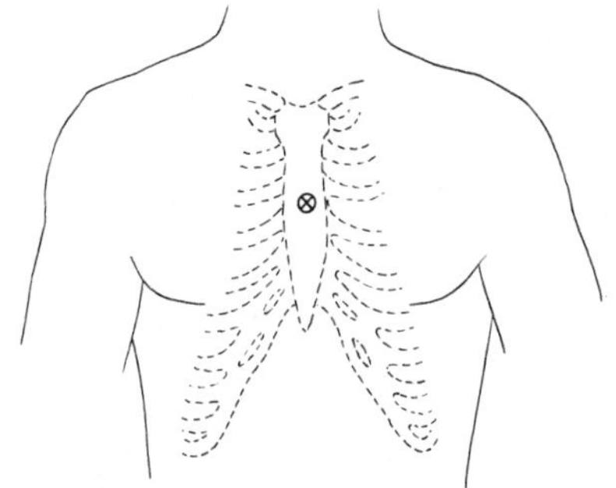

FIG. 27-4. Sternal anatomy.

5. Anesthetize the skin, subcutaneous tissue, and periosteum as described for iliac aspirations.
6. Insert a bone marrow aspiration needle. Hold the needle perpendicular to the skin. Advance the needle through the skin and subcutaneous tissue to the periosteum. After locating a site on the bone with satisfactory anesthesia, carefully penetrate the periosteum and cortical bone using a twisting motion. Steady the needle with two fingers of the other hand to prevent sudden movement. Entry into the marrow cavity is indicated by a "give." Be careful not to penetrate the posterior table of the sternum; some aspirate needles are equipped with an adjustable guard to prevent penetrating too deeply.
7. Aspirate the specimens as described for iliac aspiration. If no material is obtained, it is best to remove the aspiration needle and make another attempt at a different site.
8. Follow steps 8 to 10 of the technique for iliac aspiration.

■ TECHNIQUE FOR BONE MARROW BIOPSY

Bone marrow biopsy is usually performed in the posterior or anterior iliac crest. Sternal biopsy should never be performed because of the risk of hemothorax and cardiac injury. Generally, marrow biopsy will follow aspiration.

1. Place the patient comfortably in a prone or lateral decubitus position so that the posterior iliac crest is easily accessible.

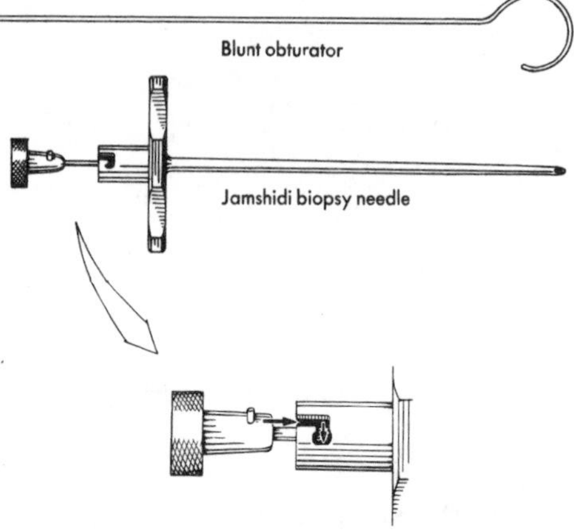

FIG. 27-5. Prepare biopsy needle.

2. Identify landmarks, locating the center of the posterior iliac spine; mark the site by indenting the skin with a coin or fingernail if desired.
3. Put on gloves.
4. Prepare the skin with an antiseptic solution and drape a biopsy site.
5. Anesthetize the skin, subcutaneous tissue, and periosteum.
6. Perform a bone marrow aspiration. (See steps 6 to 8 for iliac aspirations.)
7. It may be necessary to make a 3-mm skin incision with a number 11 scalpel blade through the skin puncture wound made by the aspiration needle to pass the biopsy needle. When aspiration has not been done first, it is always important to make this incision.
8. Prepare the biopsy needle (Fig. 27-5).
9. Insert the biopsy needle (Fig. 27-6). Hold the Jamshidi needle with the obturator in place perpendicular to skin. Advance it through the incision to the periosteum. After testing for adequate anesthesia, penetrate the cortical bone with steady rotating movements. When the

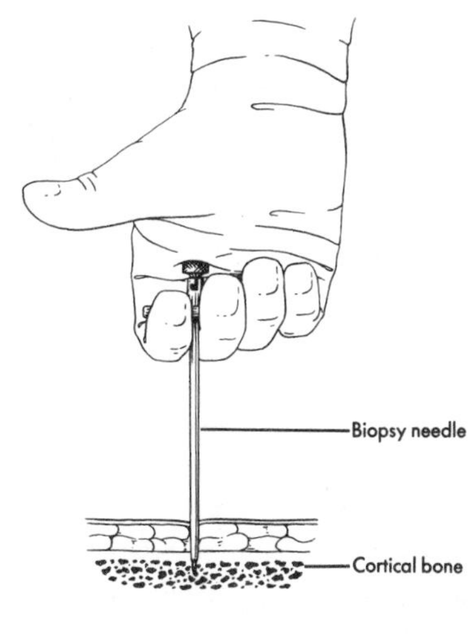

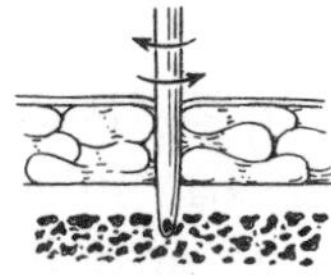

FIG. 27-6. Insert biopsy needle through incision, penetrating cortical bone with steady rotating movement.

needle is firmly lodged in cortical bone, remove the obturator without displacing the needle. Advance the needle an additional 5 to 15 mm with continued rotation. Stop if there is any question of needle tip location. Redirect the needle tip in a new direction and twist the needle in a complete 360-degree circle to break off the biopsy specimen.

10. Remove the biopsy needle with the same rotating motion used to insert it. Apply pressure to the biopsy site to control bleeding.
11. Remove the specimen from the needle (Fig. 27-7). Insert the small-caliber blunt obturator through the distal end of needle. Extrude the specimen through the hub end of the needle onto sterile gauze or a slide.
12. Prepare the specimen. Gently make two or three im-

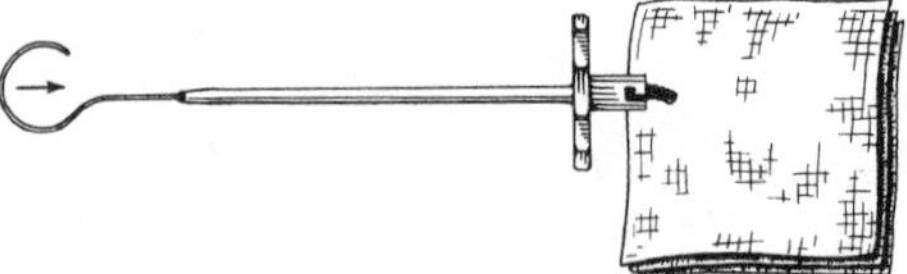

FIG. 27-7. Remove specimen from biopsy needle.

prints of the specimen (touch preparations) on 1 × 3 inches (2.5 × 7.5 cm) glass slides. Overzealous "touching" distorts the architecture. Place the specimen in a 10% formalin solution.

13. Apply a sterile sponge dressing to the puncture site after cleaning off excess antiseptic with alcohol swab.

POSTPROCEDURE CARE

1. In patients with coagulopathies, pressure should be maintained for 5 to 10 minutes after the procedure, and a pressure dressing may be required. In these patients, the wound should be checked several times during the first 24 hours after the procedure.
2. Pain or soreness at the aspiration or biopsy site is usually minor, but may rarely be severe and require analgesics.
3. Following sternal aspiration, patients should be observed for chest pain and changes in vital signs. If there is any question that the inner table of the sternum has been penetrated, patients must be closely observed for hemothorax or pericardial tamponade.

COMPLICATIONS

1. Bleeding from the puncture site. Hematomas may form in patients with thrombocytopenia or coagulopathies.
2. Pain or soreness at the puncture site may rarely be severe and require analgesics.
3. Perforation of the heart or great vessels may occur after sternal aspiration, if the needle traverses the full thickness of the sternum and enters the mediastinum. This can result in severe morbidity or death.[1] Chances of this

complication are increased when the aspiration site is too low on the sternum or when the needle is advanced abruptly, repeatedly, or carelessly.

REFERENCES

1. Bakir. F.: Fatal sternal puncture, Dis. Chest **44:**435-439, 1963.
2. Bearden, J.D., Ratkin, G.A., and Coltman, C.A.: Comparison of the diagnostic value of bone marrow biopsy and bone marrow aspiration in neoplastic disease, J. Clin. Pathol. **27:**738-752, 1974.
3. Brunning, R.D., Bloomfield, C.D., McKenna, R.W., and Peterson, L.: Bilateral trephine bone marrow biopsies in lymphoma and other neoplastic diseases, Ann. Int. Med. **82:**365-366, 1975.
4. Jamshidi, K., and Swain, K.W.: Bone marrow biopsy with unaltered architecture, J. Lab. Clin. Med. **77:**335-343, 1971.
5. Leavell, B.S., and Thorup, O.A.: Clinical hematology, ed. 4, Philadelphia, 1976, W.B. Saunders Co.
6. Rosenberg, S.A.: Bone marrow involvement in the non-Hodgkins lymphomata, Br. J. Haematol. **31**(Suppl. II):261-264, 1975.
7. Silver, R.T.: The morphology of blood and bone marrow in clinical practice, New York, 1969, Grune & Stratton, Inc.

PART EIGHT

MUSCULOSKELETAL PROCEDURES

CHAPTER 28

Joint aspiration and synovial fluid analysis

Ted M. Parris
Robert S. Gibson
John S. Davis IV

GENERAL CONSIDERATIONS

Aspiration and analysis of synovial fluid represents an important cornerstone in the diagnosis of various articular conditions.[1,3,6] It is safe, often provides immediate information, and can be done with a minimum of discomfort to the patient. Studies may prove diagnostically specific, as in septic or crystal-induced joint disease. At other times, although not specific, synovial fluid analysis can still be of great help in differentiating inflammatory from noninflammatory joint disease.

The injection of intraarticular corticosteroids[2] is considered an adjunctive therapy. Rarely does it provide primary therapy. It is useful when temporary relief of pain in an acutely inflamed joint is desired and when only a few joints are affected. The risk of introducing infection, although slight, is always present, and proper aseptic technique is essential. If used injudiciously, repeated injections of corticosteroids may accelerate cartilage destruction.

INDICATIONS FOR DIAGNOSTIC ASPIRATION[1,2,3,6]

1. For specific diagnosis of various articular conditions associated with joint effusion (Table 28-1).
2. To rule out infection or another superimposed process in an already diseased joint (e.g., infection in a rheumatoid or gouty joint and pseudogout in an osteoarthritic joint).

TABLE 28-1. SYNOVIAL FLUID ANALYSIS*

Disease	Color	Clarity	Viscosity
Group I Noninflammatory			
Normal	Straw	Transparent	High
Traumatic arthritis	Straw to bloody	Transparent to turbid	High
Osteoarthritis	Yellow	Slightly cloudy	High
Systemic lupus erythematosus	Straw	Slightly cloudy	High
Group II Inflammatory			
Rheumatic fever	Yellow	Slightly cloudy	Low
Pseudogout	Yellow	Slightly cloudy (if acute)	Low (if acute)
Gout	Yellow to milky	Cloudy	Low
Rheumatoid arthritis	Yellow to greenish	Cloudy	Low
Group III Septic			
Tuberculous arthritis	Yellow	Cloudy	Low
Septic arthritis	Grayish bloody	Turbid, purulent	Low

*From Hollander, J.L.: Bull. Rheum. Dis. **12**:264, 1961.

■ INDICATION FOR THERAPEUTIC ASPIRATION

1. Evacuation of hemarthrosis or another effusion to relieve pain caused by excessive fluid accumulation in a closed space.
2. Aspiration of infected fluid may hasten recovery in some instances.

■ INDICATIONS FOR INTRAARTICULAR INJECTION

1. Osteoarthritis.
2. Rheumatoid arthritis.

Mucin	WBC (cu mm); PMN (%)	Crystals	Bacteria
Good	<200 WBC; < 25%	0	0
Good	<2000 WBC; few to many RBC; <25%	0	0
Good	1000 WBC; <25%	0	0
Good	<5000 WBC, 10%	0	0
Good	10,000 to 20,000 WBC; 50%	0	0
Good to poor	1000 to 5000 WBC; 25% to 50%	Calcium, pyrophosphate +	0
Poor	10,000 to 30,000 WBC; 60% to 70%	Urate +	0
Poor	15,000 to 30,000 WBC; 75%	Occasional cholesterol	0
Poor	25,000 WBC; 50% to 60%	0	+
Poor	80,000 to 200,000 WBC; 75%	0	+

3. Juvenile rheumatoid arthritis.
4. Gout.
5. Pseudogout.
6. Acute traumatic arthritis.
7. Miscellaneous conditions with peripheral joint involvement (e.g., ankylosing spondylitis, psoriatic arthritis, Reiter's disease, and inflammatory bowel disease).

■ GENERAL CONTRAINDICATIONS

1. Periarticular sepsis, such as cellulitis. This is the only absolute contraindication to arthrocentesis.

2. Blood clotting disorders. In this situation, arthrocentesis can produce both intraarticular and external hemorrhage. It is, however, only a relative contraindication, particularly when acute bacterial arthritis is suspected.

■ CONTRAINDICATIONS FOR INTRAARTICULAR CORTICOSTEROID INJECTIONS

1. Joint sepsis, including tuberculous synovitis.
2. Joint instability. Instability of joints may be part of the Charcot-like arthropathy from repeated intraarticular corticosteroids. Theoretically, further injections could make the instability worse.
3. Intraarticular fracture. A corticosteroid injection will retard the healing process.
4. When joints are essentially inaccessible (e.g., spinal joints).
5. Failure to respond to prior injections.

■ EQUIPMENT AND PERSONNEL

1. A physician skilled in arthrocentesis.
2. Principal implements: an aspiration needle (18 to 23 gauge, ⅝ to 2 inches, depending on joint size and depth), a syringe (5 to 30 ml), appropriate collection tubes for cell count, chemistries, and culture, and a corticosteroid.
3. An antiseptic solution, sterile sponges and gloves, and a fenestrated drape.
4. Anesthesia: ethyl chloride spray and/or lidocaine (1%, 10 ml), a 25-gauge needle (⅝ inch), and a syringe.
5. An adhesive bandage.

■ PATIENT PREPARATION AND EVALUATION

1. Carefully examine the proposed arthrocentesis site.
2. Before injecting any medication into the joint space, obtain a careful history to rule out allergy. If previous injections were administered, determine the symptomatic response.
3. Explain the procedure to the patient, including its po-

tential complications, and obtain written informed consent.

■ TECHNIQUE[5]

1. Place the patient in a comfortable position, which depends on the joint to be aspirated.
2. Select the site for arthrocentesis. The usual approach to a joint space is the extensor surface, where major blood vessels and nerves are sparse. Avoid tendons.
3. Put on sterile gloves; prepare and drape a sterile field.
4. Anesthetize the skin overlying the site of the proposed arthrocentesis. Use either lidocaine instilled subcutaneously or topical ethyl chloride. Avoid mixing lidocaine with synovial fluid, which may confuse specimen interpretation.
5. Perform arthrocentesis. See Figs. 28-1 to 28-6 for the approach to specific joints. Use an 18- to 23-gauge needle, depending on the size of the joint. Avoid injury to articular cartilage with the needle. Obtain 10 to 20 ml of synovial fluid (if possible) for diagnostic studies. Inject medications as indicated. Remove the needle.
6. Apply an adhesive bandage over the puncture site.

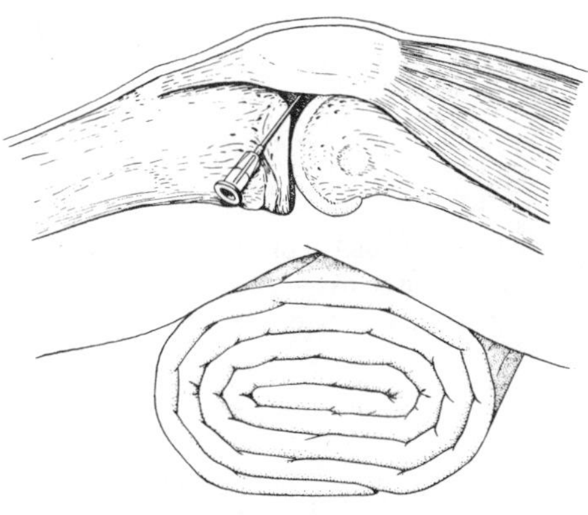

FIG. 28-1. Knee joint, anteromedial approach. Flex knee and insert needle approximately 1 cm below patella.

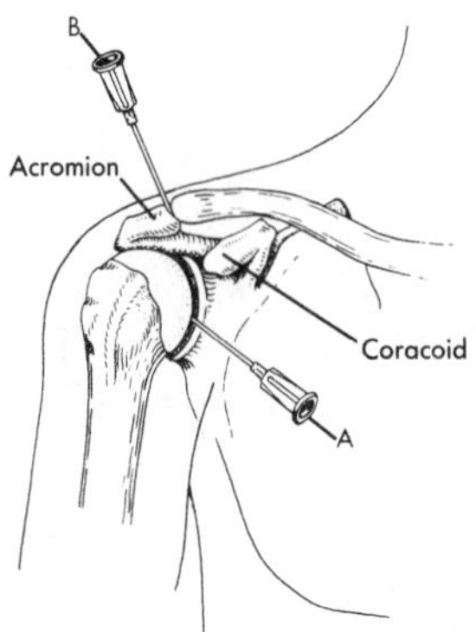

FIG. 28-2. Glenohumeral joint, anterior approach, and acromioclavicular joint, with patient in sitting position, arm at side, and hand across abdomen. Insert needle *A* lateral and inferior to coracoid. Insert needle *B* superiorly after palpating joint space.

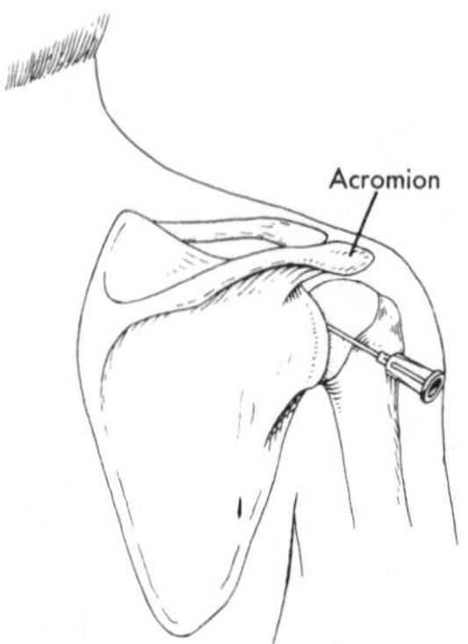

FIG. 28-3. Glenohumeral joint, posterior approach, with patient in sitting position, arm at side, and hand across abdomen. Insert needle approximately 2 cm inferior to posterior angle of acromion.

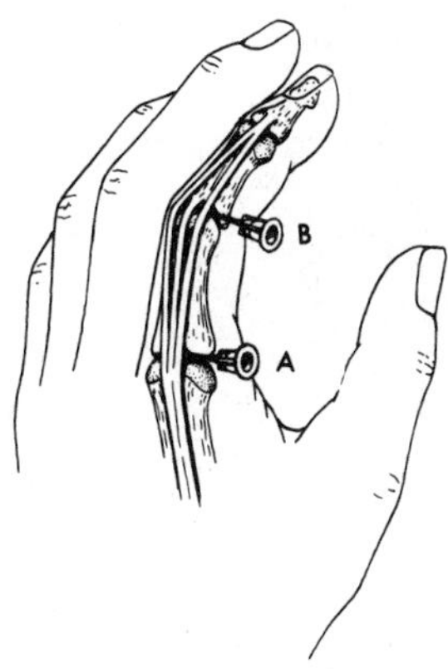

FIG. 28-4. Metacarpophalangeal and interphalangeal joints, with finger slightly flexed. Insert needles *A* and *B* dorsally and medially to extensor tendon, while applying traction to finger.

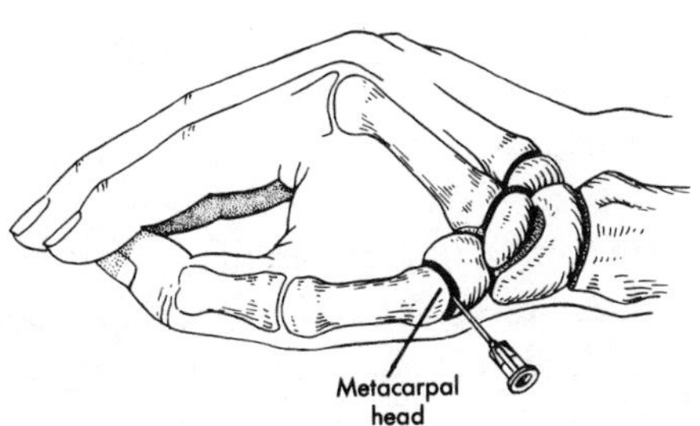

FIG. 28-5. Carpometacarpal joint with thumb opposed to little finger. Insert needle proximal to base of metacarpal head, while applying traction to thumb.

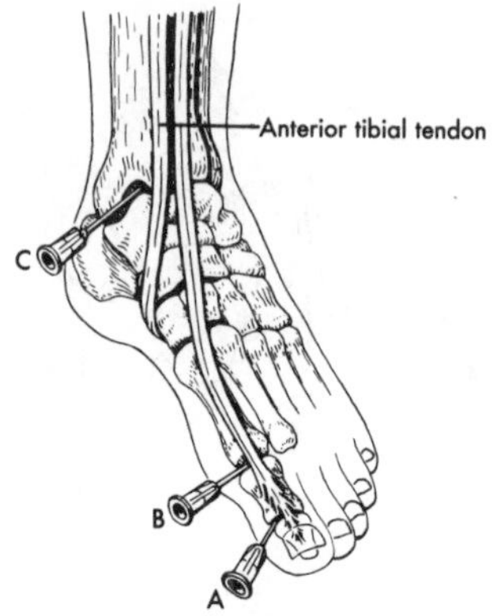

FIG. 28-6. Interphalangeal, metatarsophalangeal, and tibiotalar joint with foot and toes in plantar flexed position. Insert needles *A* and *B* dorsally and medially to extensor tendon. Insert needle *C* medially to anterior tibial tendon.

■ POSTPROCEDURE CARE

No postprocedure care is necessary.

■ SPECIMEN HANDLING

1. Obtain 2 to 5 ml of fluid for appropriate culture and microscopic examination (Gram stain or Ziehl-Neelsen stain). If gonococcal arthritis is suspected, innoculate a Thayer-Martin plate at the bedside.
2. Obtain 2 to 5 ml of fluid for a cell count, differential, and crystal examination. White blood cells are counted as in peripheral blood, using a pipette, counting chamber, and normal saline as a diluent. If many red blood cells are present, use one-fourth normal saline to lyse them. Do not use acetic acid because it will precipitate hyaluronic acid and form a mucin clot that will trap white blood cells and give falsely low counts. To examine for crystals (urate, calcium pyrophosphate, and apatite), place a drop of fresh synovial fluid on a clean glass slide and cover it with a cover slip. Examine the specimen immediately, using a polarizing microscope or a conventional binocular microscope with converting filters.

3. Obtain 5 to 10 ml of fluid for immunologic studies (rheumatoid factor test, complement), mucin clot, and assessment of viscosity. Fluid for complement determinations should be freed of clot and stored at −70° C within 2 hours of collection. To evaluate the mucin clot, add 1 or 2 ml of fluid to a test tube containing 5% acetic acid and let it stand for 1 minute. Determine the quality of the clot as "good" (a ropy clot that does not separate with shaking), "fair" (a softer mass with friable edges and some shreds in the solution), or "poor" (shreds and several small masses without a single clot). To qualitatively evaluate viscosity, allow fluid to drip from the tip of a syringe. Normal fluid will form a string (hence the term "string test") 2 or 3 inches long or longer, whereas fluid from inflamed joints will drip with little or no stringing. For quantitative analysis of viscosity, a viscometer can be used, but this is generally not considered necessary.

■ SPECIMEN INTERPRETATION (Table 28-1)

1. Gross appearance. Normal synovial fluid is straw colored and transparent. When inflammation or bleeding is present, both the color (yellow, green, grayish, or red) and the clarity (clear, turbid, grossly purulent, or bloody) will change.
2. Cell count and differential. Normal synovial fluid contains fewer than 200 white blood cells (WBC), of which less than 25% are neutrophils. Most inflammatory and septic arthritides show greater than 5000 to 10,000 WBCs and a predominance of neutrophils. Traumatic, osteoarthritic, and lupus joints often show increased WBC counts (1000 to 5000), but only 10% to 25% are neutrophils.
3. Crystal analysis. *Urate crystals* (gout) are negatively birefringent (yellow when parallel to the plane of slow vibration of the red compensator), needlelike, and may be intracellular or extracellular. During acute gouty attacks, they are more likely to be intracellular. In equi-

vocal cases, digestion of crystals by uricase can confirm the diagnosis. *Calcium pyrophosphate crystals* (pseudogout) are positively birefringent (blue when parallel to the plane of slow vibration of the red compensator), broader than urate crystals, and are often rhomboid in shape. *Apatite crystals* are shiny intracytoplasmic inclusions in white blood cells.[7]

4. Mucin clot. The quality of the clot reflects the degree of polymerization of hyaluronic acid. Since this is decreased in inflammatory and septic arthritides, the mucin clot will be poor.
5. Viscosity. Since viscosity depends on essentially the same process as mucin clot formation, synovial fluid with a poor quality clot will also have a low viscosity.
6. Synovial fluid complement. In most inflammatory conditions, synovial fluid complement is approximately half that of serum complement. It may be low in rheumatoid arthritis and is regularly elevated in Reiter's syndrome.

■ COMPLICATIONS

1. Iatrogenic infection. The incidence of iatrogenic infection is extremely low with strict aseptic technique. Arthrocentesis should never be performed through infected skin.
2. Hypersensitivity reaction. Before any medication is instilled in the joint, a careful history must be obtained to exclude allergy.
3. Radiologic deterioration of joints. Steroid-induced Charcot-like arthropathy can occur with repeated injections. Theoretically, the antianabolic effects of corticosteroids inhibit synthesis of proteoglycan and other major matrix components of cartilage, resulting in decreased cartilage stiffness. During cyclic weight bearing, cell death, fissuring, and cystic degeneration of matrix can occur.
4. Soft tissue atrophy. Soft tissue atrophy is occasionally noted when the small joints, such as the proximal interphalangeal joints of the finger, are injected. Periarticular calcifications and ecchymoses around the atrophied areas have been reported.

5. Nerve damage, such as inadvertent injection of the median nerve in carpal tunnel syndrome, can occur.
6. Postinjection flare. The intraarticular injection of corticosteroids occasionally produces a paradoxic increase in local inflammation. This may develop within a few hours of injection and last up to 48 hours. Distinguishing this reaction from an iatrogenic infection is difficult. The flare is noted more frequently with the needle-shaped corticosteroid crystals[4] and probably is caused by synovial fluid leukocytes phagocytizing the crystals and subsequently releasing lysosomal enzymes.

REFERENCES

1. Cohen, A.S.: Laboratory diagnostic procedures in the rheumatic diseases, Boston, 1975, Little, Brown & Co.
2. Hamilton, M., et al.: Simultaneous gout and pyarthrosis, Arch. Int. Med. **140**:917-919, 1980.
3. Hollander, J.L. et al.: Synovianalysis. An aid in diagnosis, Bull. Rheum. Dis. **12**:263-264, 1961.
4. Kahn, C.B. et al.: Corticosteroid crystals in synovial fluid, J.A.M.A. **211**: 807-809, 1970.
5. Pruce, A.M., Miller, J.A., Jr., and Berger, I.R: Anatomic landmarks in joint paracentesis, Clin. Sympos. **16**:19-30, 1964.
6. Rimoin, D.L., and Wennberg, J.E.: Acute septic arthritis complicating chronic rheumatoid arthritis, J.A.M.A. **196**:617-621, 1966.
7. Schumacker, H.R. et al.: Arthritis associated with apatite crystals, Ann. Int. Med. **87**:411-416, 1977.

CHAPTER 29

Intercostal nerve block

■ John C. Rowlingson

■ GENERAL CONSIDERATIONS

Injecting intercostal nerves with local anesthetics is used to block pain impulses from the chest wall, parietal pleura, and portions of the upper abdominal wall.[2,4,5,6] Anesthesia can last from 4 to 16 hours, depending on the local anesthetic used.[1]

■ INDICATIONS

1. Pain from rib fracture. An intercostal nerve block can diminish pain associated with movement of the chest and allow deeper breathing, more effective coughing, as well as increased mobility.
2. Pain following thoracic or upper abdominal surgery. Intercostal nerve blocks can decrease the need for depressant analgesic drugs, improve deep breathing and coughing, and facilitate early ambulation.
3. Neuritis or neuralgia due to trauma, metastatic cancer, acute herpes, postherpetic neuralgia, or surgical scars.
4. Costochondral pain.
5. Differentiating somatic from sympathetic-visceral pain (e.g., chest wall pain from angina).

■ CONTRAINDICATIONS

1. Infection at the site of needle insertion.
2. Septicemia.
3. Anticoagulation or hemorrhagic diathesis.
4. Inability to palpate rib margins.
5. Lack of resuscitation equipment.

PATIENT EVALUATION AND PREPARATION

1. Explain the procedure to the patient and obtain written informed consent.
2. A mild sedative (diazepam, 2 to 10 mg) or analgesic (meperidine, 10 to 25 mg) may be given intravenously, especially if multiple nerves will be blocked.

PERSONNEL AND EQUIPMENT

1. A physician trained to perform intercostal nerve block and a nurse or other health care professional to assist with the equipment and comfort the patient.
2. Alcohol swabs, sterile gloves, 4 × 4 inch gauze pads.
3. Lidocaine, 1% to 1.5%, with or without 1:200,000 epinephrine or bupivacaine, 0.25% to 0.5%, with or without 1:200,000 epinephrine. (See Table 2-1 for duration of effect and maximum doses of each agent.[1])
4. Needles (25 gauge, ¾ inch; 22 gauge, 1½ inches) and syringes (3 ml, 10 ml).
5. Resuscitation equipment is desirable.

TECHNIQUE

1. Place the patient in a sitting position, leaning forward onto a table (Fig. 29-1). If unable to sit up, place the

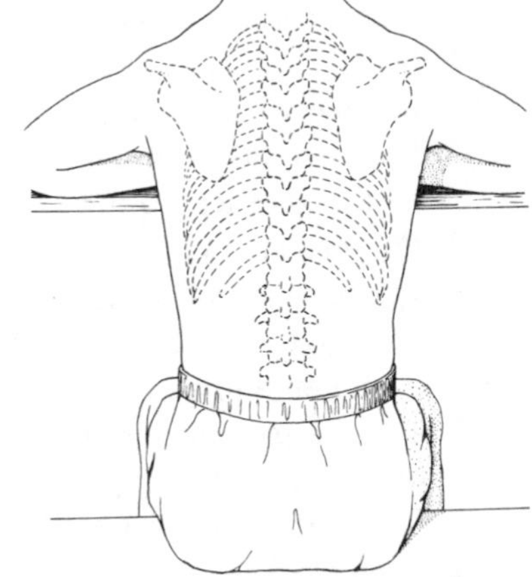

FIG. 29-1. Patient position.

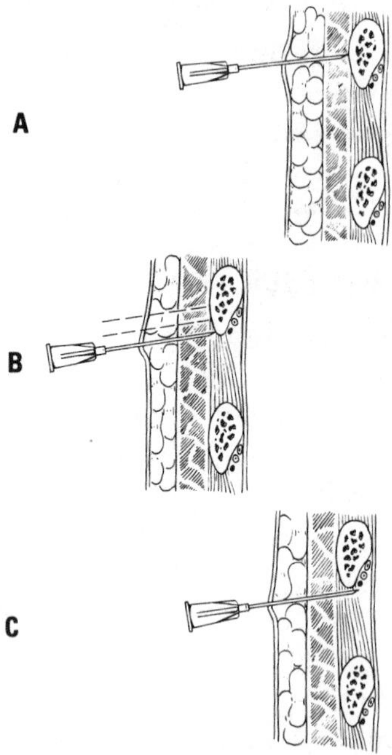

FIG. 29-2. Needle insertion. A, Needle inserted toward center of rib in slightly cephalad direction. **B,** Needle "walked" to lower border of rib. **C,** Needle advanced to level of intercostal nerve.

patient prone with the back arched and arms extended in the cephalad direction to elevate the scapula.

2. Select the nerve(s) to be blocked. Place a fingertip on the lower border of the rib at a site along the rib that is between the painful lesion and the spine. Place a mark on the skin with a fingernail at this point.
3. Put on sterile gloves and prepare the skin with alcohol.
4. Inject ½ ml of local anesthetic into the skin with a 25-gauge needle and 3-ml syringe to raise a wheal at each nerve to be blocked.
5. Tell the patient that it is vitally important not to move during the rest of the procedure.
6. Relocate the lower border of the rib where the nerve is to be blocked.

7. Insert the 22- or 23-gauge needle (attached to the 10-ml syringe filled with local anesthetic solution) through the skin wheal and advance it toward the center of the rib with a slightly cephalad direction (Fig. 29-2, *A*).
8. Move the needle gradually down the rib until it reaches the rib's lower border (Fig. 29-2, *B*).
9. Advance the needle 2 or 3 mm farther from the depth at which the bone was last contacted (Fig. 29-2, *C*). (The rib is approximately 7 mm thick.) Avoid moving the needle if the patient suddenly coughs or strains.
10. Aspirate through the needle to ascertain if an intercostal vessel has been entered. If so, reposition the needle.
11. Inject 2 to 4 ml of local anesthetic while moving the needle 0.5 to 1 mm in and out.
12. Remove the needle and wipe the skin clean.
13. Repeat steps 2 to 12 if more nerves are to be blocked. (See Chapter 2 for guidelines to the maximal dose of each drug allowed.)
14. This block can be repeated as needed.

■ POSTPROCEDURE CARE

1. Observe for a decrease in the patient's pain. Local anesthetics that have a long duration of action take longer to produce their full effects.
2. Observe the patient for a toxic reaction to the local anesthetic. Symptoms such as light headedness, tinnitus, perioral numbness, slurring of speech, or drowsiness usually precede the onset of convulsions, cardiovascular collapse, and respiratory arrest.
3. Observe for symptoms and signs of a pneumothorax, such as dyspnea, chest pain, and decreased breath sounds. A pneumothorax may not become apparent for several hours after the procedure because a small needle is used to perform intercostal nerve block. If a pneumothorax is suspected, obtain a posteroanterior expiratory chest roentgenograph. It may be necessary to observe a patient who has developed symptoms for several hours

even if the roentgenograph is initially negative. On discharge, it is essential to provide the patient (and caregivers) with a careful explanation of the symptoms of a pneumothorax and what to do should one occur.

■ COMPLICATIONS

1. Pneumothorax. The frequency of this is approximately 0.5% to 2%. The onset may be delayed, and treatment ranging from careful observation to the placement of a chest tube may be necessary.
2. Toxic reaction to the local anesthetic as described may occur, particularly after multiple nerves are blocked.[2] Potentially dangerous blood levels of anesthetics are related to the number of blocks performed, the proximity of intercostal vessels to the injection, and the high blood flow of the intercostal muscles.[3] Appropriate measures to assure the patient's airway (oxygen by mask or intubation), circulation (body position, intravenous fluids, vasopressors), and overall safety (harm from convulsions) must be taken.
3. Injection of a local anesthetic into the epidural or subarachnoid space (as when an intercostal nerve block is attempted too close to the spinal column) may produce either widespread sensory or motor loss or a high spinal block that require cardiovascular and pulmonary support until the local anesthetic effect disappears.
4. Rupture of an intercostal artery is rare.
5. Air embolus is rare.
6. Vasovagal syncope from fear or pain is possible.
7. Neuritis or breaking a needle are rare problems.

REFERENCES

1. Covino, B.G.: New local anesthetics in regional anesthesia: advances and selected topics, Int. Anesthesiol. Clin. **16**(4):10-11, 1978.
2. Lofstrom, B.: Intercostal nerve block. In Eriksson, E., editor: Illustrated handbook in local anaesthesia, Philadelphia, 1980, W.B. Saunders Co.
3. Mather, L.E., and Tucker, G.T.: Local anesthetic kinetics in regional anesthesia, Int. Anesthesiol. Clin. **16**(4):40-41, 1978.
4. Moore, D.C.: Regional block, Springfield, Ill., 1975, Charles C Thomas, Publisher.

5. Moore, D.C., Bush, W.H., and Scurlock, J.E.: Intercostal nerve block: a roentgenographic anatomic study of technique and absorption in humans, Anesth. Analg. **59:**815-825, 1980.
6. Scott, D.B.: Intercostal nerve blocks in regional anesthesia, Int. Anesthesiol. Clin. **16**(4):135-147, 1978.

CHAPTER 30

Trigger point injection

■ John C. Rowlingson

■ GENERAL CONSIDERATIONS

A trigger point is a discrete area of a muscle or ligament that is painful to palpation.[3] It can result from either injury to the muscles or ligaments or from tension, fatigue, or postural abnormalities. Trigger points also occur as part of the myofascial syndrome, which may include headaches, stiff neck, sore shoulders, anterior chest wall pain, back pain, abnormal posture with secondary muscle spasm, splinting, and decreased range of motion of joints.[2,4]

The pathophysiology of trigger points is not well understood. It was first believed that trigger points were localized areas of chronic inflammation,[5] but recent histologic evidence reveals a preponderance of myofibrillar degeneration and mucopolysaccharide accumulation.[1] It is also not well understood why injections of local anesthetics are effective treatment. It appears that these injections interrupt the cycle of pain which precipitates secondary muscular and vascular spasm, which in turn aggravates the original pain. Many physicians also inject corticosteroids for their antiinflammatory effect, although there are little scientific data available to support the use of corticosteroids.

■ INDICATION

A trigger point is an indication for injection.

■ CONTRAINDICATIONS

The contraindications are the same as the first four contraindications given for intercostal nerve block in Chapter 29.

■ PATIENT EVALUATION AND PREPARATION

Explain the procedure to the patient and obtain written informed consent.

PERSONNEL AND EQUIPMENT

1. A physician familiar with the technique.
2. Alcohol swabs and 4 × 4 inch gauze pads.
3. Lidocaine, 1% to 1.5%, 0.25% bupivacaine, and water-soluble corticosteroid preparations are sometimes used.
4. Needles (25 gauge, ¾ inch; 22 gauge, 1½ inches) and a syringe (10 ml).

TECHNIQUE

1. Place the patient in a comfortable position that allows easy access to the trigger point (Fig. 30-1).
2. Prepare the skin overlying the trigger point with alcohol.

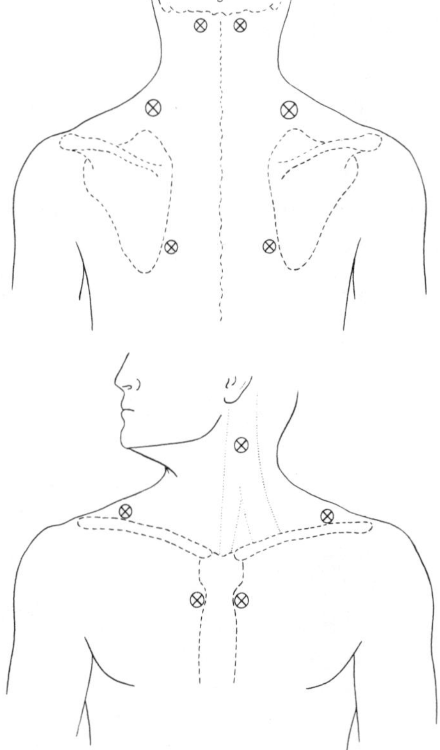

FIG. 30-1. Common trigger points.

3. Place a skin wheal of 0.5 ml of local anesthetic with the 25-gauge needle on the syringe. Then remove the needle from the syringe.
4. Attach the 22-gauge needle (depending on the depth of the trigger point) to the syringe and insert the needle through the skin wheal into the trigger point.
5. Aspirate through the needle; if a vessel has been entered, reposition the needle.
6. Inject 2 to 4 ml of local anesthetic, with or without 1 or 2 ml of the corticosteroid in a fanwise fashion.
7. Remove the needle and wipe the skin clean.
8. The block can be repeated as needed. If, however, corticosteroids are injected, the interval between injections should probably be at least 1 week.

■ POSTPROCEDURE CARE

1. Observe the patient for a change in symptoms and document any changes in the record. The patient may experience more pain for several hours after the block.
2. Observe the patient for vasovagal syncope or an unusual reaction to the local anesthetic, such as giddiness, excitation, oral numbness, or tinnitus.

■ COMPLICATIONS

1. Local irritation from the needle puncture or the drugs injected.
2. A toxic reaction to the local anesthetic is rare.
3. Significant bleeding is rare.
4. Cervical root block could occur when injecting scapulohumeral trigger points.
5. A pneumothorax is a remote possibility when injecting the chest wall.

REFERENCES

1. Brown, B.: Diagnosis and therapy of common myofascial syndromes. J.A.M.A. **239:**646-648, 1978.
2. Grosshandler, S., and Burney, R.: The myofascial syndrome, N.C. Med. J. **40:**562-565, 1979.
3. Levy, B.A.: Diagnostic, prognostic, and therapeutic nerve blocks, Arch. Surg. **112:**870-879, 1977.

4. Simons, D.G.: Electrogenic nature of palpable bands and "jump sign" associated with myofascial trigger points, Adv. Pain Res. Ther. **1**:913-926, 1976.
5. Travell, J., and Rinzler, S.H.: The myofascial genesis of pain, Postgrad. Med. **11**:425-434, 1952.

PART NINE

NEUROLOGIC PROCEDURE

CHAPTER 31

Lumbar puncture

■ Robert S. Gibson

■ GENERAL CONSIDERATIONS

Lumbar puncture and examination of the cerebrospinal fluid (CSF) is one of the simplest, yet most informative, tests that a physician can perform. It is the definitive test for meningitis and subarachnoid hemorrhage (SAH). It is hazardous to perform, however, when intracranial pressure is elevated, particularly when there is an expanding lesion in the posterior fossa.

■ DIAGNOSTIC INDICATIONS

1. Suspected meningitis (bacterial, viral, tuberculous, fungal, amebic, or syphilitic).
2. Suspected subarachnoid hemorrhage.
3. Suspected Guillain-Barré syndrome, multiple sclerosis, leptomeningeal carcinomatosis and other central and peripheral nervous system diseases of obscure etiology.
4. To observe the results of meningitis therapy, such as changes in cell count; protein or glucose level; culture for bacteria, tuberculosis, or fungus; VDRL (Venereal Disease Research Laboratory) titer, and cryptococcal antigen titer.
5. To inject air (pneumoencephalogram), contrast media (myelogram), or radioactive substances, such as indium or radioactive-iodinated serum albumin (RISA).

■ THERAPEUTIC INDICATIONS

1. To administer intrathecal antimicrobial or antineoplastic therapy.
2. To administer spinal anesthesia.
3. Occasionally it may be used for the symptomatic treatment of severe headache of SAH and to lower the CSF pressure in SAH and pseudotumor cerebri.

■ CONTRAINDICATIONS

All contraindications are relative, especially when the risk of missing meningitis is high. Sepsis is not a contraindication, nor is anticoagulant therapy.

1. Local tissue suppuration, such as cellulitis, furunculosis, or epidural abscess in or near the needle entry site. When this situation exists, one can obtain CSF via the cisterna magna or lateral cervical puncture route.
2. Papilledema, or other signs of increased intracranial pressure, or focal neurologic signs until a mass lesion is ruled out.
3. Suspected intracranial mass lesions, including posterior fossa tumors, brain abscess, and subdural hematoma.[6,10]

■ PATIENT EVALUATION AND PREPARATION

1. Neurologic and fundoscopic examination.
2. Explain the procedure to the patient, including potential complications, and obtain a written informed consent.

■ PERSONNEL AND EQUIPMENT

1. A physician trained in lumbar puncture and an assistant to hold the patient in the proper position.
2. Principal implements: two spinal needles with stylets (18 and 20 gauge, each 3½ inches long), a three-way stopcock, a manometer, and four sterile specimen collection tubes with screw tops.
3. Disinfection and sterile field: sterile sponges, a disinfectant solution, sterile gloves and gown, a mask and hair cap, draping towels with a window, and towel clips.
4. Anesthesia: lidocaine (1%, 10 ml), a syringe (3 ml), a 23-gauge needle (1 inch).
5. Dressing: an adhesive bandage.

■ TECHNIQUE

1. Position the patient in the lateral decubitus position (Fig. 31-1). The patient's knees should be drawn toward the chest and the head flexed to widen the space between the spinous processes. The shoulders, back,

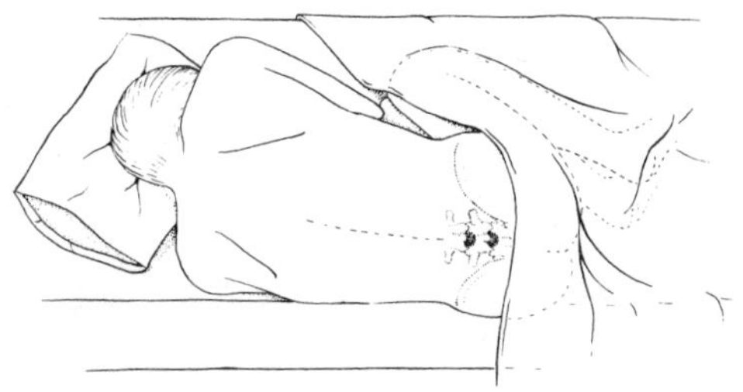

FIG. 31-1. Lateral decubitus position.

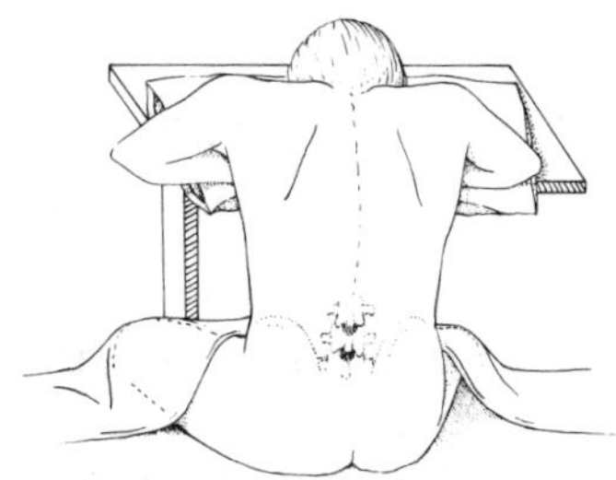

FIG. 31-2. Sitting position.

and hips should be perpendicular to the floor. In patients with massive obesity, ankylosing spondylitis, degenerative or rheumatoid spinal arthritis, a sitting position (Fig. 31-2) may be used. Have the patient sit on the edge of a bed, bend forward, and rest the upper extremities and head on a bedside tray table placed just above the nipple line.

2. Select a puncture site. Any vertebral interspace below L2 can be used in the adult, although we suggest either the L4 to L5 or L5 to S1 interspace (the iliac crest is at the level of the L4 spinous process). Mark the interspinous space by indenting the skin with a coin or fingernail.
3. Put on a mask, hair cap, sterile gloves, and gown.
4. Prepare the skin with a disinfectant solution and form a sterile field with draping towels.

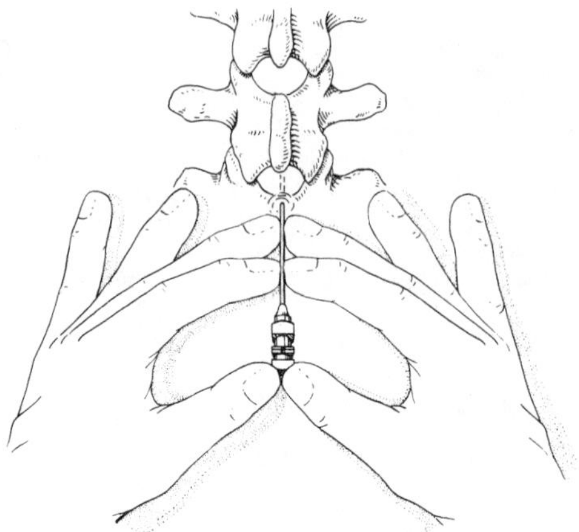

FIG. 31-3. Insert spinal needle into subcutaneous tissue and advance needle into subarachnoid space.

5. Anesthetize the skin by raising a subcutaneous wheal with lidocaine; infiltrate deeper tissue to the level of the longitudinal ligament and periosteum.
6. Set up the manometer and familiarize yourself with the operation of the stopcock.
7. Insert the spinal needle and stylet into the subcutaneous tissue (Fig. 31-3). The needle should enter the interspinous space perpendicular to the long axis of the spine and pointed toward the umbilicus.
8. Advance the needle into the subarachnoid space slowly, until a "give" is felt, which indicates that the ligamentum flavum has been penetrated. Remove the stylet to check for CSF flow. If no CSF flows out the needle, rotate the needle, because the beveled tip may be blocked. If still no CSF appears, replace the stylet and advance the needle farther. Remove the stylet at approximately 2-mm intervals and check for CSF flow. Repeat this sequence until CSF appears.
9. Attach the manometer and three-way stopcock to the needle and measure opening pressure (Fig. 31-4). The normal range is 60 to 180 mm of CSF with the patient lying in the lateral decubitus position. Before measur-

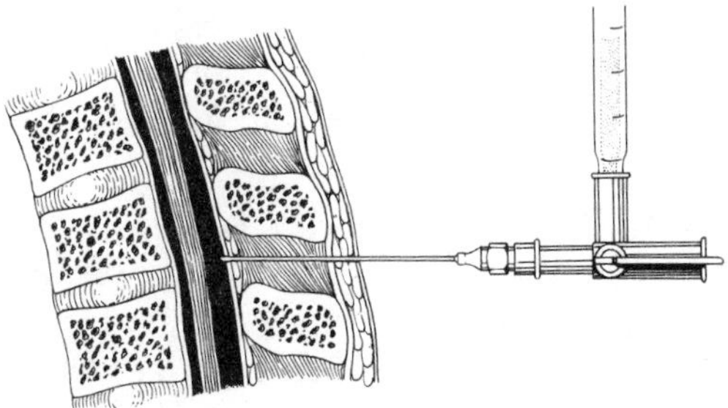

FIG. 31-4. Measure opening pressure. Note position of stopcock.

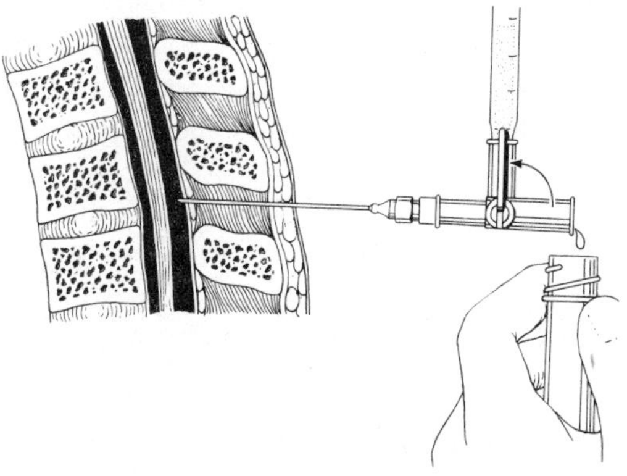

FIG. 31-5. Collect cerebrospinal fluid.

ing the pressure, the patient's legs and head should be straightened. Do not allow the patient to hyperventilate, since this may falsely lower an elevated pressure. In the sitting position, the level of CSF in the manometer normally does not rise above the external occipital protuberance. If an obstruction of the spinal subarachnoid space is suspected, the operator can perform a Queckenstedt test by transiently occluding both the external and internal jugular veins bilaterally by hand. Normally, the CSF pressure should rise rapidly and, with release of the veins, fall to the precompression baseline within 20 seconds. Either a slow rise or fall is considered an abnormal result. This test is of no value in the diagnosis of intracranial disease and is contraindicated in the presence of increased intracranial pressure.

10. Collect CSF for diagnostic studies. Adjust the three-way stopcock and obtain separate samples as indicated (Fig. 31-5). Separate samples should be obtained for cell counts and cell differentials (tube number 1), culture and Gram stain (tube number 2), protein and glucose (tube number 3), and special studies (tubes 4 and 5), such as cytological examination, VDRL test, protein electrophoresis, cryptococcal antigen, sequential red blood cell (RBC) count to differentiate a traumatic tap from SAH, and lactic acid level.[3] Collect 1 or 2 ml for tubes 1 to 3. Usually, 2 to 4 ml is adequate for most special studies.
11. Measure the closing pressure, detach the manometer, reinsert the stylet, and remove the needle.
12. Apply an adhesive bandage.
13. Instruct the patient to remain flat in bed for 12 to 24 hours.

■ SPECIMEN EXAMINATIONS AND INTERPRETATIONS (Table 31-1)

1. Gross appearance.[1,2] CSF is normally water clear. It is best inspected by comparing it to tap water against a white background. Visible haziness appears when the cell count is between 200 to 500 cells/mm^3. More than 500 cells/mm^3 produce a definite cloudy or purulent appearance. If cells are present in the fluid, remove the supernatant fluid and reinspect it for color. Yellow discoloration of the CSF is called xanthochromia and is due to the presence of bilirubin, oxyhemoglobin, or methemoglobin. Bilirubin may be present if the CSF protein is increased, in jaundiced patients, and 2 or 3 days after SAH. Oxyhemoglobin may be found within 2 hours after the clinical onset of intracranial hemorrhage[2]. Methemoglobin may be present if blood is encapsulated as within a subdural or intracerebral hematoma or cyst.

TABLE 31-1. TYPICAL SPINAL FLUID FINDINGS

Condition	Appearance	Cell count (mm^3)	Protein (mg/dl)	Sugar (mg/dl)	Pressure (mm CSF)
Normal	Clear, colorless	0 to 5 (lymphocytes)	15 to 45	45 to 100	60 to 180
Acute bacterial meningitis	Hazy to purulent	500 to 20,000 (chiefly polymorphonuclear leukocytes)	50 to 500	Low or absent	200 to 500
Tuberculous meningitis	Hazy	10 to 2000 (chiefly lymphocytes)	50 to 500	Moderately decreased	200 to 500
Viral meningitis	Clear or slightly cloudy	10 to 2000 usually <200 (chiefly lymphocytes)	45 to 200	Normal; may be low with specific viruses	Normal or moderately increased
Multiple sclerosis	Clear	Normal or 10 to 50 lymphocytes	Normal to 45 to 150 in some cases	Normal	Normal
Subarachnoid hemorrhage	Bloody or xanthochromic	Many erythrocytes	50 to 1000	Normal	Normal to > 500
Cerebral thrombosis	Clear	Usually normal	Normal or slightly increased	Normal	Usually normal
Cerebral hemorrhage	Bloody or xanthochromic	Increased, chiefly erythrocytes	Usually increased	Normal	Usually increased
Carcinomatous meningitis	Often clear	Variable	Usually increased	Low or absent	Usually increased

2. Cell counts and differential. Cell counts and differential must be done within the first hour after collection of CSF. After an hour, the cells begin to disintegrate. Cells can be counted by manual hemacytometry or with an electronic cell counter. The normal number of white blood cells (WBC) in CSF is 0 to 5 lymphocytes per cubic mm. If the CSF contains RBCs, one must distinguish accidental contamination due to a traumatic tap from SAH. In a traumatic tap the RBC count will be less in tube 4 than in tube 1, whereas with SAH the count will not change. Xanthochromia in the supernatant fluid favors SAH and is against a traumatic tap. When blood is found in CSF, one can normally expect to find approximately 1 WBC for each 800 red blood cells. An approximate differential WBC count can be done in the hemacytometer chamber, but it is best to study a well-prepared stained film. When the total WBC count is under 500, it is necessary to centrifuge the CSF and make the smears from the concentrated sediment.
3. Microbiology. The second tube is reserved for culture (bacteria, viruses, cryptococci, fungi, tubercle bacilli, etc). When infection is suspected, appropriate smears and stains (Gram, india ink, potassium hydroxide, Kenyon, Ziehl-Neelsen, etc.) must be prepared and meticulously inspected for organisms to guide initial antimicrobial therapy.
4. CSF glucose level. Obtain a blood glucose level immediately before or after lumbar puncture. A normal CSF glucose level is 45 to 100 mg/dl or not less than two thirds of the blood value. A low CSF glucose level is commonly seen in bacterial, mycobacterial, fungal, and even viral (especially mumps) meningitis. Leptomeningeal carcinomatosis is associated with low CSF glucose levels in 38% of patients on the first lumbar puncture and 72% if subsequent taps are performed.[9] When cultures are persistently negative, carcinomatous meningitis should be considered.
5. CSF serologic test. The quantitative VDRL test is the

CSF serologic test of choice for central nervous system syphilis.[7] Presently, the Center for Disease Control recommends that the fluorescent treponemal antibody absorbed (FTA-ABS) test not be done on CSF.

6. Special studies. CSF immunoglobulin analysis by electroimmunodiffusion remains a reliable test for the diagnosis of multiple sclerosis.[11] Newer tests on CSF protein levels that may prove to be clinically useful for diagnosing this disease include the finding of oligoclonal bands in agarose electrophoresis[8] and myelin basic protein (MBP).[4] The former test can be done using readily available commercial reagents and is of great help in evaluating the early symptom of optic neuritis. It has the potential of evaluating atypical multiple sclerosis. The value of finding MBP is that it is released into the CSF during acute attacks of demyelination and may serve as a marker of activity. The CSF cryptococcal antigen titer has both diagnostic and prognostic value in cryptococcal meningitis.[5] Recently, Brooks and co-workers[3] have reported the usefulness of measuring CSF lactic acid levels and suggest it may be helpful in distinguishing bacterial and tuberculous meningitis from meningitis due to nonbacterial causes.

■ POSTPROCEDURE CARE

1. Instruct the patient to lie prone in bed for at least 12 hours to help avoid postlumbar puncture headache.
2. If CSF pressure is elevated, perform serial neurologic evaluations and look for signs of herniation.

■ COMPLICATIONS

1. Headache.[12] Headache occurs in up to 20% to 30% of patients. It is most frequently seen after multiple puncture attempts and when the patient is ambulated too early. The headache is precipitated or made worse by sitting up or standing. Its onset is usually within 24 to 48 hours but may be delayed as long as 7 days after lumbar puncture. The headache may be severe, accom-

panied by nausea and vomiting, and require intravenous fluids and analgesics. It generally lasts 2 to 8 days and rarely longer.

2. Transtentorial or tonsillar herniation. These types of herniation are most frequently due to inadequate preprocedure evaluation. Lumbar puncture should not be done in patients who have papilledema, other signs of increased intracranial pressure, or focal neurologic signs, until a mass lesion has been excluded. Herniation may not occur until 24 to 36 hours after lumbar puncture. Herniation requires immediate recognition and treatment with corticosteroids, mannitol, and hyperventilation[13] while awaiting neurosurgical consultation.
3. Septic meningitis and epidural or subdural empyema. These are due to faulty aseptic technique, such as a contaminated needle, inadequate skin preparation, or puncture in the presence of local tissue suppuration.
4. Backache. Backache may be caused by injuries to the spinal ligaments, periosteum, or annulus fibrosus.
5. Vascular trauma. Blood vessels arising from the perivertebral plexus of veins and those which accompany nerve roots may be perforated during lumbar puncture. Injury to the former may cause an epidural hematoma or, if the blood gains access to the subarachnoid space, signs of meningitis. Damage to the latter may cause ischemia of nerve roots.
6. Intraspinal epidermoid cyst. An intraspinal epidermoid cyst is due to introduction of viable epithelial cells into the spinal canal. It can be avoided by introducing the spinal needle with stylet in place.

REFERENCES

1. Barrows, L.J., Hunter, F.T., Banker, B.Q.: The nature and clinical significance of pigments in the cerebrospinal fluid, Brain **78**:59-80, 1955.
2. Bell, W.E., Joynt, R.J., and Sahs, A.L.: Low spinal fluid pressure syndromes, Neurology **10**:512-521, 1960.
3. Brooks, I. et al.: Measurement of lactic acid in cerebrospinal fluid of patients with infections of the central nervous system, J. Infect. Dis. **137**:384-390, 1978.

4. Cohen, S.R., et al.: Cerebrospinal fluid myelin basic protein and multiple sclerosis, Adv. Exp. Med. Biol. **100:**513-519, 1978.
5. Diamond, R.D., and Bennett, J.E.: Prognostic factors in cryptococcal meningitis, Ann. Intern. Med. **80:**176-181, 1974.
6. Garfield, J.: Management of supratentorial intracranial abscess. Review of 200 cases, Br. Med. J. **2:**7-11, 1969.
7. Jaffe, H.W.: The laboratory diagnosis of syphilis, Ann. Int. Med. **83:**846-850, 1975.
8. Johnson, K.J. et al.: Agarose electrophoresis of CSF in multiple sclerosis, Neurology **27:**273-277, 1977.
9. Olson, M.E., Chernik, N.L., and Posner, J.B.: Infiltration of the leptomeninges by systemic cancer, Arch. Neurol. **30:**122-137, 1974.
10. Samson, D.S., and Clark, K.: A curent review of brain abscess, Am. J. Med. **54:**201-210, 1973.
11. Schneck, S.A., and Claman, H.N.: CSF immunoglobulins in multiple sclerosis and other neurologic diseases, Arch. Neurol. **20:**132-139, 1969.
12. Wolff, H.G.: Headache and other head pain, New York, 1950, Oxford University Press.
13. Zervas, N.T., and Hedley-Whyte, J.: Successful treatment of cerebral herniation in five patients, N.Engl. J. Med. **286:**1075-1077, 1972.

PART TEN

OPHTHALMIC PROCEDURE

CHAPTER 32

Tonometry

Steven A. Newman
Robert S. Gibson

GENERAL CONSIDERATIONS[1,5,6]

Pressure within the eye is maintained by a balance between aqueous humor produced by the ciliary body and absorption in the trabecular mesh. When absorption is unequal to production, intraocular pressure rises. Any pressure elevation may potentially damage the optic nerve. When optic nerve damage occurs in the setting of increased intraocular pressure, we refer to it as glaucoma.

Glaucoma is generally categorized as narrow angle or open angle. This refers to the proximity of the iris to the cornea and trabecular mesh (visible on gonioscopy). Open-angle glaucoma is further divided into simple or secondary (following trauma, hemorrhage, or inflammation). Patients with narrow-angle glaucoma may complain of acute, severe ocular pain, blurred vision, ocular injection, nausea and vomiting, or halos around lights. Chronic simple glaucoma, on the other hand, tends to be an insidious asymptomatic disease, leading to eventual blindness if not treated.

Tonometry is the determination of intraocular pressure by means of an instrument that measures the amount of corneal identation (or flattening) produced by a given weight. It is the single most important screening test for chronic simple glaucoma and will detect the vast majority of patients who are at risk for glaucomatous loss of optic nerve fibers. It should be part of the general physical examination performed by internists and general practitioners.

INSTRUMENTATION

The Schiøtz indentation tonometer[8] is the most commonly used device because it is relatively inexpensive, easy to use, and durable. The instrument (Fig. 32-1) consists of a foot plate curved to fit the average normal cornea with a metal plunger in the center for holding various gram weights. On top of the plunger is a short curved arm with a lever whose long arm is a pointer for reading positions on the scale. When the ocular end of the plunger fits flush with the curved foot plate resting on the cornea, the pointer is at 0 on the scale. As the plunger indents the cornea, the scale reading increases according to the resistance encountered. Each instrument is accompanied by a calibration table to convert the scale reading into millimeters of mercury of intraocular pressure.

The Goldmann aplanation tonometer measures the force required to flatten 3.06 mm of the central corneal surface,[1] and is more accurate than Schiøtz tonometry. These instruments, however, require magnification, either built into the machine or used in conjunction with a slit-lamp microscope. Although widely used by ophthalmologists, the equipment is impractical for the general practitioner because it requires training for its use and is very expensive. Other methods of ocular pressure analysis include the use of mechanical transducers (Mackay-Marg tonometer) or air tonometry. The air tonometer is quite expensive but may be used by a technician without difficulty. Because of cost, we recommend Schiøtz tonometry for general medical use by the nonophthalmologist.

■ INDICATIONS[4,5]

1. All patients over the age of 40, when undergoing routine examination, should have tonometric screening. The incidence of elevated ocular pressure in this age group is between 1% and 2%.
2. Special attention should be given to any patient with a family history of serious visual loss or diabetes, treated glaucoma, unexplained headaches, or pain about the eyes.
3. Patients who are high hyperopes (farsighted) or have congenitally small eyes are also at risk for angle-closure attacks.
4. Any patient with a history of iritis, trauma, hyphema,

uveitis, or with a dislocated lens carries a long-term increased glaucoma risk.

CONTRAINDICATIONS

1. Conjunctivitis, blepharitis, or other superficial infection.
2. Corneal damage, including abrasions or exposure.
3. Inability of the patient to relax and cooperate (squeezing of the lids will give a false elevation of ocular pressure).
4. Ocular pain. (See Indications for Referral to an Ophthalmologist.)

PATIENT PREPARATION

1. Explain the purpose of the procedure and assure the patient that there will be no discomfort.
2. Instruct the patient to cooperate by looking straight up at a ceiling target during the procedure, holding the eyes steady, and avoiding squeezing the lids. This ensures reliable intraocular pressure measurements and lessens the chance of injuring the cornea with the footplate.

EQUIPMENT

1. Schiøtz tonometer and measured weights (5.5, 7.5, and 10 g). Before using the tonometer, ensure that the plunger slides easily in the barrel. The instrument should be frequently cleaned; ideally by disassembling it (it can be safely placed under running water). The footplate should be thoroughly wiped with an appropriate disinfectant solution, such as alcohol or benzalkonium chloride (Zephiran).
2. A topical anesthetic. We prefer to use 0.5% proparacaine.

TECHNIQUE

1. Instill one drop of topical anesthetic into each eye. Inform the patient in advance that this drop will burn transiently.

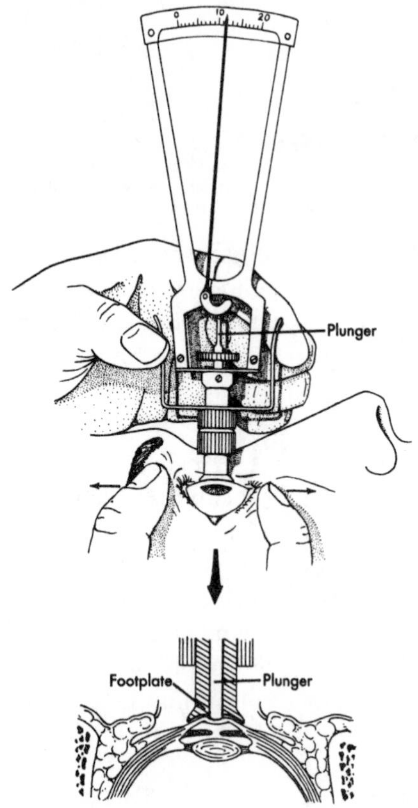

FIG. 32-1. Technique of Schiøtz tonometry.

2. Place the patient in a semirecumbent position. Have the patient relax both eyelids and gaze at the ceiling.
3. Gently separate the eyelids, avoiding digital pressure on the globe (Fig. 32-1).
4. Slowly lower the tonometer over the cornea, keeping it vertical. The curved footplate fits smoothly over the corneal surface. The tonometer must rest completely and stably on the cornea. Allow the plunger to exert its full weight on the corneal surface (Fig. 32-1).
5. Obtain a scale reading and determine intraocular pressure by referring to the calibration table (Table 32-1) that converts the scale reading to millimeters of mer-

TABLE 32-1. STANDARD CONVERSION TABLE*

Tonometer reading	5.5-g weight	7.5-g weight	10-g weight	15-g weight
4.0	20.6	30.4	43.4	71.0
4.5	18.9	28.0	40.2	66.2
5.0	17.3	25.8	37.2	61.8
5.5	15.9	23.8	34.4	57.6
6.0	14.6	21.9	31.8	53.6
6.5	13.4	20.1	29.4	49.9
7.0	12.2	18.5	27.2	46.5
7.5	11.2	17.0	25.1	43.2
8.0	10.2	15.6	23.1	40.2
8.5	9.4	14.3	21.3	38.1
9.0	8.5	13.1	19.6	34.6
9.5	7.8	12.0	18.0	32.0
10.0	7.1	10.9	16.5	29.6
10.5	6.5	10.0	15.1	27.4
11.0	5.9	9.0	13.8	25.3
11.5	5.3	8.3	12.6	23.3
12.0	4.9	7.5	11.5	21.4
12.5	4.4	6.8	10.5	19.7
13.0	4.0	6.2	9.5	18.1
13.5		5.6	8.6	16.5
14.0		5.0	7.8	15.1
14.5		4.5	7.1	13.7
15.0		4.0	6.4	12.6

*From Kronfeld, P.C. Published with permission from The American Journal of Ophthalmology **45**:308-312. Copyright by the Ophthalmic Publishing Company.

cury. Begin by using the standard 5.5-g weight. Check the scale reading. If it reads less than 4, the next heavier weight should be added. The 7.5-g weight is placed on top of the 5.5-g weight. If this is insufficient, the 7.5-g weight should be removed and replaced by the 10-g weight. Record pressure in the second eye in the same fashion. If the patient squeezes the lids, intraocular pressure will rise, creating a falsely high pressure.

■ POSTPROCEDURE CARE

Instruct the patient to avoid rubbing the eyes for 15 to 30 minutes after tonometry, because this could scuff the anesthetized cornea without the patient feeling it.

INTERPRETATION

1. Intraocular pressures are said to be "normal" up to 20 mm Hg. Pressures higher than this may also be normal but suggest that further analysis and follow-up are required. Pressures in the 20s indicate only a 10% chance of glaucomatous damage but the risk rises with the pressure. In fact, there is a significant variability in the sensitivity of the optic nerve to increased pressure, and some individuals may tolerate pressures in the 30s without ever developing damage.
2. Ocular pressure, like blood pressure, is not a fixed number and tends to have a diurnal variation. Therefore a single pressure reading, even when in the normal range, does not exclude the possibility of glaucoma. This is particularly true in patients who have acute or angle-closure glaucoma. In these patients, intermittent block of the trabecular mesh can be produced either mechanically or by inflammation. Any patient with symptoms or fundoscopic findings suggestive of glaucoma deserves additional study beyond a single normal pressure reading.
3. Absolute accuracy of intraocular pressure measurement depends on an assumed scleral rigidity. Unfortunately, this is not constant and may lead to inaccuracies, particularly in patients with odd ocular shapes (high nearsightedness) following eye surgery or simply with aging.

COMPLICATIONS

1. Immediate complication. Corneal abrasions as a complication of tonometry are uncommon. The patient, however, may not recognize there has been a problem until the anesthetic begins to wear off (15 to 30 minutes). At this point, the patient will complain of a sharp sticking or foreign body sensation in the eye aggravated by light or moving the lids.
2. Delayed complication. Infection may be transmitted by contaminated tonometers. This is relatively uncommon; most cases of epidemic conjunctivitis are probably spread by the fingers of the examining physician. It be-

hooves all concerned that the physician clean not only the instrument but the hands.

INDICATIONS FOR REFERRAL TO AN OPHTHALMOLOGIST[2,3]

1. Pressure above 20 mm Hg. Patients who have even transiently elevated pressures need further evaluation. This should include gonioscopy (measurement of the chamber angle), Goldmann fields (one of the earliest manifestations of optic nerve damage is loss of visual fields), and measurement of the optic cup (best done dilated with binocular indirect observation or stereophotography).
2. Severely elevated pressures. Pressures in the 60s and above may cause occlusion of the central retinal artery and should be treated as a medical emergency with immediate referral.
3. Ocular pain. Although ocular pain may be a symptom of acute angle closure, other possible causes, including uveitis and endophthalmitis, must be excluded by biomicroscopic examination.
4. Complications of tonometry. Although corneal abrasions usually heal rapidly if patched, the possibility of infection and the current medicolegal atmosphere warrants referral.

REFERENCES

1. Armaly, M.F.: The Des Moines population study of glaucoma, Invest. Ophthalmol. **1**:618-628, 1962.
2. Armaly, M.F.: Ocular pressure and visual fields, Arch. Ophthalmol. **81**:25-40, 1969.
3. Armaly, M.F.: The visual field defect and ocular pressure level in open angle glaucoma, Invest Ophthalmol. **8**:105-124, 1969.
4. Davanger, M., and Holter, O.: The statistical distribution of intraocular pressure in the population, Acta. Ophthalmol. **43**:314-322, 1963.
5. Fisher, R.F.: Value of tonometry and tonography in the diagnosis of glaucoma, Br. J. Ophthalmol. **56**:200-204, 1972.
6. Kolker, A.E., and Hetherington, J.Jr.: Becker-Shaffer's diagnosis and therapy of the glaucomas, ed. 4, St. Louis, 1976, The C.V. Mosby Co.
7. Kronfeld, P.C.: The new calibration scale for Schiøtz tonometers. Am. J. Ophthalmol. **45**:308, 1958.
8. Schiøtz, H.: Tonometry, Br. J. Ophthalmol. **4**:201-210, 1920.

PART ELEVEN

PULMONARY PROCEDURES

CHAPTER 33

Arterial puncture

A. Ross Hill

GENERAL CONSIDERATIONS

Arterial puncture is a simple and repeatable method for obtaining arterial blood samples. The analysis of arterial Po_2, Pco_2, and pH level provides invaluable information about respiratory and cardiovascular function and acid-base status.

INDICATIONS

1. Respiratory failure, both acute and chronic. Arterial blood gas analysis is essential in assessing the nature and severity of respiratory failure, as well as in guiding therapy with oxygen and mechanical ventilation.
2. Cardiopulmonary arrest.
3. Acid-base derangements, as may occur with shock, diabetic ketoacidosis, toxin ingestion, and renal failure.
4. Suspected pulmonary embolism.
5. Evaluation of respiratory disability for occupational health and compensation purposes.
6. Determination of right-to-left cardiovascular shunts, pulmonary shunt fraction, and cardiac output by the Fick principle.
7. Clinical research.
8. Occasionally arterial blood samples are required for other purposes, such as lactic acid measurement.

CONTRAINDICATIONS

1. Bleeding diathesis. Mild elevations of coagulation screen values pose no threat; major abnormalities create a relative contraindication, as during therapeutic anticoagulation (especially with heparin).[13] Any severe hemostatic defect, whether of coagulation or of platelet number or

function, may result in a serious bleeding hazard and make the procedure inadvisable. Examples include disseminated intravascular coagulation, thrombolytic therapy, and extreme thrombocytopenia.
2. Arterial abnormality at the proposed puncture site, such as a reduced pulse or bruit, an aneurysm, or arteritis.
3. Infection along the needle path.

SELECTION OF ARTERY FOR PUNCTURE

The radial, brachial, and femoral arteries can usually be entered with equal ease. The radial artery is preferred because of its convenient and superficial location, ready compressibility against underlying bone, and because the hand usually receives collateral circulation through the ulnar artery.[1] Brachial and femoral punctures are safe in most individuals but should be avoided when there is a bleeding diathesis; hematomas are difficult to control at these sites and can cause compression neuropathies.[13] The femoral artery also suffers from frequent atherosclerosis in older patients. It is often useful, however, during cardiopulmonary resuscitation, since it is the easiest of the three to palpate in hypotensive patients.

PATIENT EVALUATION AND PREPARATION

1. If a bleeding tendency may be present, obtain a prothrombin time, partial thromboplastin time, and platelet count.
2. Note the inspired oxygen concentration if the sample is for blood gas analysis. If this has just been changed, allow time for equilibration (10 minutes without lung disease, up to 30 minutes with lung disease).[15]
3. Explain the procedure to the alert patient.

PERSONNEL AND EQUIPMENT

1. One physician, nurse, or technician trained in arterial puncture. An assistant should be available to compress the artery after the procedure.
2. Principal implements: 5-ml glass syringe with a plunger

that slides freely,* 21- to 23-gauge needles, a rubber or steel syringe cap, and heparin (1000 units/ml solution).

3. A disinfectant swab and 2-inch gauze pad.
4. Lidocaine, 1%, 1 or 2 ml, a 3-ml syringe, and a 25-gauge needle.
5. A cup containing ice water to hold the specimen.

■ TECHNIQUE FOR RADIAL ARTERY PUNCTURE

1. Place the patient in a comfortable position, either seated or supine. The Po_2 is normally lower in the supine, as compared with upright, posture and may vary substantially between the two lateral decubitus positions when asymmetric lung disease is present.[17]
2. Place the patient's arm on a flat surface.
3. Extend the wrist 30 to 45 degrees (a rolled towel under the wrist may be helpful).
4. Palpate the artery and note its course 1 or 2 cm proximal to the wrist crease (Fig. 33-1).
5. Cleanse the overlying skin with an antiseptic swab.
6. Anesthetize the skin at the puncture site, using approximately 0.5 ml of lidocaine solution and taking care not to inject into the vessel (Fig. 33-2). Arterial punc-

*Plastic syringes may be used for blood gas determinations, although gas diffusion through the syringe wall can produce an unacceptable error if the Po_2 is very high or if sample analysis is delayed.[2,8] In addition, the tight-fitting plunger impedes spontaneous blood flow into the syringe, and small air bubbles may be harder to expel than from a glass syringe.[16]

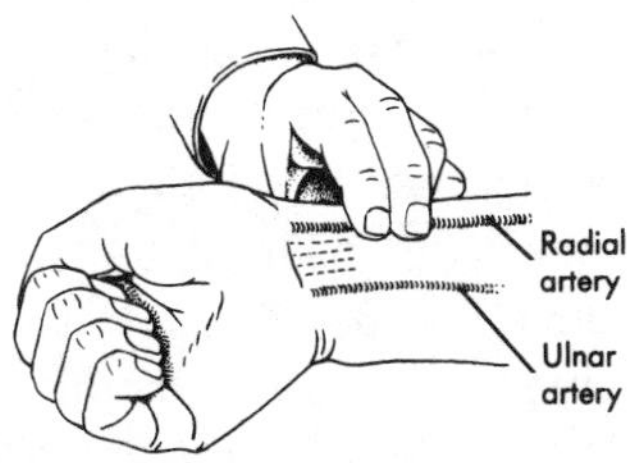

FIG. 33-1. Radial artery puncture technique. Localization of artery by palpation.

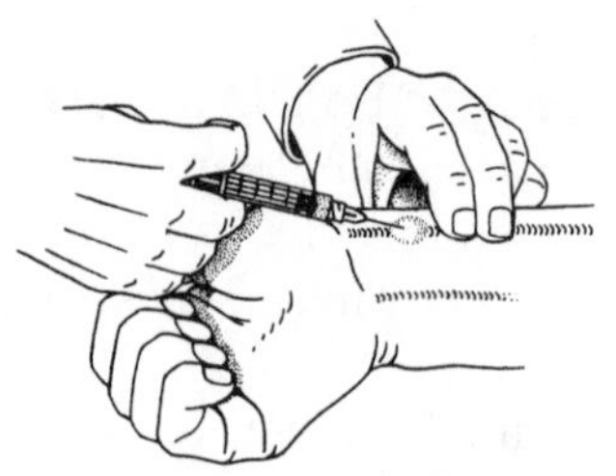

FIG. 33-2. Local infiltration with anesthetic.

ture without anesthesia causes relatively mild discomfort, provided the needle enters the artery in one deft pass. The procedure becomes more painful when, as commonly happens, this is not achieved. Most patients who have had repeated arterial puncture prefer local anesthesia. Another suggested advantage of anesthesia is that it might reduce any tendency of the patient to hyperventilate or breath hold in response to pain or apprehension; however, two studies have failed to show a change of P_{CO_2} during unanesthetized punctures.[3,11]

7. Draw 1 ml of heparin solution into the syringe, wet the entire inner surface of the barrel, then point the needle upward, and expel air and heparin until only the dead space of the syringe and needle remains filled. Heparin solution alters blood gas values by dilution and ideally should be limited to the minimum volume needed to prevent coagulation.[4,5,8] The expected changes include a reduction of P_{CO_2}, a rise in P_{O_2} (a decrease if the true P_{O_2} exceeds 200 torr), and a slight reduction of pH level. These errors become negligible if at least 3 ml of blood are added to a properly prepared syringe.
8. Hold the syringe like a pencil with the needle at 45 degrees to the skin, pointed proximally and aligned with the artery (Fig. 33-3).
9. Pierce the skin and advance steadily toward the vessel until blood enters the syringe (Fig. 33-3).
10. If the syringe does not fill, despite adequate penetration, withdraw the needle slowly and watch for blood

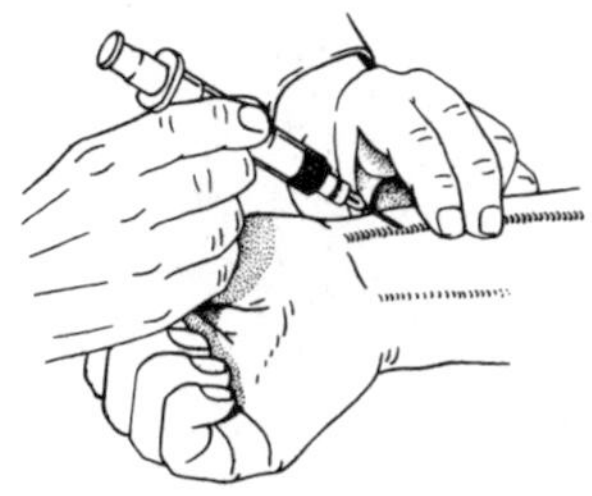

FIG. 33-3. Collection of arterial sample.

return. Should this fail, remove the needle and relocate the pulse. Then check that the needle contains no clot and try again. Avoid pulling on the syringe plunger, because this may spoil the syringe with aspirated venous blood or air.

11. Collect 3 to 5 ml of arterial blood. Although 1 or 2 ml provides an adequate volume for contemporary blood gas analyzers, the larger sample minimizes the effect of heparin solution on blood gas results and permits duplicate analysis of the same sample when desired.
12. Expel any air bubbles from the syringe while holding its tip upward. Small bubbles will not affect results if removed before the sample is agitated or stored.[7,12]
13. Cap the syringe tightly and immerse it immediately in ice water. This inhibits the metabolic consumption of oxygen in the sample and is particularly important when leukocyte or platelet counts are markedly elevated.[2,6]
14. Send the sample for prompt analysis.

TECHNIQUE FOR BRACHIAL ARTERY PUNCTURE

Position the patient with the arm fully extended at the elbow. Locate the artery just proximal to the elbow crease and medial to the biceps tendon (Fig. 33-4). The technique is otherwise the same as for radial puncture.

TECHNIQUE FOR FEMORAL ARTERY PUNCTURE

Have the patient lie supine with the leg mildly abducted and externally rotated. Locate the artery 2 cm distal to the

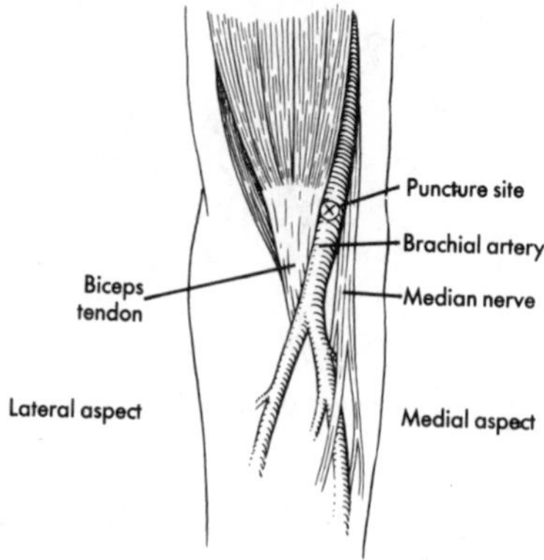

FIG. 33-4. Anatomic site for brachial artery puncture. Approximate point of entry into vessel is indicated with *X*.

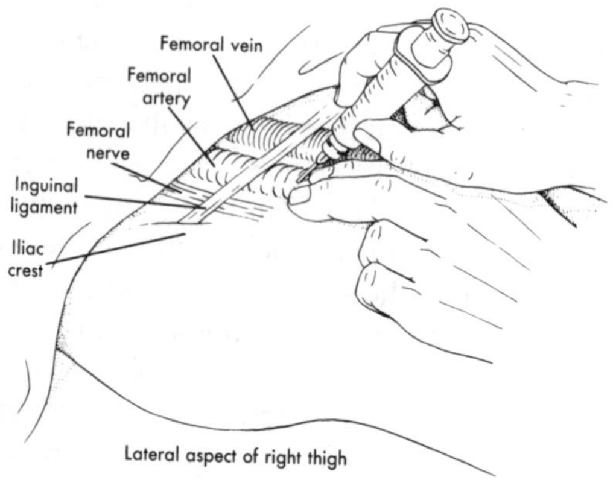

FIG. 33-5. Technique of femoral artery puncture. First two fingers of free hand are used to palpate femoral artery.

inguinal ligament (Fig. 33-5). The technique is otherwise the same as for arterial puncture.

■ POSTPROCEDURE CARE

Either an assistant or the patient should exert moderate pressure over the puncture site for 3 to 5 minutes (vessel occlusion should be avoided). Longer compression is required in patients with a bleeding tendency.

■ COMPLICATIONS

Arterial puncture is a remarkably safe procedure when carefully performed; important complications are seldom encountered.[9,14]

1. Hematoma. Deep hematomas are rare but can develop insidiously in patients with bleeding disorders and cause pain, muscle ischemia, or peripheral nerve damage.[13] Superficial hematomas occur more commonly but are unimportant.
2. Thrombosis.
3. Distal embolization of a dislodged thrombus or plaque.
4. Vasovagal reaction (rare).
5. Hypersensitivity reaction to local anesthetic (rare).
6. Infection (rare, associated with repeated punctures and hematoma formation).
7. Aneurysm formation (a possible but rare sequela of repeated puncture, reported once in a radial artery that was also cannulated).[10]

REFERENCES

1. Coleman, S.S., and Anson, B.J.: Arterial patterns in the hand based upon a study of 650 specimens, Surg. Gynecol. Obstet. **113:**409-424, 1961.
2. Fletcher, G., and Barber, J.L.: Effect of sampling technique on the determination of P_{AO_2} during oxygen breathing, J. Appl. Physiol. **21:**463-468, 1966.
3. Glauser, F.L., and Morris, J.F.: Accuracy of routine arterial puncture for the determination of oxygen and carbon dioxide tensions, Am. Rev. Respir. Dis. **106:**776-779, 1972.
4. Hamilton, R.D., Crockett, A.J., and Alpers, J.H.: Arterial blood gas analysis: potential errors due to the addition of heparin, Anaesth. Intensive Care **6:**251-255, 1978.
5. Hansen, J.E., and Simmons, D.H.: A systematic error in the determination of blood P_{CO_2}, Am. Rev. Respir. Dis. **115:**1061-1063, 1977.
6. Hess, C.E., Nichols, A.B., Hunt, W.B., and Suratt, P.M.: Pseudohypoxemia secondary to leukemia and thrombocytosis, N. Engl. J. Med. **301:**361-363, 1979.
7. Ishikawa, S., Fornier, A., Borst, C., and Segal, M.S.: The effects of air bubbles and time delay on blood gas analysis, Ann. Allergy **33:**72-77, 1974.
8. Janis, K.M., and Fletcher, G.: Oxygen tension measurements in small samples, Am. Rev. Respir. Dis. **106:**914-916, 1972.
9. Lindesmith, L.A., Winga, E.R., Goodnough, D.E., and Paradise, R.A.: Arterial punctures by inhalation therapy personnel, Chest **61:**83-84, 1972.
10. Mathieu, A., Dalton, B., Fischer, J.E., and Kumar, A.: Expanding aneu-

rysm of the radial artery after frequent puncture, Anesthesiology **38:**401-403, 1973.

11. Morgan, E.J., Baidwan, B., Petty, T.L., and Zwillich, C.W.: The effects of unanesthetized arterial puncture on Pco_2 and pH, Am. Rev. Respir. Dis. **120:**795-798, 1979.
12. Mueller, R.G., Lang, G.E., and Beam, J.M.: Bubbles in samples for blood gas determinations, Am. J. Clin. Pathol. **65:**242-249, 1976.
13. Neviaser, R.J., Adams, J.P., and May, G.I.: Complications of arterial puncture in antigoagulated patients, J. Bone Joint Surg. **58-A:**218-220, 1976.
14. Petty, T.L., Bigelow, B., and Levine, B.E.: The simplicity and safety of arterial puncture, J.A.M.A. **195:**693-695, 1966.
15. Sherter, C.B., Jabbour, S.M., Kovnat, D.M., and Snider, G.L.: Prolonged rate of decay of arterial Po_2 following oxygen breathing in chronic airways obstruction, Chest **67:**259-261, 1975.
16. Winkler, J.B., Huntingtion, C.G., Wells, D.E., and Befeler, B.: Influence of syringe material on arterial blood gas determinations, Chest **66:**518-521, 1974.
17. Zack, M.B., Pontoppidan, H., and Kazemi, H.: The effect of lateral positions on gas exchange in pulmonary disease, Am. Rev. Respir. Dis. **110:** 49-55, 1974.

CHAPTER 34

Endotracheal intubation

■ Paul M. Suratt
Robert S. Gibson
John W. Hoyt

■ GENERAL CONSIDERATIONS

Insertion of an endotracheal tube allows a patient to receive positive pressure ventilation with a hand-held bag or a mechanical ventilator and to have the airway suctioned and protected from aspiration.

■ INDICATIONS

1. Cardiopulmonary arrest.
2. Respiratory failure necessitating mechanical ventillation. The indications for mechanical ventilation will vary with each patient.[5] One general indication for ventilation is an acutely elevated pCO_2 and a lowered pH level in an exhausted, somnambulant, or weak patient. This will include patients with asthma or chronic obstructive pulmonary disease who have become fatigued while struggling to breath, patients with muscle weakness or drug overdose, and postoperative patients who still have drug-related respiratory tract depression. Another general indication for ventilation is when a patient's pO_2 falls to less than 55 mm Hg despite the administration of 50% oxygen. This may occur in patients with overwhelming pneumonia or pulmonary edema.
3. The poorly responsive patient who may vomit and aspirate.
4. Temporary need for bronchial suctioning to remove secretions.

CONTRAINDICATIONS (RELATIVE)

1. Upper airway foreign bodies.
2. Laryngeal trauma.
3. Laryngeal edema with acute laryngitis.
4. Nasotracheal intubation is contraindicated in basilar skull fractures.

PATIENT EVALUATION AND PREPARATION

Explain the procedure if the patient is conscious.

PERSONNEL AND EQUIPMENT

1. One physician trained and experienced in endotracheal intubation and one assistant familiar with the equipment.
2. Principal implements: an endotracheal tube, a laryngoscope, a stylet, a 10-ml syringe to inflate the cuff, a lubricant, an oral airway, and Magill forceps.
3. Suction apparatus.
4. An oxygen source and resuscitation equipment, including a bag and mask for ventilation.
5. Lidocaine, 1%, 10 ml, in a spray apparatus if the patient is conscious.

ROUTE OF INSERTION AND TUBE SELECTION

The choice of tube size and insertion site is based on the considerations listed in Table 34-1. Choose the tube with the largest diameter that the patient can tolerate comfortably. To decrease tracheal injury, select a tube with a soft cuff that exerts little pressure on the tracheal mucosa.

TECHNIQUE FOR ORAL TRACHEAL TUBE INSERTION[1,4]

1. Clear the airway of secretions, vomitus, dentures, etc.
2. Ventilate the patient with 100% oxygen using a bag and mask if the patient is apneic, hypoxic, or hypercarbic.
3. Select an endotracheal tube and check the balloon cuff for leaks. Deflate the cuff and lubricate the distal end, including the cuff.

TABLE 34-1. ADVANTAGES AND DISADVANTAGES OF NASOTRACHEAL AND OROTRACHEAL INTUBATION

Tube	Usual size	Advantage	Disadvantage
Nasotracheal	7	Tolerated better by patient; when secured with tape, it is less likely to pull out accidentally	Increased resistance to airflow because of longer length and narrower diameter
		Mouth care easier to administer	Contraindicated with basilar skull fracture because insertion may push bacteria into subarachnoid space
			Higher frequency of bacteremia[2] and sinusitis
Orotracheal	8	Less resistance to airflow because of shorter length and diameter	May kink behind tongue or occlude if patient clenches teeth without bite block
		Can perform fiberoptic bronchoscopy through tube if it is a number 8 or larger size	Initially less comfortable for patient

4. Anesthetize the pharynx and larynx if the patient is awake.
5. Position the patient's head on a 4-inch (10-cm) pillow or pad in a slightly extended position (Fig. 34-1).
6. Open the mouth by extending the jaw with your right hand. Hold the laryngoscope with your left hand and insert the blade in the right side of the mouth so that it pushes the tongue to the left. Advance the blade until the epiglottis appears. If the blade has been advanced deep into the throat, yet the epiglottis is still not visible, the blade may have passed the epiglottis and entered the esophagus. In this case, pull back slowly on the blade and the epiglottis may flop into view. When using a curved blade, place it in the space between the epiglottis and the base of the tongue known as the vallecula (Fig. 34-1). When using a straight blade, place it just beyond the epiglottis (Fig. 34-2).

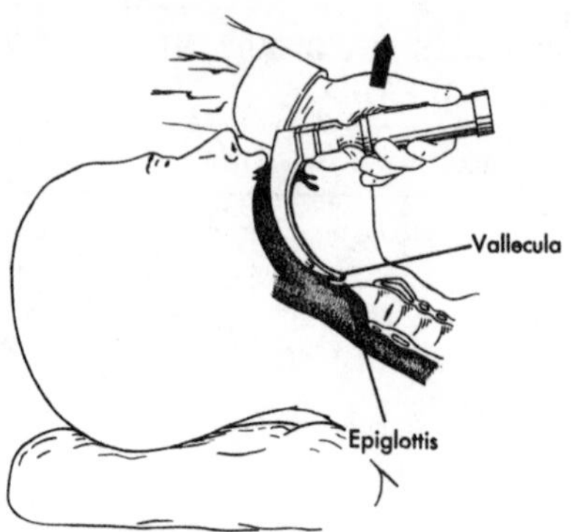

FIG. 34-1. Proper head position for intubation. Tip of curved laryngoscope blade placed in vallecula. Arrow shows direction laryngoscope should be lifted to expose larynx.

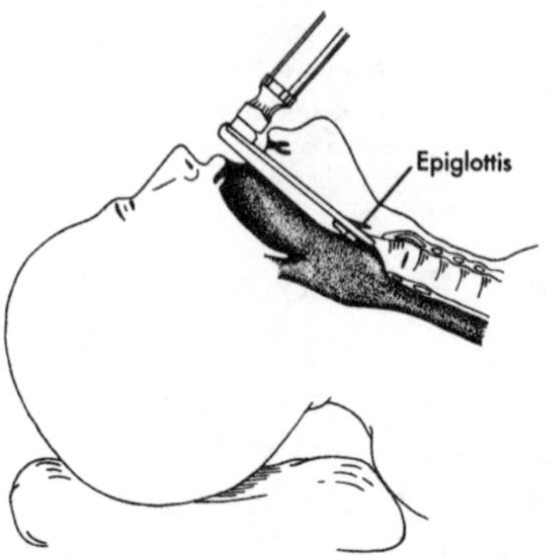

FIG. 34-2. Placement of tip of straight laryngoscope blade.

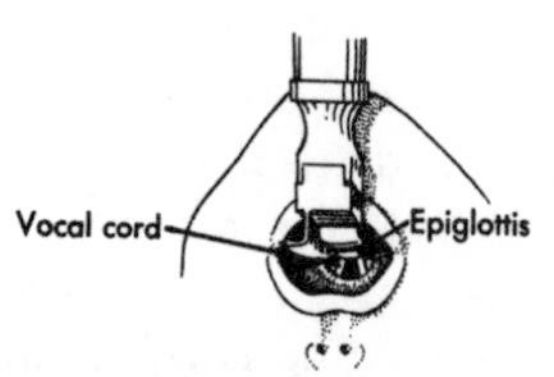

FIG. 34-3. View of larynx from mouth.

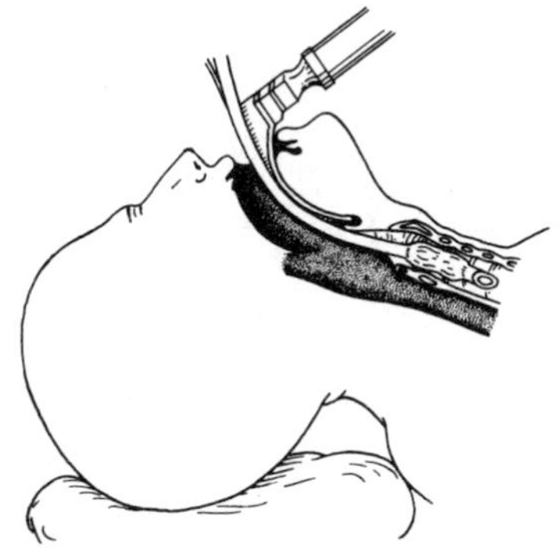

FIG. 34-4. Insertion of endotracheal tube.

7. Expose the larynx (Fig. 34-3) by lifting the laryngoscope handle with your left arm and shoulder upward and forward (Fig. 34-1). Hold your wrist rigid during this maneuver and do not rotate the tip of the blade upward while using the teeth as a fulcrum. If the larynx cannot be seen despite proper head and blade position, have an assistant push down on the thyroid cartilage; this will usually bring the larynx into view.
8. Place the endotracheal tube into the trachea by holding it in your right hand with its tip pointed up and toward the right. Insert it in the mouth and slide it along the right side into the trachea until the cuff just disappears beyond the larynx (Fig. 34-4). If the tube cannot be inserted because the tip flexes in the wrong direction in the pharynx, remove the tube and insert the stylet in it. Bend the tube and the stylet in the proper curvature, usually the natural curvature of the tube, and try again.
9. Attach a ventilation bag to the endotracheal tube and resume ventilation immediately.
10. Inflate the cuff just enough so that no leak is heard when auscultating the neck during ventilation.
11. Auscultate the patient's chest for bilateral equality of breath sounds.
12. Slide a bite block over the tube if the patient is agitated and may bite and occlude the tube.

13. Tape the tube securely in place to prevent it from sliding out of the trachea or down into a mainstem bronchus.

■ TECHNIQUE FOR NASOTRACHEAL TUBE INSERTION

1. Clear the airway of secretions and vomitus and remove dentures.
2. Ventilate the patient with 100% oxygen using a hand-held bag and mask if the patient is apneic, hypoxic, or hypercarbic.
3. Select an endotracheal tube and check the balloon cuff for leaks. Deflate the cuff and lubricate the distal end, including the cuff.
4. Spray the nostril with 0.5% phenylephrine and with lidocaine (Xylocaine) if the patient is awake.
5. Hold the tube so that its curvature conforms to the curvature of the nose and throat.
6. Insert the tip of the tube in the nose and advance it gently but firmly. When the tube enters the nasopharynx one can usually feel it pop and will hear more air moving through it.
7. Extend the head and hold it in the midline.
8. Advance the tube only during inspiration while listening to breath sounds through the tube. If breath sounds become fainter the tube may be in a piriform sinus or the esophagus. Withdraw the tube, rotate it, and try again. When the tube touches the epiglottis the patient will cough, indicating that it is properly positioned. After the cough the patient will inspire and at that time firmly push the tube into the trachea. Breath sounds will be louder through the tube when it is in the trachea. Advance the tube approximately 4 cm farther. If the trachea cannot be entered, try rotating the patient's head to the left or right or flexing the head. If the trachea still cannot be entered, use a laryngoscope to visualize the larynx and pass the tube with Magill forceps.
9. Resume ventilation with a hand-held bag immediately.
10. Inflate the cuff just enough so that no leak is heard

when auscultating the patient's neck during ventilation.

11. Auscultate the patient's chest for bilateral equality of breath sounds.
12. Tape the tube in place to prevent displacement upward out of the trachea or downward into a mainstem bronchus.

■ TUBE REMOVAL

Have a laryngoscope present in case the tube needs to be reinserted. Suction the patient thoroughly and provide hyperventilation with 100% oxygen using a hand ventilation bag. Deflate the cuff and remove the tube during inspiration. Administration of nebulized or humidified air or oxygen following extubation may decrease laryngeal edema.

■ POSTPROCEDURE CARE

1. Obtain a chest roentgenogram to ensure that the tip of tube is 2 or 3 cm above the carina.
2. Write orders for nurses to check the tube position and cuff inflation about every hour. Also specify the frequency of endotracheal suctioning.

■ COMPLICATIONS DURING INTUBATION[3]

1. Traumic lacerations of the mouth, pharynx, larynx, or esophagus, and broken or dislodged teeth.
2. Endobronchial or esophageal intubation.[7]
3. Aspiration.
4. Cardiac arrhythmias.

■ COMPLICATIONS WITH TUBE IN PLACE

1. Tracheal necrosis, which may lead to tracheal stenosis. Necrosis is related to the pressure in the cuff, the number of days it is in place, the peak inspiratory pressure, and the characteristics of the cuff.[3,6]
2. Laryngeal trauma.

■ LATE COMPLICATIONS

Tracheal stenosis may occur as a late complication.

REFERENCES

1. Applebaum, E.L., and Bruce, D.L.: Tracheal intubation, Philadelphia, 1976, W.B. Saunders Co.
2. Berry, F.A., Blankenbaker, W.L., and Ball, C.G.: A comparison of bacteremia occurring with nasotracheal and orotracheal intubation, Anesth. Analg. **52**:873-876, 1973.
3. Blanc, V.F., and Tremblay, N.A.G.: The complications of tracheal intubation, Anesth. Analg. **53**:202-213, 1974.
4. Dripps, R.D., Eckenhoff, J.E., and Vandam, L.D.: Introduction to anesthesia. Principles of safe practice, Philadelphia, 1977, W.B. Saunders Co.
5. Sykes, M.K., McNicol, M.W., and Campbell, E.J.M.: Respiratory failure, Oxford, 1976, Blackwell Scientific Publications, Inc.
6. Weber, A.L., and Grillo, H.C.: Tracheal stenosis. An analysis of 151 cases. Radiol. Clin. North Am. **16**:291-308, 1978.
7. Zwillich, C.W., Pierson, D.J., Creagh, C.E., Sulton, F.D., Schatz, E., and Petty, T.L.: Complications of assisted ventilation. A prospective study of 354 consecutive episodes,Am. J. Med. **57**:161-170, 1974.

CHAPTER 35

Esophageal obturator airway insertion

John W. Hoyt
Robert S. Gibson
Paul M. Suratt

GENERAL CONSIDERATIONS

The esophageal obturator airway (EOA) is used to rapidly establish an airway in nonbreathing unconscious patients. Its design prevents aspiration of stomach contents and gastric dilation during ventilation (Fig. 35-1).[1-5,7-10] Since insertion of the EOA requires less skill than endotracheal intubation, the EOA can be used by specially trained paramedical personnel. The trachea cannot be suctioned through an EOA; therefore an EOA should be used only until skilled personnel are available who can insert an endotracheal tube.

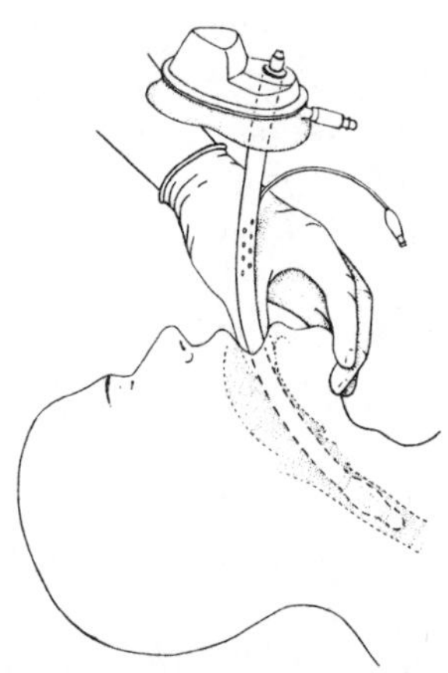

FIG. 35-1. Assembled EOA, proper head position, lifting jaw up and out with thumb, and EOA insertion.

■ INDICATION

Esophageal obturator airway insertion is indicated when a skilled person is not available to insert an endotracheal tube in an unconscious patient in respiratory or cardiorespiratory arrest.

■ CONTRAINDICATIONS

1. Adults less than 5 feet (150 cm) tall, since there is only one size EOA, and, in such a patient, it might be inflated in the stomach. Also smaller people might be more prone to develop esophageal perforation from the EOA cuff.
2. Children because they have a small esophagus.
3. Patients who have ingested a corrosive liquid such as lye.
4. Patients with known esophageal disease, such as cancer, stenosis, or varices.

■ PATIENT EVALUATION AND PREPARATION

None are necessary, since insertion of an EOA is an emergency procedure.

■ PERSONNEL AND EQUIPMENT

1. Trained medical or paramedical personnel.
2. Principal implements; an EOA with an inflatable mask, a syringe (35 ml), and a sterile lubricant.
3. Suction apparatus.
4. A hand ventilation bag with oxygen source.

■ TECHNIQUE FOR INSERTION

1. Attach the face mask to the proximal 15-mm adapter of the EOA (Fig. 35-1).
2. Lubricate the obturator tip.
3. Check the hand ventilation bag for oxygen flow and ability to hold pressure.
4. Check the inflation of the EOA mask.
5. Open the mouth of the unconscious patient and clear the upper airway of secretions, vomitus, dentures, etc.

6. Place the head in a neutral position. *Do not hyperextend head,* since this will disrupt the natural curves of the pharynx and increase the risk of accidental tracheal intubation.
7. Put your left thumb on the patient's lower teeth with your fingers under the chin; lift the jaw up and out.
8. Insert the EOA into the mouth and over the tongue (Fig. 35-1). Advance it gently by feel into the pharynx and down the esophagus until the mask is flush with the face. The EOA should glide smoothly into the esophagus; if it does not, do not attempt a second insertion without first performing mouth-to-mouth ventilation.
9. Place your left hand on the mask with your thumb on top, your index finger on the bottom, and your other fingers under the chin. Maneuver the mask up and down and to the side until a good tight fit is achieved.
10. Deliver a large breath through the 15 mm adapter and watch the chest for a moment. If a rise and fall is not observed, remove the EOA immediately, since it may be in the trachea instead of the esophagus. Before attempting insertion again, perform mouth-to-mouth ventilation.
11. If the chest does expand, attach the 35-ml syringe filled with air to the one-way valve and inflate the EOA cuff (Fig. 35-2). Disconnect the syringe from the one-way valve.

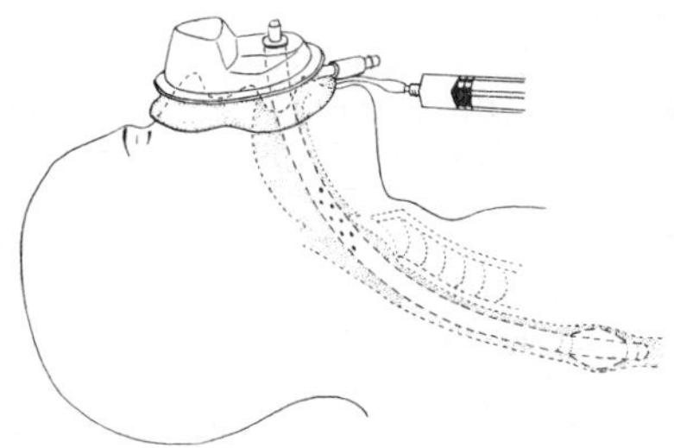

FIG. 35-2. Inflating EOA when tube and mask are properly positioned.

12. Begin hand ventilation, watching for chest expansion. The mask must fit well for this technique to work.

■ TECHNIQUE FOR REMOVAL

1. If the patient is not alert, an endotracheal tube should be placed before the EOA is removed to protect the airway from reflex vomiting. The mask is removed and the obturator slid to the *left* side of the mouth. A laryngoscope is inserted into the *right* side of the mouth to visualize the trachea. After the endotracheal tube has been passed, inflate its cuff to protect the airway. The EOA cuff may now be deflated and the obturator removed without risk of aspiration.
2. If the patient becomes alert and does not need assisted ventilation, the EOA should be removed. This can be dangerous because EOA removal may cause regurgitation and aspiration. The EOA should only be removed with the *patient on the side* and *suction available.* Remember to deflate the EOA cuff before pulling it out of the esophagus.

■ COMPLICATIONS

1. Insertion of the obturator into the trachea instead of the esophagus.[10]
2. Aspiration of gastric contents during removal of the EOA.
3. Perforation of the esophagus, usually associated with removal of the EOA before deflating the cuff.[8,11,12]

REFERENCES

1. Don Michael, T.A.A., and Gordon, A.S.: Esophageal obturator airway: a new adjunct for artificial ventilation. Read before the National Conference on Standards for Cardiopulmonary Resuscitation and Emergency Cardiac Care, Washington, D.C., May 16, 1973.
2. Don Michael, T.A., Lambert, E.H., and Mehran, A.: Mouth to lung airway for cardiac resuscitation, Lancet **2:**1329, 1968.
3. Fairley, M.: The esophageal obturator airway, Respir. Ther. **3:**95-99, 1973.
4. Greenbaum, D., Poggi, J., and Grace, W.J.: Esophageal obstruction during oxygen administration: a new method for use in resuscitation, Chest **65:**188-191, 1974.

5. Johnston, K.R., Genovesi, M.G., and Lassar, K.H.: Esophageal obturator airway: use and complications, JACEP **5:**36-39, 1976.
6. Scholl, D.G., and Tsai, S.H.: Esophageal perforation following the use of esophageal obturator airway, Radiology **122:**315-316, 1977.
7. Schotferman, J., Dill, P., and Lewis, A.J.: The esophageal obturator airway: a clinical evaluation, Chest **69:**67-71, 1976.
8. Smock, S.: Esophageal obturator airway: preferred CPR technique, JACEP **4:**232-233, 1975.
9. Standards for cardiopulmonary resuscitation (CPR) and emergency cardiac care (ECC), National Conference on Cardiopulmonary Resuscitation (CPR) and Emergency Cardiac Care, J.A.M.A. **227:**837-868, 1974.
10. Standards and guidelines for cardiopulmonary resuscitation (CPR) and emergency cardiac care (ECC), National Conference on Cardiopulmonary Resuscitation (CPR) and Emergency Cardiac Care, J.A.M.A. **224:** 453-509, 1980.
11. Strate, R.G., and Fischer, R.P.: Midesophageal perforations by esophageal obturator airways, J. Trauma **16:**503-509, 1976.
12. Walloch, Y., Zer, M., and Dintsman, M., et al.: Iatrogenic perforations of the esophagus, Arch. Surg. **108:**357-360, 1974.

CHAPTER 36

Emergency treatment of the obstructed airway

■ Richard F. Edlich

■ GENERAL CONSIDERATIONS

Early recognition of acute extrathoracic airway obstruction is mandatory. In most cases, there is a clear-cut history of foreign body, allergic reaction, trauma, or tumor that accounts for the problem. In the conscious victim, airway obstruction by a *foreign body* is generally recognized when a victim who is eating becomes unable to speak or cough.[2,4] The victim attempts to breathe using accessory muscles of respiration without significant air exchange. The victim who has seen the universal distress signal for airway obstruction will clutch the neck over the laryngotracheal complex between the thumb and index finger, thereby signaling for help. An observer should ask "Are you choking?" The victim will be unable to speak but will usually nod yes. Without treatment the victim will quickly become cyanotic and then lose consciousness.

In the *unconscious supine patient* airway obstruction may occur when a relaxed tongue falls against the posterior larynx. To detect airway obstruction in an unconscious patient, listen and feel for air movement at the mouth as well as look for movement of the chest. Movement of the chest is not as reliable a sign of adequate ventilation as hearing and feeling air movement, since with complete airway obstruction the victim may expand and compress his chest without moving air.

Trauma can cause airway obstruction by a number of mechanisms. Wounds of the mouth, pharynx, or larynx may cause hemorrhage that obstructs airflow. Blunt trauma to the neck, especially the "clothesline" injury, can cause damage to the laryngotracheal complex, major vessels, or spinal trauma without breaking the skin. Cervical spine injuries with vertebral subluxation and retropharyngeal hematoma also result in airway obstruction. Shotgun and missile injuries may result in extensive damage to the upper airway and major vessels, as well as overlying skin. Aspiration of a foreign body during the accident must always be considered as a cause of airway obstruction.

Laryngeal edema is usually heralded by stridor, a coarse high pitched rasping sound heard usually during inspiration. When laryngeal edema occurs as part of anaphylaxis the patient may be hypotensive and have urticaria.

Tumors may also cause airway obstruction but the onset of obstruction is usually over days or weeks. Hemoptysis may occur with this condition. The presence of stridor and hoarseness for a long period of time is consistent with the diagnosis of tumor. The treatment of tumors is beyond the scope of this book and will not be discussed.

Infections are an uncommon cause of airway obstruction in adults in contrast to children.

■ INDICATIONS FOR TREATMENT

1. Complete airway obstruction. A conscious patient with complete airway obstruction will be unable to speak and may grasp the throat between the thumb and index finger. In an unconscious patient one will be unable to hear or feel air movement at the mouth and there may be no movement of the chest.
2. Incomplete airway obstruction with inadequate ventilation. Stridor with inability to cough are the signs of this condition.

■ CONTRAINDICATIONS

If the patient is alert and can talk or cough effectively, it can be assumed that the patient has no ventilatory disturbance which imposes an immediate threat to life.

■ TECHNIQUE FOR PARTIAL AIRWAY OBSTRUCTION WITH ADEQUATE VENTILATION

Allow the patient to cough and expel the foreign body.

■ TECHNIQUE FOR COMPLETE OR PARTIAL AIRWAY OBSTRUCTION WITH INADEQUATE VENTILATION AND NO TRAUMA[2,4]

1. Manual thrusts are indicated in the conscious patient with complete airway obstruction resulting in respiratory distress. They increase intrathoracic pressure and "blow" the obstruction out of the airway. In a pregnant woman, patients with a suspected abdominal injury, and children below the age of 8, go to step 8. In the unconscious patient go to step 4.
2. For an abdominal thrust, position yourself behind the standing patient and wrap your arms under the victim's axilla and around the waist. Place the thumb side of one fist against the victim's upper abdomen, between the navel and rib cage. Grasp your fist with your other hand (Fig. 36-1) and press your fist four times into the victim's abdomen with quick inward and upward thrusts. It may be necessary to repeat the abdominal thrust as many as six times, each time with increasing force, to dislodge the obstructing object from the airway. The first thrust is often a tentative one, whereby you gauge the force that is necessary to dislodge the foreign body.
3. If the foreign body is unresponsive to these manual thrusts and the victim becomes unconscious, gently position the patient supine on a hard surface.
4. Perform the head-tilt neck-lift maneuver by placing one hand on the forehead and applying firm backward pressure with the palm and the other hand beneath the neck to lift and support it (Fig. 36-2). If the patient is not breathing (listen, feel, look) attempt to ventilate the patient (four times) by pinching the nose, taking a deep breath, and blowing it into the mouth (Fig. 36-3). If a self-inflating bag mask ventilator connected to an oxygen outlet is available, use it rather than mouth-to-mouth ventilation.
5. If air cannot be blown into the subject's mouth, the airway is still obstructed and a head-tilt and chin-lift

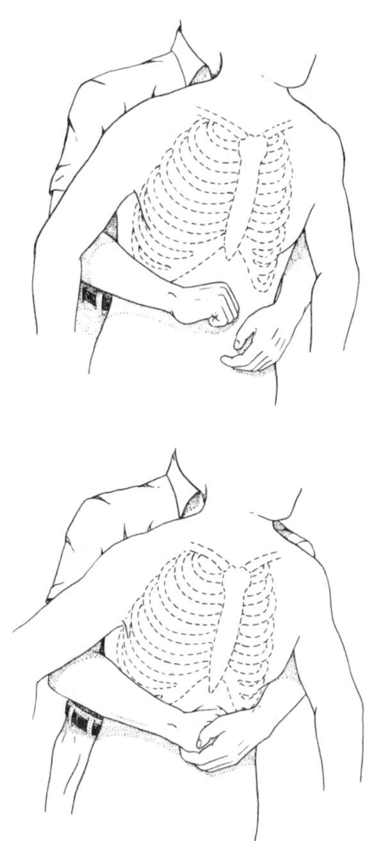

FIG. 36-1. Abdominal thrust.

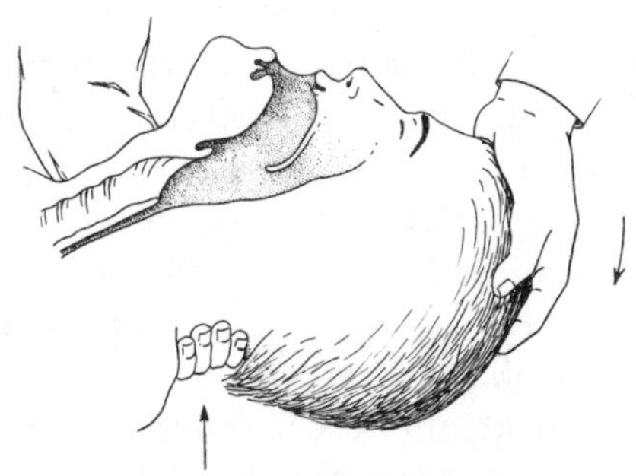

FIG. 36-2. Head-tilt neck-lift maneuver.

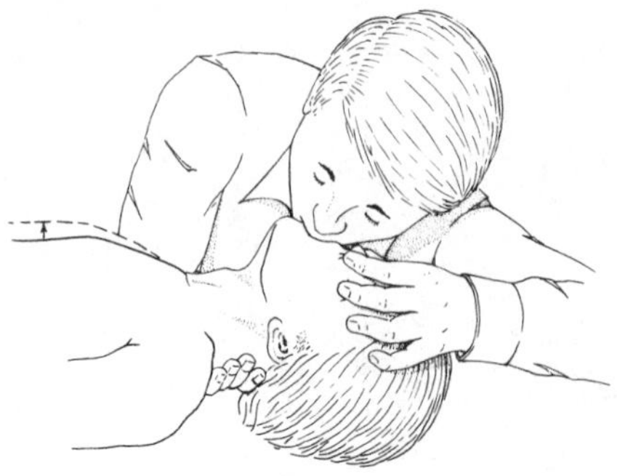

FIG. 36-3. Mouth-to-mouth ventilation. Look to see whether chest rises with ventilation.

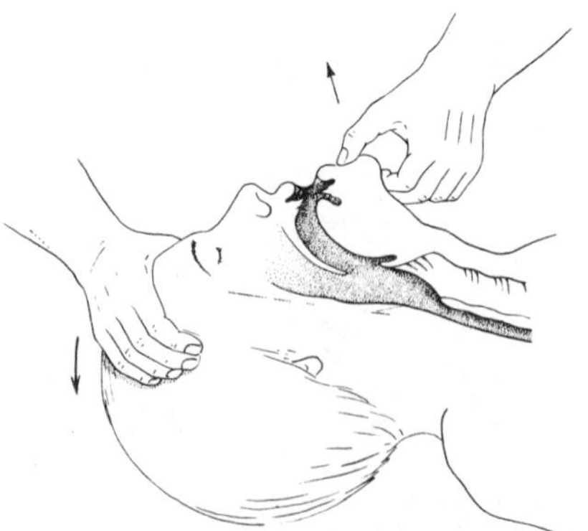

FIG. 36-4. Head-tilt chin-lift maneuver.

maneuver should be performed. Tilt the head with one hand and with the fingers of the other hand lift the chin until the teeth are almost touching (Fig. 36-4). If necessary, use your thumb to keep the lips open. Again attempt to administer four quick breaths.

6. If the patient still cannot be ventilated, kneel astride the victim's hip and place the heel of one hand against the victim's abdomen, slightly above the navel and below the xiphoid. After placing your other hand on top of your first hand, press into the abdomen with a quick upward thrust. Repeat this manual thrust four times.

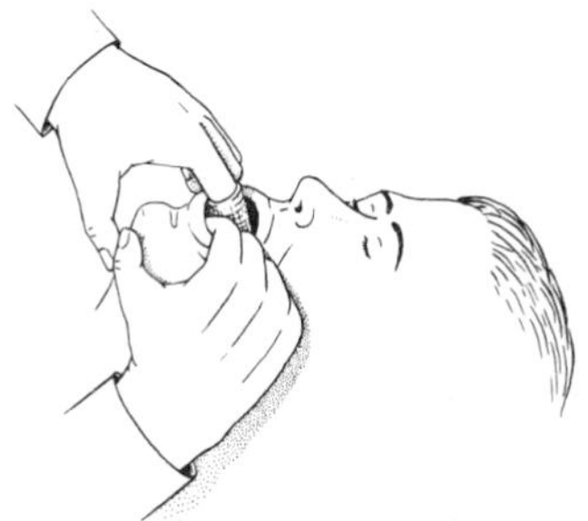

FIG. 36-5. Tongue-jaw lift maneuver.

7. Use the tongue-jaw lift maneuver to remove any foreign body that may have been expelled from the airway. Open the victim's mouth by grasping both the tongue and lower jaw between your thumb and index finger of one hand and lift the tongue and mandible anteriorly (Fig. 36-5). This maneuver draws the tongue away from the pharynx and allows the index finger of your hand to sweep the back of the throat in an effort to remove or dislodge the foreign body. We recommend removal of dentures to facilitate the performance of this technique.
8. A chest-thrust maneuver, rather than an abdominal thrust should be performed in a pregnant woman, patients with a suspected abdominal injury, and children below the age of 8. Position yourself behind the patient, placing your arms under the victim's axilla and around the chest. Place the thumb side of one fist on the middle of the sternum. Then grasp your fist with your other hand and exert backward thrusts with the intent of relieving the obstruction. This is similar to the abdominal thrust (Fig. 36-1) except that the thrust is delivered to the sternum. If the victim loses consciousness, position the victim in a supine position on a hard surface. After opening the airway using the head-neck tilt and/or head-neck lift technique, ventilate the patient with four quick breaths. If the patient cannot be ventilated, kneel close to the side of the body and posi-

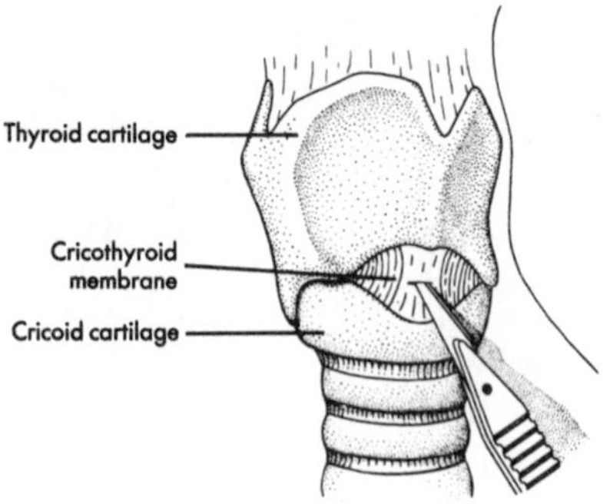

FIG. 36-6. Stab cricothyroid membrane with knife blade.

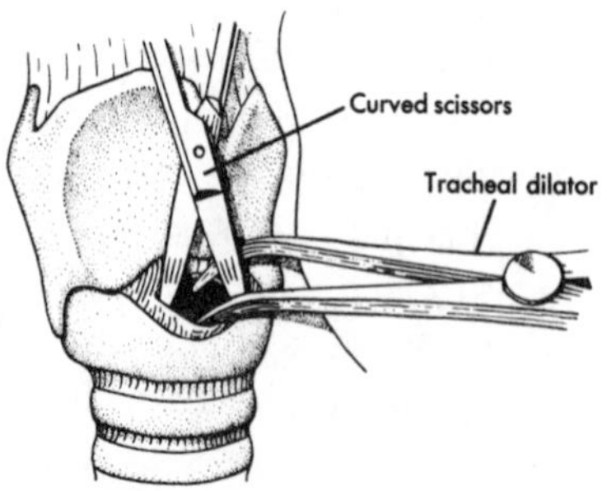

FIG. 36-7. Tracheal dilator spread in caudal-cephalad direction, while curved scissors are spread transversely to widen opening.

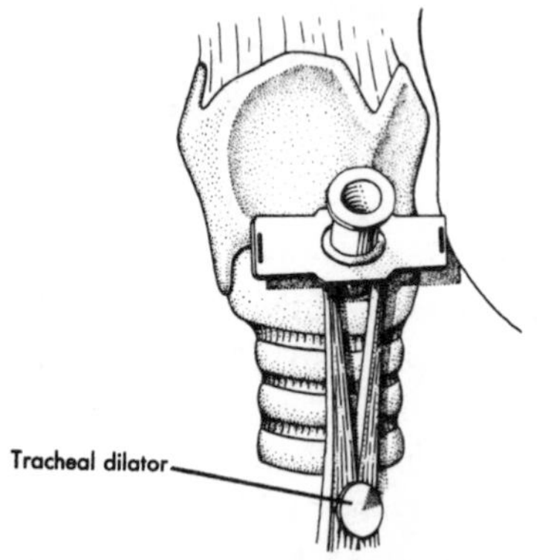

FIG. 36-8. Dilator rotated and tracheostomy tube inserted.

tion your hands on the lower half of the sternum in the same manner as that used to apply external cardiac compression (Fig. 13-3). Then press down four times.

9. If the combined use of the manual thrusts and finger sweep fail to open the airway and a laryngoscope is available, visualize the larynx directly. If a foreign body is identified, it can usually be grasped with a Magill forceps and removed.
10. If the obstruction persists despite these previous interventions, a *cricothyroidotomy* should probably then be performed.[1]
11. Identify the cricothyroid membrane, which is located between the thyroid and cricoid cartilages (Fig. 36-6). The cricothyroid membrane is easily palpable, regardless of how fat the patient's neck is.
12. Hold the skin taut over the cricothyroid membrane and make a stab wound with a number 11 knife blade (Fig. 36-6). An ordinary penknife can even be used to perform the procedure. Even if the knife goes too deep, it will stop harmlessly against the posterior aspect of the cricoid cartilage.
13. Guide a tracheal dilator along the knife blade.
14. After the knife is removed, spread the dilator in a caudal-cephalad direction to separate the two cartilages (Fig. 36-7).
15. Insert curved scissors between the jaws of the dilator and spread them transversely to widen the opening (Fig. 36-7).
16. Rotate the dilator so that its blades are parallel to the trachea (Fig. 36-8).
17. Insert a tracheostomy tube between the blades. Once the tube is in place, it is firmly held in place with cotton tapes that are tied around the neck.
18. In the nonhospital setting it has been suggested that cricothyroidotomy be performed by cutting the cricothyroid membrane with a knife and then inserting a ball-point pen or other tube or even a finger to keep the airway open.[5] We have not, however, found any information that documents the effectiveness of this

method. It has also been suggested that large-bore needles be inserted through the cricothyroid membrane into the trachea. Reports indicate that patients may maintain themselves for several minutes breathing spontaneously through an 11-gauge needle but that if a 14- or 16-gauge needle is used, high-pressure oxygen ventilation is required, and even then some patients will develop carbon dioxide retention.[3]

■ TECHNIQUE FOR TRAUMATIC EXTRATHORACIC AIRWAY OBSTRUCTION

1. Because the patient may have a spinal cord injury, stabilize the head and attempt to open the airway using the jaw thrust without the head-tilt technique. This maneuver is the safest approach to opening the airway, since it usually can be done without extending the neck. Place your index, long, ring, and small fingers of both hands posterior to the angles of the mandible with your thumbs touching the lower lip (Fig. 36-9). By lifting the angles of the mandible, the mandible is elevated anteriorly. If the victim's lips are closed, your thumbs should retract the lower lip, opening the victim's mouth.
2. If this measure does not restore ventilation, factors other than simple airway obstruction should be suspected as the cause of inadequate ventilation. These include severe neurologic injury, thoracic trauma, or extrathoracic

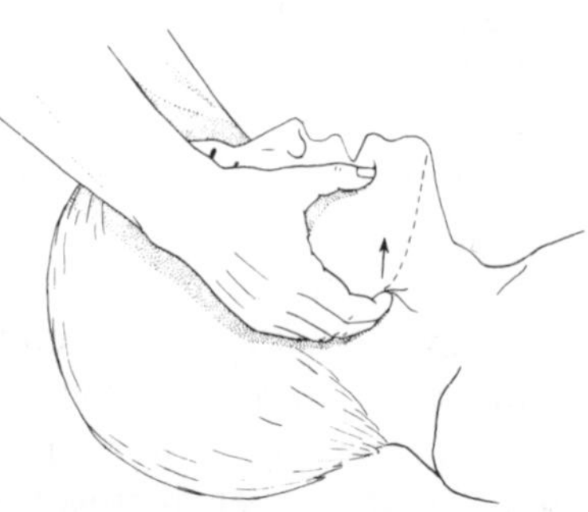

FIG. 36-9. Jaw thrust without head tilt.

airway obstructions. Deliver four quick breaths to the patient, preferably with a self-inflating bag mask ventilator connected to an oxygen outlet, or, if this is not available, with mouth-to-mouth resuscitation. Insertion of an oropharyngeal airway will facilitate maintenance of the airway during ventilation with a bag mask. If you are still unsuccessful in ventilating the unconscious patient, gently reposition the victim's head and try to ventilate again.

3. If the air exchange is still poor, endotracheal intubation should be attempted to establish a patent airway. Suctioning the patient's mouth with a tonsil sucker prior to and during intubation is frequently necessary to remove fluids and debris that limit visualization of the vocal cords and trachea. The pharynx and larynx should be inspected for foreign bodies with Magill forceps close at hand. Partial or complete dentures should be removed prior to intubation. Intubation may be unsuccessful with wounds of the mouth, pharynx, or larynx with severe hemorrhage, since visualization of the upper larynx may be impossible. Fractures of the larynx may cause life-threatening airway obstruction, and orotracheal intubation may occasionally worsen the situation by displacing a mucocartilaginous fragment into the upper trachea. Cervical spine injuries with vertebral subluxation and retropharyngeal hematoma often result in upper airway obstruction that defies management by endotracheal intubation. Foreign bodies in the larynx also preclude intubation for establishment of an airway.
4. If intubation is unsuccessful, a cricothyroidotomy should be performed, providing that the anatomic landmarks are not obscured by swelling or soft tissue injury. In the presence of significant soft tissue swelling, it may be difficult to identify the trachea by palpation or inspection.
5. In such cases, direct a number 13 plastic needle assembly attached to a syringe to the midline at an angle of 95 degrees. During insertion of the needle, negative

pressure is applied to the syringe. Entrance of air within the syringe signifies that the needle is in the trachea.

6. Then insert a knife with a number 11 blade by a "stab" maneuver into the trachea immediately below the needle. The opening in the trachea is lengthened caudally to a point, 1 or 2 cm above the suprasternal notch without division of the thyroid isthmus.
7. Guide a tracheal dilator along the knife blade. After the knife is removed, spread the dilator in a transverse direction to allow insertion of a tracheostomy tube of suitable size into the trachea.

■ LARYNGEAL EDEMA

1. Administer 0.3 mg of epinephrine subcutaneously. This may be repeated every 10 minutes, not to exceed 1 mg in 40 minutes.
2. If the patient is experiencing great difficulty breathing or is becoming cyanotic, insert an endotracheal tube as described in Chapter 34.
3. If intubation cannot be performed, a cricothyroidotomy should be done if the patient becomes unconscious.

REFERENCES

1. Brantigan, C.O., and Grow, J.B., Sr.: Cricothyroidotomy. Elective use in respiratory problems requiring tracheostomy, J. Thorac. Cardiovasc. Surg. **71**:72-81, 1976.
2. Heimlich, H.J., and Uhley, M.H.: Clinical symposia Ciba. The Heimlich maneuver, **31**(3):1-32, 1979.
3. Linscott, M.S., and Horton, W.C.: Management of upper airway obstruction, Otolaryngol. Clin. North Am. **12**:351-373, 1979.
4. National Conference on Cardiopulmonary Resuscitation and Emergency Cardiac Care, J.A.M.A. **244**:453-508, 1980.
5. Oppenheimer, R.P.: Airway . . . instantly, J.A.M.A. **230**:76, 1974.

CHAPTER 37

Nasotracheal suctioning

■ Linda L. Martin
Paul M. Suratt

■ GENERAL CONSIDERATIONS

Nasotracheal suctioning is a method of removing secretions from the trachea and major bronchi. It is particularly useful in patients who do not cough effectively because of weakness or pain associated with coughing. It can be hazardous because suctioning removes air from the bronchi causing a fall in Po_2. It is also an extremely uncomfortable procedure for alert patients. Nasotracheal suctioning is frequently given in concert with chest physiotherapy, since the latter can dislodge secretions in distal airways that can then be removed through the suction catheter.

■ INDICATIONS

1. For the patient with an ineffective cough who cannot clear bronchial secretions and who has developed or is at risk of developing hypoxemia, atelactasis, or pneumonia.
2. To obtain sputum for diagnostic studies, such as a Gram stain and culture. Sputum obtained this way, however, will be contaminated with nasopharyngeal flora.

■ CONTRAINDICATIONS

1. Hypoxemia that cannot be corrected with oxygen, since suctioning lowers Po_2.
2. The patient with a full stomach, since aspiration may occur.

3. The unconscious patient, since risk of aspiration is higher in the patient without a gag reflex.
4. Myocardial infarction or irritability because of the higher risk of arrhythmias.
5. Hemorrhagic diathesis.
6. Facial fracture.
7. Recent surgery of the airway or esophagus.

PATIENT EVALUATION AND PREPARATION

1. Explain the procedure to the patient and ask for assistance. This is an uncomfortable procedure and helping the patient understand why it is done is important.
2. Attach a cardiac monitor to the patient to observe for arrhythmias.

PERSONNEL AND EQUIPMENT

1. A physician, nurse or paramedical person trained in endotracheal suctioning and one assistant familiar with the procedure.
2. A suction catheter, size 14 or 16 French for all adults. If the patient is large and the secretions are extremely tenacious, an 18 French may be used. Three types of catheters are generally used:
   a. A "whistle-tip" catheter has two or three vents on alternate sides of the catheter to prevent the catheter from collapsing when touching the tracheal wall and to decrease suction injury to the wall.[7] Some whistle-tip catheters are stiffer than rubber catheters and may cause more trauma to the nasopharynx and larynx during insertion.
   b. A rubber catheter.
   c. A Coudé catheter (Fig. 37-1) has a slightly angled tip to facilitate placing it in the left mainstem bronchus.[3]
3. Principal implements: a Y connector if a rubber catheter is used, a water-soluble lubricant, sterile saline, a 10-ml syringe, and a suction trap if collecting a specimen for Gram stain and culture.
4. Sterile gloves.

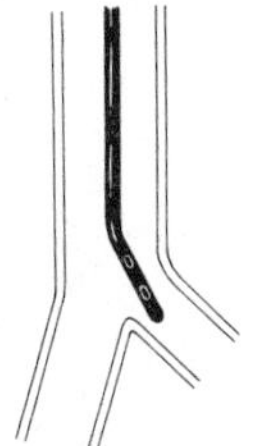

FIG. 37-1. Coudé catheter entering left mainstem bronchus.

5. A suction source and tubing with adaptor to attach to suction catheter.
6. An oxygen source and tubing with an adapter to attach to the suction catheter.

■ TECHNIQUE

1. Place the patient upright or, if this is not possible, in a semiupright position. The head and jaw should be jutting slightly forward as if to sniff a flower, with the head supported by a pillow (Fig. 37-2).
2. Open the catheter package while leaving the catheter on one half of the sterile package and lubricate the catheter tip.
3. Turn on the suction to 80 to 100 mm Hg.
4. Attach the oxygen tubing to the oxygen source and turn on the oxygen to approximately 6 L/min.
5. Oxygenate the patient by holding the oxygen catheter in front of the patient's nose and mouth.
6. Put on sterile gloves. Keep your dominant hand glove sterile and consider the other clean.
7. Hold the catheter with the sterile glove.
8. Attach the Y connector to the suction catheter if you are using a rubber catheter. A Y connector is not necessary when using a whistle-tip catheter.
9. Insert the suction catheter into the nostril and pass it through the nasopharynx.
10. Grasp the patient's tongue with a 4 × 4 inch gauze pad using your clean hand and hold the tongue out so the

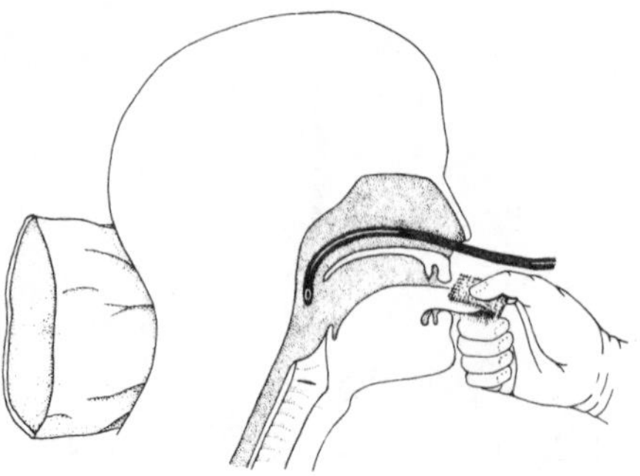

FIG. 37-2. Head position, pulling tongue out.

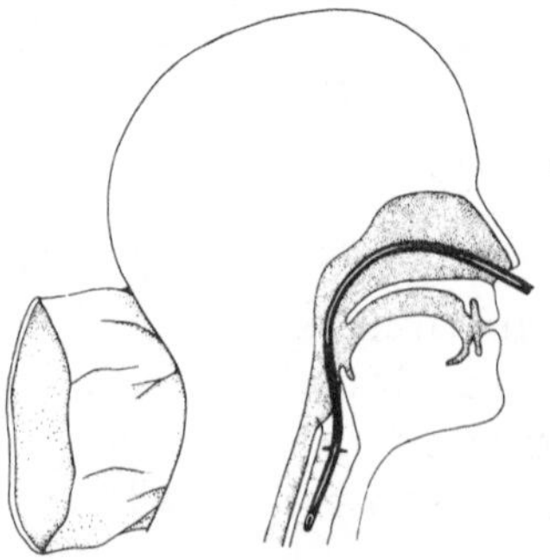

FIG. 37-3. Catheter in trachea.

catheter will not hit it and enter the mouth (Fig. 37-2).

11. Tell the patient to take a deep breath and, as the breath is taken, quickly insert the catheter into the trachea (Fig. 37-3). This may take several tries. When the catheter is in the trachea, the patient will generally cough and have difficulty talking because the vocal cords cannot be opposed. Also air can be heard moving in and out of the catheter with respirations. If there is difficulty deciding whether the catheter is in the trachea or esophagus, instill about 5 ml of saline into the catheter. If the patient coughs, the catheter is probably in the trachea.
12. Oxygenate the patient for at least 30 seconds while the

catheter is in the trachea by attaching the oxygen tubing to the Y connector and placing your thumb over the open end of the Y.

13. Remove the oxygen tubing from the Y connector and replace it with the suction tubing with the clean gloved hand.
14. Apply suction by placing your thumb over the open end of the Y and rotate the catheter for not more than 10 seconds.
15. Remove the suction tubing, attach the oxygen tubing, and administer oxygen again for 30 to 60 seconds.
16. If the secretions are thick and difficult to remove, quickly instill about 5 ml of sterile normal saline through the catheter to liquefy the secretions.
17. Repeat suctioning and oxygenation until the airways sound clear. Always oxygenate the patient following suctioning and watch the monitor for arrhythmias.
18. Withdraw the catheter and administer oxygen to the patient for 30 to 60 seconds.

■ POSTPROCEDURE CARE

1. Observe for signs of hypoxemia, such as agitation, cyanosis, and arrhythmias.
2. Ausculate the chest to determine whether there has been any improvement in breath sounds.
3. Record the quantity, color, and thickness or thinness of the secretions and how the patient tolerated the procedure.

■ COMPLICATIONS

1. Hypoxemia.[2,6,7]
2. Arrhythmias.[1,6,7]
3. Hypotension.[1,6,7]
4. Aspiration.
5. Trauma to the tracheobronchial mucosa.[1,5-7]
6. Death.[4]

REFERENCES

1. Bendixen, H.H., Egbert, L.D., Hedley-Whyte, J., Laver, M.B., and Pontoppidan, H.: Respiratory care, St. Louis, 1965, The C.V. Mosby Co.

2. Fell, T., and Cheney, F.W.: Prevention of hypoxia during endotracheal suction, Ann. Surg. **174**:24-28, 1971.
3. Kirimli, B., King, J.E., and Pfaeffle, H.H.: Evaluation of tracheobronchial suction techniques, J. Thorac. Cardiovasc. Surg. **59**:340-344, 1970.
4. Marx, G.F., Steen, S.N., Arkins, R.E., Foster, E.S., Joffe, S., Kepes, E.R., and Soapira, M.: Endotracheal suction and death, N.Y. State J. Med. **68**: 565-566, 1968.
5. Sackner, M.A., Landa, J.F., Greeneltch, N., and Robinson, M.J.: Pathogenesis and prevention of tracheobronchial damage and suction procedures, Chest **64**:284-290, 1973.
6. Shapiro, E.A., Harrison, R.A., and Trout, C.A.: Clinical application of respiratory care, Chicago, 1975, Year Book Medical Publishers, Inc.
7. Sorensen, K.C., and Luckman, J.: Basic nursing: a psychophysiologic approach, Philadelphia, 1979, W.B. Saunders Co.

CHAPTER 38

Transtracheal aspiration

■ Paul M. Suratt
James K. Pohl

■ GENERAL CONSIDERATIONS

Transtracheal aspiration is a method of obtaining secretions from the tracheobronchial tree without incurring oropharyngeal contamination. A 14-gauge needle punctures the cricothyroid membrane, a catheter is inserted through the needle into the trachea, and secretions are aspirated through the catheter.[4,6]

■ INDICATIONS

This procedure should be performed whenever secretions are needed from the lower respiratory tract that are uncontaminated by oropharyngeal flora. This procedure is probably not indicated in previously healthy individuals with uncomplicated pneumonia. The need for uncontaminated secretions has been recommended in the following situations:

1. An immunocompromised host with pneumonia (an individual with alcoholism, malnutrition, or malignancy) who is predisposed to pulmonary infections with unusual organisms such as gram-negative bacteria, anaerobic bacteria, or staphylococci.[1,2,4,8] If the sputum Gram stain shows a clear predominance of an identifiable organism, a transtracheal aspiration is probably not necessary.
2. A severely ill patient with pneumonia who is unable to raise sputum spontaneously.[2,4]
3. A patient with an undiagnosed infiltrate on a chest roentgenogram that could represent either pneumonia or a nonbacterial process, such as atelectasis, who is

unable to produce sputum. A false negative sterile transtracheal aspirate may result, however, if the infected lung is distal to an obstructing endobronchial lesion.[8]

■ CONTRAINDICATIONS

1. Bleeding diathesis, including patients with azotemia who have impaired platelet function.[4,10]
2. Hypoxemia that cannot be corrected by oxygen administration.[10]
3. Anatomic deformities of the neck that prevent access to the cricothyroid cartilage.
4. An uncooperative patient.
5. A severe cough, which is a relative contraindication.[10]

■ PATIENT EVALUATION AND PREPARATION

1. Obtain a prothrombin time, partial thromboplastin time, platelet count, blood urea nitrogen or creatinine levels, and bleeding time if platelet dysfunction is suspected.
2. Arterial blood gases if the patient might be hypoxic.
3. Explain the procedure to the patient and obtain written informed consent.

■ PERSONNEL AND EQUIPMENT

1. A physician trained in transtracheal aspiration.
2. Principal implements: a 14-gauge intracatheter kit (I-CATH), a 30-ml syringe, and nonbacteriostatic saline.
3. An antiseptic solution, sterile gloves, 4 × 4 inch gauze pads, and sterile towels.
4. Lidocaine, 1%, 5 ml, a 3-ml syringe, and a 25-gauge needle.
5. Culture tubes and glass slides.

■ TECHNIQUE

1. Place the patient supine with the neck hyperextended; placing a pillow under the shoulders helps hyperextend the neck.
2. Locate the thyroid cartilage, cricothyroid membrane, cricoid cartilage, trachea, and thyroid gland. The punc-

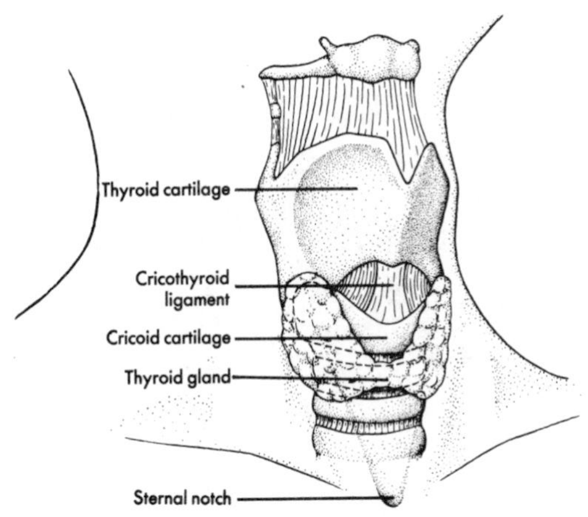

FIG. 38-1. Anatomy.

ture site is the skin overlying the cricothyroid membrane, exactly in the midline (Fig. 38-1).

3. Put on sterile gloves, prepare the skin with an antiseptic solution, and form a sterile field with towels.
4. Anesthetize the skin and cricothyroid membrane, but do not inject the anesthetic into the trachea, since local anesthetics are often bacteriostatic.
5. Puncture the skin and crycothyroid membrane with the intracatheter needle perpendicular to the membrane and in the midline (Fig. 38-2). Proceed with caution because too much force may lacerate the posterior portion of the trachea and underlying esophagus.
6. Point the needle slightly caudally, with its bevel anterior, and thread the catheter through the needle and into the trachea. Do not pull back the catheter, since it may catch on the needle and sever.
7. Withdraw the 14-gauge needle and sheath it with the needle guard supplied with the kit (Fig. 38-3).
8. To aspirate secretions, attach the 30-ml syringe to the catheter and pull back on the plunger. If no sputum is aspirated, check the posterior pharynx to rule out

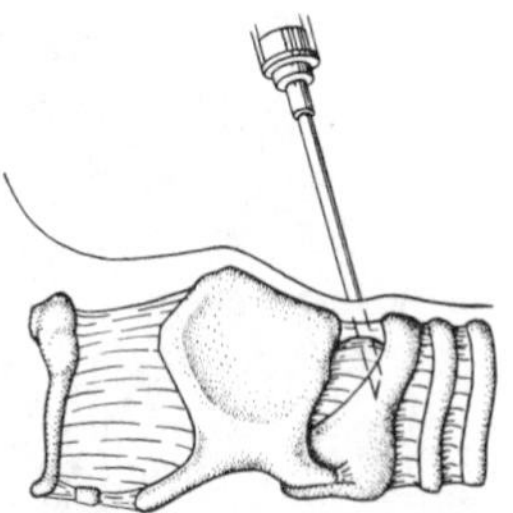

FIG. 38-2. Needle inserted through cricothyroid ligament.

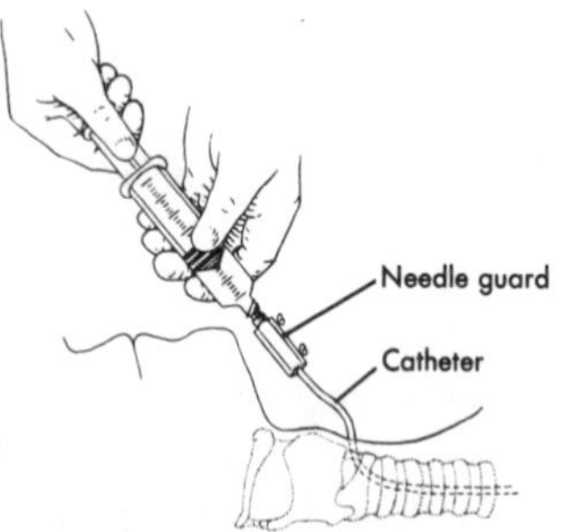

FIG. 38-3. Aspirating secretions.

cephalad placement of the catheter; then flush 2 to 4 ml of nonbacteriostatic saline through the catheter and aspirate again.

9. Remove the catheter from the trachea and skin site, making sure the entire length of the intracatheter is recovered. Apply pressure to the puncture site for 3 mintues.
10. Innoculate the appropriate culture tubes and make at least one smear for staining.

■ POSTPROCEDURE CARE

1. Observe patients closely who have had blood-streaked sputum during the procedure.
2. Avoid procedures, such as intermittent positive pressure breathing, for 24 hours that stimulate coughing and that

may aggravate subcutaneous and mediastinal emphysema.

SPECIMEN EXAMINATION

1. A Gram stain should always be performed on the aspirated secretions. Other stains, such as a Ziehl-Neelsen stain, should be performed when *Mycobacterium tuberculosis* or nonbacterial infections are suspected.
2. Culture for aerobic and anaerobic bacterial organisms. Culture for nonbacterial organisms when clinically indicated.

COMPLICATIONS

1. Death, 0.26%.[3]
2. Blood-streaked sputum during the procedure. This is reported to occur in approximately half the patients.[2,4]
3. Severe endotracheal hemorrhage. Severe endotracheal hemorrhage is rare and has been reported in patients who were uremic or had an aberrant branch of the superior thyroid artery pass through the cricothyroid cartilage.[9] It also occurred in an uncooperative patient in whom air could not be aspirated through the catheter and multiple punctures were performed, one of which was shown at autopsy to have perforated the thyroid.[11]
4. Subcutaneous emphysema. Subcutaneous emphysema limited to the anterior neck has been reported to occur after 19% of procedures.[7] In another study, 2% of patients developed subcutaneous emphysema that involved their neck, shoulders, and chest wall.[4]
5. Mediastinal emphysema. Mediastinal emphysema occurred in 2% of patients; it is said to occur more commonly in patients with severe cough.[4] In one patient it progressed to pneumothorax.[5]
6. Respiratory arrest. Respiratory arrest occurred in hypoxic patients who were not given supplemental oxygen during the procedure.[10,11]
7. Violent coughing from the procedure led to aspiration of gastric contents and death in one alcoholic jaundiced

patient.[10] In another patient uncontrolled coughing was believed to cause rupture of esophageal varices and death.[3]

8. Cardiac arrhythmias have caused at least two deaths.[3]

9. Paratracheal infection, 0.23%.[3]

REFERENCES

1. Bartlett, J.C., Rosenblatt, J.E., and Finegold, S.M.: Percutaneous transtracheal aspiration in the diagnosis of anaerobic pulmonary infection, Ann. Int. Med. **79:**535-540, 1973.
2. Hahn, H.H., and Beaty, H.N.: Transtracheal aspiration in the evaluation of patients with pneumonia, Ann. Int. Med. **72:**183-187, 1970.
3. Jay, S.J.: Getting the most out of transtracheal aspiration, J. Respir. Dis., pp. 13-21, Feb., 1981.
4. Kalinske, R.W., Parker, R.H., Brandt, D., and Hoeprich, P.D.: Diagnostic usefulness and safety of transtracheal aspiration, N. Engl. J. Med. **276:**604-608, 1967.
5. Parsons, G.H., Price, J.E., and Auston, P.W.: Bilateral pneumothorax complicating transtracheal aspiration, West J. Med. **125:**73-75, 1976.
6. Pecora, D.V.: A comparison of transtracheal aspiration with other methods of determining the bacterial flora of the lower respiratory tract, N. Engl. J. Med. **269:**664-666, 1963.
7. Pratter, M.R., and Irwin, R.S.: Transtracheal aspiration, guidelines for safety, Chest **76:**518-520, 1979.
8. Ries, K., Levison, M.E., and Kaye, D.: Transtracheal aspiration in pulmonary infection, Arch. Int. Med. **133:**453-458, 1974.
9. Schillaci, R.F., Iacovoni, V.E., and Conte, R.S.: Transtracheal aspiration complicated by fatal endotracheal hemorrhage, N. Engl. J. Med. **295:**488-490, 1976.
10. Spencer, C.D., and Beaty, H.N.: Complications of transtracheal aspiration, N. Engl. J. Med. **286:**304-306, 1972.
11. Unger, K.M., and Moser, K.M.: Fatal complications of transtracheal aspiration, Arch. Int. Med. **132:**437-439, 1973.

CHAPTER 39

Thoracentesis

Paul M. Suratt
Cary Fishburne

GENERAL CONSIDERATIONS

Thoracentesis is a method of removing pleural fluid from a needle inserted through the skin and chest wall. It is performed when the cause of a pleural effusion is unknown and fluid is needed for diagnostic laboratory tests or when a large volume of pleural fluid collapses the lung and contributes to respiratory embarrassment.

DIAGNOSTIC INDICATION

Pleural effusion of unknown cause.

THERAPEUTIC INDICATIONS

1. Respiratory function critically impaired by a pleural effusion.
2. To instill sclerosing or chemotherapeutic agents to prevent a reoccurrence of neoplastic effusion.

CONTRAINDICATIONS

1. Uncorrectable hemorrhagic diathesis or anticoagulation therapy.
2. A patient who is unable to tolerate a pneumothorax.
3. A patient receiving positive pressure ventilation. A bronchopleural fistula and tension pneumothorax may result from lung laceration and positive pressure ventilation. This is a relative contraindication.

PATIENT EVALUATION AND PREPARATION

1. Obtain a chest roentgenogram: posteroanterior, lateral, and decubitus views.
2. Obtain a prothrombin time, partial thromboplastin time, and platelet count.

3. Explain the procedure to the patient, including potential complications, and obtain written informed consent.

PERSONNEL AND EQUIPMENT

1. This procedure can be performed entirely by one physician. It is easier, however, if an assistant is present to hand the physician items during the procedure.
2. Principal implements: needles (16 and 18 gauge, 3 inches; 20 gauge, 1½ inches; and 25 gauge, ¾ inch), syringes (10 ml for anesthesia and 30 or 50 ml for aspirating fluid), a three-way stopcock, 4 × 4 inch gauze pads, and sterile towels.
3. Lidocaine, 1%, 10 ml.
4. An antiseptic solution and sterile gloves.
5. Fluid collection materials: a purple-top tube for hematologic analysis, a red-top tube for chemical analysis, a culture tube, a glass bottle with 0.5 ml of heparin per 50 ml of effusion for cytologic studies, a heparinized syringe, and an ice bucket for pH studies and sterile gloves.
6. Optional—14-gauge intracatheter set.

TECHNIQUE

1. Have the patient sit erect with the arms resting comfortably on a table placed in front (Fig. 39-1) or on the back of a chair.
2. Locate the fluid by percussing the chest and identifying the superior margin of dullness. If fluid is loculated and cannot be localized using this technique, it can usually be found by echography or fluoroscopy. The site for needle insertion is usually two rib interspaces below the superior margin of dullness in the posterior lateral chest, but the site may vary, depending on where the fluid is located. Mark the site with a fingernail or other object that will indent the skin and not be removed by the antiseptic.
3. Open the thoracentesis tray and put on sterile gloves. Inspect the tray to ensure that all necessary items are

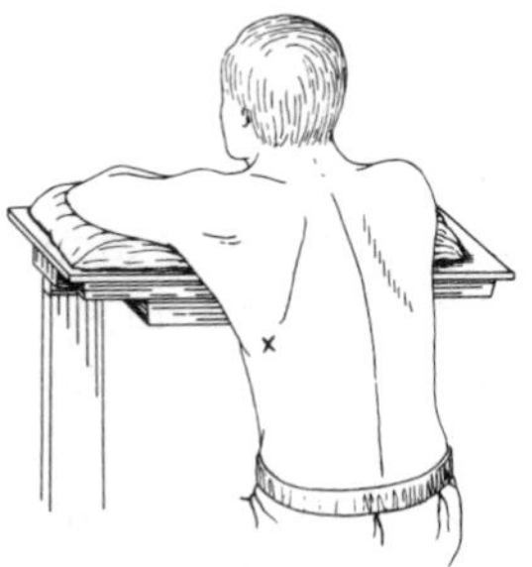

FIG. 39-1. Patient position.

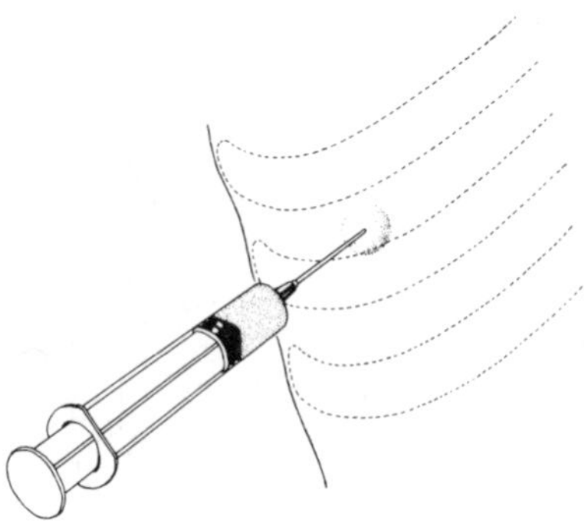

FIG. 39-2. Anesthetic injection.

present. Familiarize yourself with the operation of the stopcock.

4. Disinfect and drape the puncture site.
5. Anesthetize the skin over the biopsy site with the 25-gauge needle on the 10-ml syringe. Then put the 20-gauge needle on the syringe and slowly penetrate the skin at the superior border of the rib and anesthetize liberally (aspirating before each injection to ensure that you are not injecting directly into a vessel) (Fig. 39-2). If the periosteum is reached, it too should be anesthetized. Then point the needle just above the rib and advance the needle, slowly aspirating and anesthetizing until fluid enters the syringe. If no fluid is obtained, try having the patient lean back toward the needle.

6. When pleural fluid enters the syringe, mark the depth of the needle with a clamp (Fig. 39-3) and remove the needle.
7. Attach the 18- or 16-gauge, 3-inch thoracentesis needle to the stopcock and the 50-ml syringe, clamp the needle at the depth noted previously and insert it at the same site to the same depth into the pleural space (Fig. 39-4). Some physicians prefer to insert a 14-gauge intracatheter needle into the pleural space, thread in the catheter, and then withdraw the needle. This is believed to decrease the risk of a pneumothorax, but we can find no data to support or refute this claim.

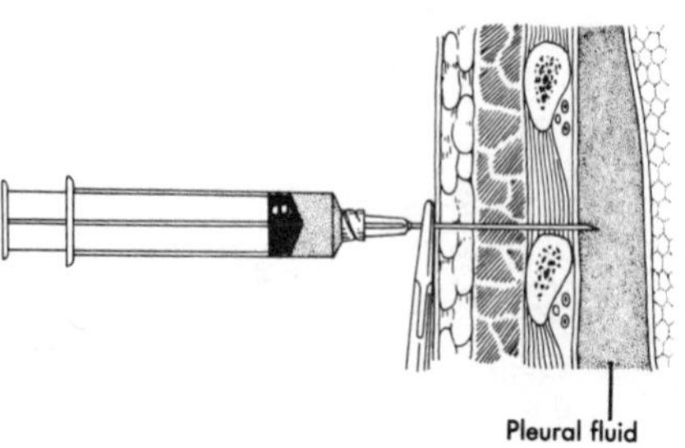

FIG. 39-3. Anesthetic needle in pleura, clamp attached.

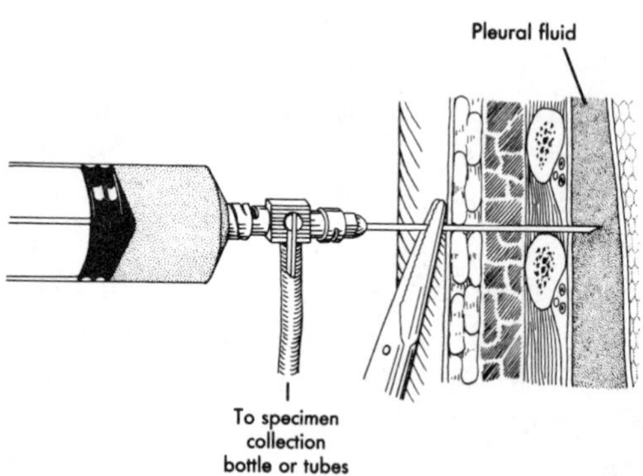

FIG. 39-4. Fluid removal through thoracentesis needle and three-way stopcock.

8. Aspirate fluid into the syringe and then express it through the stopcock into the collection tubes.
9. If a pleural biopsy is planned later, leave pleural fluid as a buffer zone between the lung and the pleura.
10. Do not remove more than 1 L of fluid at a sitting. It has been suggested that more than 1 L may be removed safely if pleural pressure is carefully measured and does not fall below −20 cm H_2O during the thoracentesis.[8] Further study is necessary to confirm this.

■ POSTPROCEDURE CARE

1. Percuss and auscultate the area of thoracentesis, searching for a pneumothorax.
2. Obtain a posteroanterior expiratory chest roentgenogram to look for a pneumothorax.

■ SPECIMEN EXAMINATION

1. Chemistries: glucose, protein, lactic dehydrogenase (LDH), amylase, triglycerides, and pH level (place the latter in a lightly heparinized syringe and put it in ice).
2. Hematologic examination includes white cell and differential counts, red cell count, and hematocrit value.

TABLE 39-1. PLEURAL TRANSUDATES AND EXUDATES[1,9]

Condition	Physiologic cause	Disease
Transudate*	Low colloid osmotic pressure	Hypoproteinemia
	Increased pulmonary capillary hydrostatic pressure	Congestive heart failure
Exudate*	Pleural inflammation or injury	Infections
		Pulmonary embolism or infarctions
		Malignancies
		Connective tissue disease, such as lupus erythematosus and rheumatoid arthritis
		Gastrointestinal disorders, such as pancreatitis, subphrenic abscess and esophageal rupture
	Lymphatic obstruction	Thoracic duct interruption

*See Table 39-2 for definitions of transudate and exudate.

3. Cytologic examination.
4. Cultures include aerobic and anaerobic bacteria, *Mycobacterium tuberculosis* and a Gram stain.
5. C-4 if rheumatoid arthritis or lupus erythematosus is a possibility.[4]

■ SPECIMEN INTERPRETATION

Classification of pleural fluid as a transudate or exudate will indicate which categories of disease have caused it (Table 39-1). Other specific laboratory tests will frequently narrow down the diagnostic possibilities (Table 39-2).

TABLE 39-2. PLEURAL FLUID TESTS

Test	Result	Significance	
Protein	Pleural fluid–to–serum ratio greater than 0.5	Exudate, 70% cases[9]	With all these characteristics there is 97% chance of fluid being exudate; with none there is 97% chance of it being transudate
LDH	Pleural fluid–to–serum ratio greater than 0.6	Exudate, 70% cases[9]	
	Pleural fluid value greater than 200 units	Exudate, 70% cases[9]	
Red blood cell count	Greater than 100,000 mm^3	Suggests trauma, malignancy, or pulmonary infarction[7]	
White blood cell count	Greater than 10,000 mm^3	Occurs in pneumonia, pulmonary embolism, tuberculosis, malignancy, pancreatitis, and collagen vascular disease	
Lymphocytes	Greater than 50% lymphocytes	In an exudate this suggests tuberculosis or a malignancy[7]	
Glucose	Less than 60 mg/dl	May occur in pneumonia (the lower the value, the larger the likelihood of empyema), rheumatoid pleural effusion, tuberculosis, and malignancy[6]	
Amylase	Higher than normal	Occurs in pancreatitis, esophageal rupture, and malignancy[6]	
pH	Less than 7.20	Suggests empyema; may also occur in malignancy rheumatoid arthritis, tuberculosis, or esophageal rupture[3,5]	
Triglycerides	Higher than 100 mg/dl	Suggests thoracic duct interruption due to malignancy, particularly lymphoma, surgery, or trauma[10]	
C-4	Less than 10 units × 10^{-5}/g protein	Present in most patients with rheumatoid arthritis and in many with lupus erythematosus[4]	

■ COMPLICATIONS

1. Pneumothorax.
2. Hemothorax may occur if an intercostal artery is lacerated.
3. Unilateral pulmonary edema and/or sudden death are rare but have occurred after removal of more than 1L of pleural fluid at one sitting.[11]
4. Vasovagal attack.
5. Hypoxemia generally occurs following thoracentesis but can be prevented by oxygen administration. The degree of hypoxemia is directly related to the volume of fluid removed.[2]

REFERENCES

1. Black, L.F.: The pleural space and pleural fluid, Mayo Clin. Proc. **47:**493-506, 1972.
2. Brandstetter, R.D., and Cohen, R.P.: Hypoxemia after thoracentesis, J.A.M.A. **242:**1060-1061, 1979.
3. Good, J.T., Jr., Taryle, D.A., Maulitz, R.M., Kaplan, R.L., and Sahn, S.A.: The diagnostic value of pleural fluid pH, Chest **78:**55-59, 1980.
4. Halla, J.T., Schrohenloher, R.E., and Volanakis, J.E.: Immune complexes and other laboratory features of pleural effusions, Ann. Int. Med. **92:**748-752, 1980.
5. Light, R.W.: Evaluating the patient with pleural effusions, J. Respir. Dis. **2**(3):89-100, 1981.
6. Light, R.W., and Ball, W.C.: Glucose and amylase in pleural effusions, J.A.M.A. **225:**257-260, 1973.
7. Light, R.W., Erozan, Y.S., and Ball, W.C., Jr.: Cells in pleural fluid: their value in differential diagnosis, Arch. Int. Med. **132:**854-860, 1973.
8. Light, R.W., Jenkinson, S.G., Minh, V., and George, R.B.: Observations on pleural fluid pressures as fluid is withdrawn during thoracentesis, Am. Rev. Respir. Dis. **121:**799-804, 1980.
9. Light, R.W., MacGregor, M.I., Luchsinger, P.C., and Ball, W.C., Jr.: Pleural effusions: the diagnostic separation of transudates and exudates, Ann. Int. Med. **77:**507-513, 1972.
10. Staats, B.A., Ellefson, R.D., Budahn, L.L., Dines, D.E., Prakash, U.B.S., and Offord, K.: The lipoprotein profile of chylous and nonchylous pleural effusions, Mayo Clin. Proc. **55:**700-704, 1980.
11. Trapnell, D.H., and Thurston, J.G.B.: Unilateral pulmonary edema after pleural aspiration, Lancet **1:**1367-1369, 1970.

CHAPTER 40

Pleural biopsy

■ Paul M. Suratt
James K. Pohl

■ GENERAL CONSIDERATIONS

This technique is used to diagnose pleural granulomatous disease, particularly tuberculosis and pleural malignancy.[1-6] The diagnostic yield in pleural tuberculosis has been reported to be 71%; in pleural carcinoma it is 40%.[5] To achieve these results a second biopsy must be performed if the first biopsy does not produce a diagnosis. The technique is usually performed when pleural fluid is present, although it can be done when pleural fluid is absent.[5]

■ INDICATION

Unexplained pleural disease, particularly an exudative effusion, that could be due to a granulomatous disorder or carcinoma is an indication for a pleural biopsy.

■ CONTRAINDICATIONS

1. Uncorrectable bleeding diathesis.
2. Inability of the patient to tolerate a pneumothorax.
3. A patient receiving positive pressure ventilation, since a bronchopleural fistula and tension pneumothorax may result from lung laceration. This is a relative contraindication.
4. An uncooperative patient.

■ PATIENT EVALUATION AND PREPARATION

1. Obtain a history and physical examination.
2. Obtain a prothrombin time, partial thromboplastin time, and platelet count. A bleeding time is needed if platelet dysfunction is suspected.
3. Obtain chest roentgenograms: posteroanterior, lateral, and decubitus views.

4. Explain the procedure and its potential complications to the patient and obtain written consent.

PERSONNEL AND EQUIPMENT

1. A physician trained in the procedure; an assistant will be helpful, although not absolutely necessary.
2. Principal implements: a pleural biopsy needle (we prefer the Abrams needle[1] because in our experience it is easier to obtain pleural tissue with it than with the Cope needle[3]), a scalpel with a number 11 blade, and a Kelly clamp.
3. An antiseptic solution with a cup to hold it, sterile gloves, 4 × 4 inch gauze pads, and sterile towels.
4. Lidocaine, 1%, 20 ml, syringes (2 and 10 ml), and needles (25 gauge, ¾ inch; 20 gauge, 1½ inch).
5. Specimen containers, 10% formalin solution, and liquid culture medium for *Mycobacterium tuberculosis*.

TECHNIQUE USING ABRAMS NEEDLE WITH PLEURAL FLUID PRESENT

1. Have the patient sit erect with the arms resting comfortably on a table in front or on a chair back (Fig. 40-1).
2. Select an intercostal space that is below the top of the pleural fluid, using the chest roentgenogram and chest physical examination as guides. Palpate the lower rib

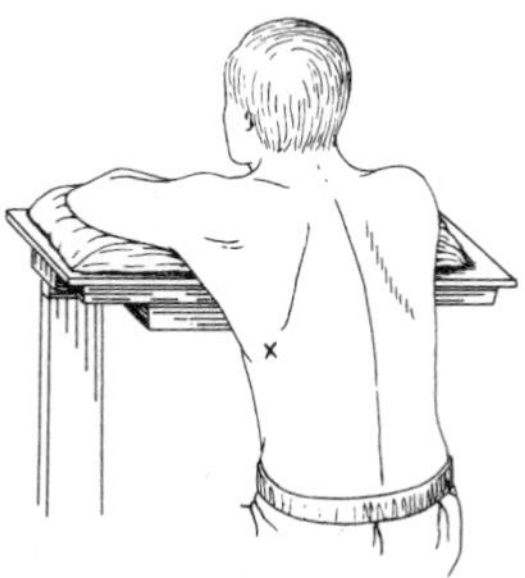

FIG. 40-1. Patient position.

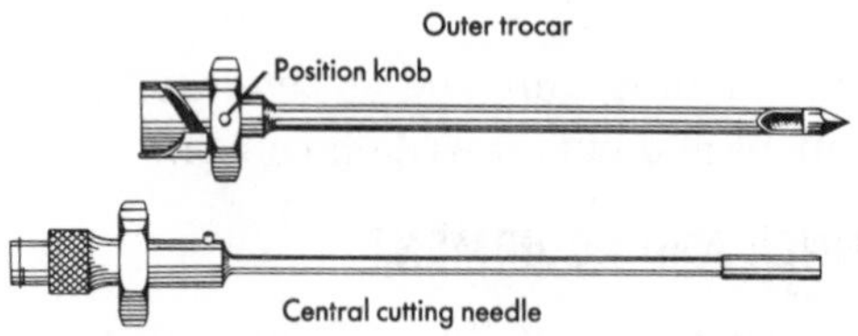

FIG. 40-2. Abrams needle, unassembled.

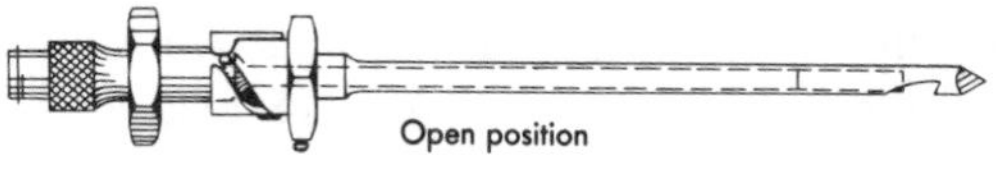

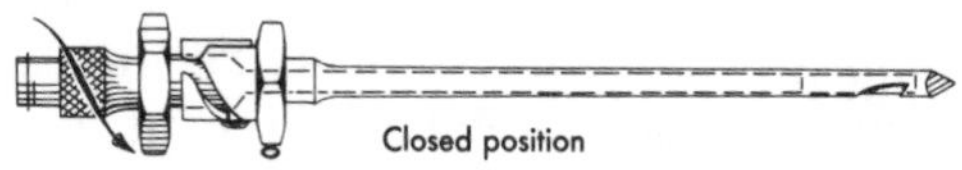

FIG. 40-3. Abrams needle, assembled.

and indent the skin with a fingernail just above the edge of this rib.

3. Put on sterile gloves and assemble the Abrams pleural biopsy needle (Figs. 40-2 and 40-3). Slide the central cutting needle into the outer trocar tube and connect it to a closed 10-ml syringe. Do not insert the inner trocar. Familiarize yourself with the open and closed positions. The knob on the outer trocar indicates the position of the cutting surface.
4. Disinfect the skin and form a sterile field with draping towels.
5. Anesthetize the skin over the biopsy site with the 25-gauge needle on a 10-ml syringe. Then attach the 20-gauge needle to the syringe and slowly penetrate the skin just above the rib and anesthetize liberally (Fig. 40-4). Aspirate before each injection to ensure that you are not injecting directly into a vessel. Pointing the needle just above the rib, advance the needle slowly while aspirating and anesthetizing until fluid enters

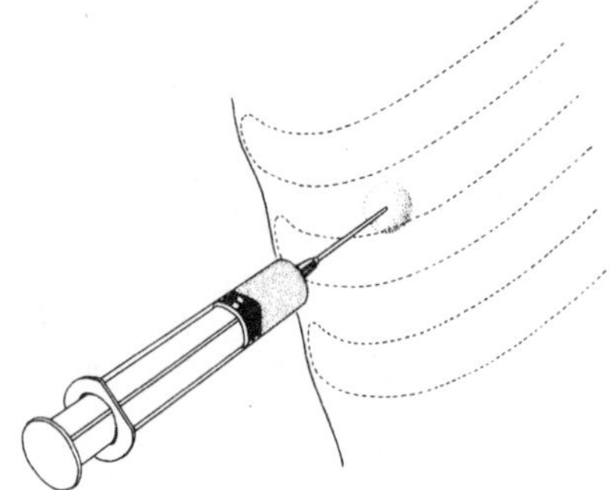

FIG. 40-4. Injecting anesthetic.

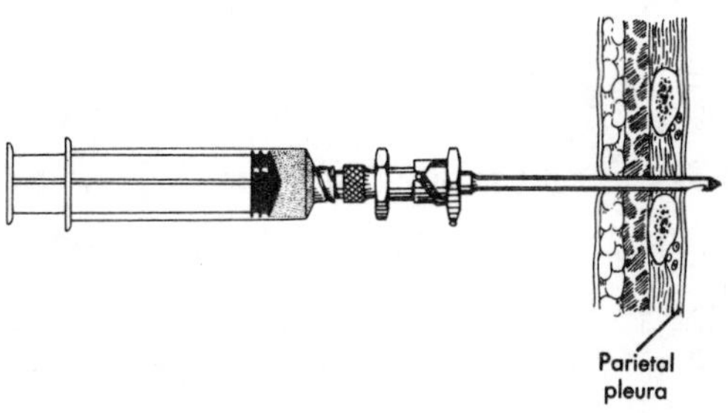

FIG. 40-5. Abrams needle in pleura, aspirating fluid to document position.

the syringe. This verifies the presence of fluid and gives the depth of needle penetration required to enter the pleural cavity. Remove the needle.

6. With the scalpel make a 3-mm incision through the skin at the previous puncture site.
7. Advance the Abrams needle in the closed position through the incision with a firm twisting motion. Advance while twisting the needle so that it just clears the superior aspect of the rib until a popping sensation is felt. This signifies that the pleural cavity has been entered. Turn the apparatus to the open position and aspirate with the syringe (Fig. 40-5). The return of fluid verifies that the cutting surface is in the pleural cavity.
8. Position the cutting surface at the 6-o'clock position.

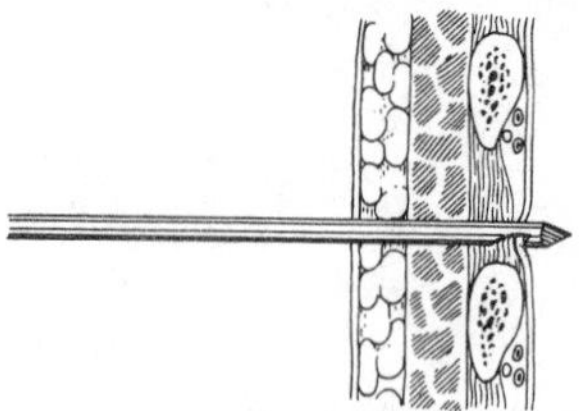

FIG. 40-6. Catching pleura in open Abrams needle.

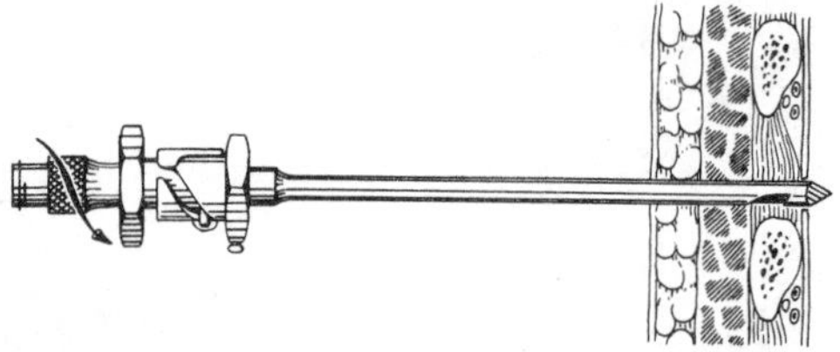

FIG. 40-7. Twisting central cutting needle to cut off pleura.

Pull back, while exerting pressure on the cutting side, until the surface of parietal pleura is caught by the cutting surface (Fig. 40-6). Then twist the central cutting needle to the closed position (Fig. 40-7) and withdraw the entire apparatus.

9. Open the biopsy apparatus on a sterile towel and pick out the tissue biopsy materials with a small needle. Parietal pleura is light gray; skeletal muscle is red. Place one specimen in broth for *Mycobacterium tuberculosis* and fungal culture; others should be placed in 10% formalin for histologic examination.

10. Repeat this procedure five times with the cutting surface of the needle directed downward between the 2-o'clock and 10-o'clock positions. The surface of the cutting needle should not be directed upward, since this could damage the intercostal nerves and vessels.

11. If you wish to remove pleural fluid, a thoracentesis needle can be inserted into the hole and the fluid removed, or fluid can be removed through the Abrams needle.

12. An adhesive bandage and, occasionally, a suture should be used to close the puncture site.

▪ TECHNIQUE USING ABRAMS NEEDLE WITH NO PLEURAL FLUID

The risk of a pneumothorax may be higher when the biopsy is performed in the absence of pleural fluid. The technique is the same as just described, except for the differences listed below.[5] The biopsy site is the area of maximal pleural involvement as determined by the chest roentgenogram and percussion. The Abrams needle is advanced through the chest wall until there is a sudden and appreciable decrease in resistance, indicating that the needle has penetrated the pleura.

▪ TECHNIQUE USING COPE NEEDLE WITH PLEURAL FLUID PRESENT[3]

1. Seat the patient erect with the arms resting comfortably on a table in front or on a chair back (Fig. 40-1).
2. Select an intercostal space below the level of the pleural fluid, using the chest roentgenogram and chest physical examination as guides. Palpate the lower rib and indent the skin with a fingernail just above the edge of this rib.
3. Put on sterile gloves and familiarize yourself with the Cope needle (Figs. 40-8 to 40-10). Assemble the Cope needle by placing the pointed trocar in the outer cannula (Fig. 40-9). Attach a 10-ml syringe to the pointed trocar and to the biopsy trocar.
4. Disinfect the skin and form a sterile field with draping towels.
5. Anesthetize the skin over the biopsy site with the 25-gauge needle. Then, using the 20-gauge needle, slowly penetrate the skin just above the rib and anesthetize liberally; do not inject more than the maximum allowable dose (Fig. 40-4). Aspirate before each injection to ensure that you are not injecting directly into a vessel. Pointing the needle just above the rib, advance the needle slowly while aspirating and anesthetizing until fluid enters the syringe. Remove the needle.

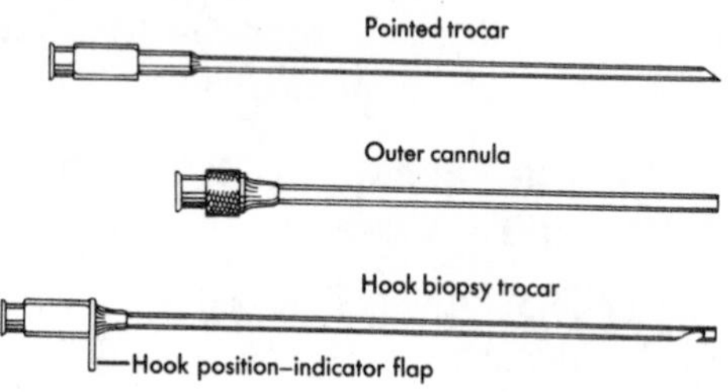

FIG. 40-8. Cope needle components.

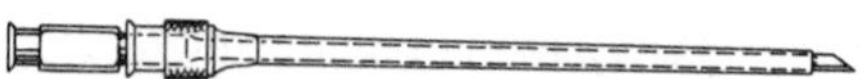

FIG. 40-9. Cope needle, assembly for penetration into pleural space.

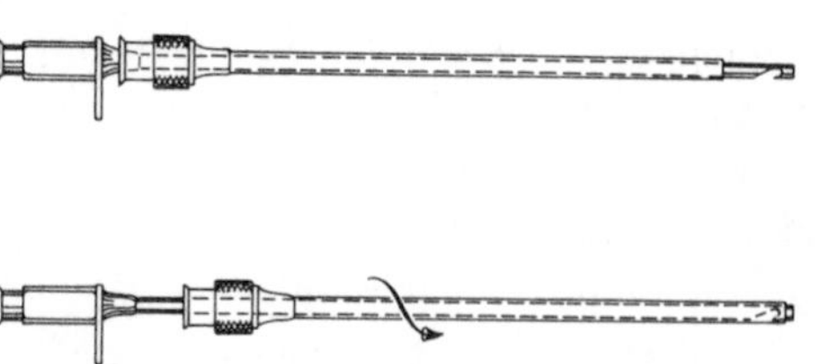

FIG. 40-10. Cope needle with hooked biopsy trocar in outer cannula.

6. With a scalpel make a 3-mm incision through the skin at the previous puncture site.
7. Advance the pointed trocar within the outer cannula with a twisting motion until fluid is aspirated.
8. Remove the pointed trocar from the outer cannula and insert the hook biopsy trocar within the outer cannula (Fig. 40-11). To prevent air from entering the pleural space when the trocars are removed from the outer cannula, instruct the patient to bear down and hold his breath whenever a trocar is removed. Also place your thumb over the open end of the outer cannula.
9. Position the cutting edge of the hook biopsy trocar between the 2-o'clock and 10-o'clock positions (not point-

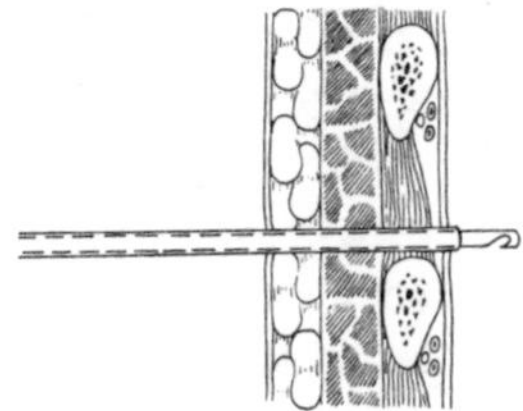

FIG. 40-11. Hooked biopsy trocar in outer trocar.

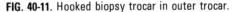

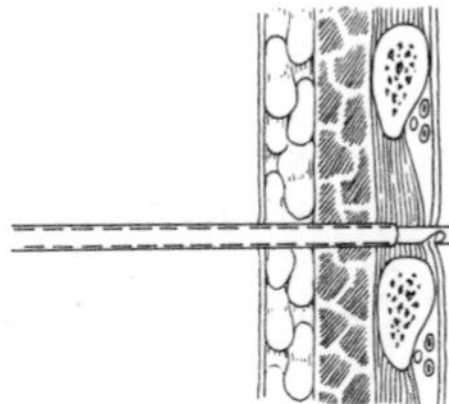

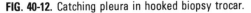

FIG. 40-12. Catching pleura in hooked biopsy trocar.

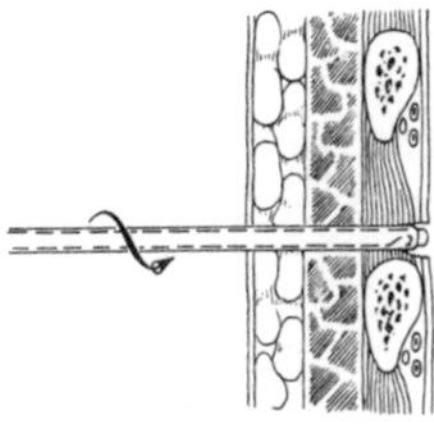

FIG. 40-13. Twisting and advancing outer cannula to cut off pleura.

ing up), using the metal flap at the proximal end of the biopsy trocar as a guide.

10. Slowly withdraw the biopsy trocar and the outer cannula together while exerting pressure on the hook side, until the hook catches (Fig. 40-12).
11. Advance the outer cannula into the chest with a twisting motion, while exerting steady traction on the biopsy trocar. The outer cannula will thus cut off pleural tissue that has been hooked by the biopsy trocar (Fig. 40-13).

12. Withdraw the biopsy trocar from the outer cannula and remove the biopsy specimen. The biopsy trocar can be reinserted into the outer cannula and additional biopsies obtained. Three to six specimens should be obtained by pointing the biopsy hook in different directions (but not up). Place one tissue specimen in broth for *Mycobacterium tuberculosis* and fungal culure; others should be placed in 10% formalin for histologic examination.
13. If you wish to remove pleural fluid, withdraw it through the outer cannula.
14. Close the puncture site with an adhesive bandage or, if necessary, a suture.

■ POSTPROCEDURE EVALUATION

1. Percuss and auscultate the chest, observing for signs of a pneumothorax.
2. Obtain a posteroanterior expiratory chest roentgenogram, also looking for a pneumothorax.

■ COMPLICATIONS

1. Pneumothorax, 3.1% frequency.[2]
2. Hemorrhage, 1.3% frequency.[2]
3. Damage to intercostal nerves with residual pain or sensory deficit.
4. Subcutaneous abscess following biopsy of empyema, occurred in two of five patients with empyema.[5]
5. Tuberculous nodule at the biopsy site.[5]

REFERENCES

1. Abrams, L.D.: Pleural biopsy punch, Lancet **1**:30-31, 1958.
2. Boutin, C., Arnaud, A., Farisse, P., Viallat, J., Choux, R., Aimard, A., and Belnet, M.: Les biopsies pleurales: incidents et rentabilite actuelle de la biopsie a l'aiguille d'Abrams. A propos de 1000 prelevements. Interet de la biopsy pleuroscopique, Poumon. Coeur **31**:317-321, 1975.
3. Cope, C., and Bernhardt, H.: Hook-needle biopsy of pleura, pericardium, peritoneum and synovium, Am. J. Med. **35**:189-195, 1963.
4. Deluccia, V.C., and Reyes, E.C.: Percutaneous needle biopsy of parietal pleura, N.Y. State J. Med. **77**:2058-2061, 1977.
5. Scerbo, J., Keltz, H., and Stone, D.J.: A prospective study of closed pleural biopsies, J.A.M.A. **218**:377-380, 1971.
6. VonHoff, D.D., and Livolsi, V.: Diagnostic reliability of needle biopsy of the parietal pleura, Am. J. Clin. Pathol. **64**:200-203, 1975.

CHAPTER 41

Chest tube insertion

George R. Minor
Paul M. Suratt

GENERAL CONSIDERATIONS

A fenestrated catheter or "chest tube" is inserted into the pleural space to remove either air or fluid.[5,6] Large quantities of air or fluid can be evacuated quickly and continuously as they reform over a period of several days.

INDICATIONS

1. Pneumothorax. Any pneumothorax over 20% probably should be decompressed with a chest tube.[5] If the patient requires mechanical ventilation, a tube should be inserted regardless of the size of the pneumothorax.
2. Hemothorax. Continued bleeding or drainage of a total of 2000 ml within 6 hours probably calls for exploration.
3. Empyema. Pus in the pleural space should be removed, even if sterilized by antibiotics, since it will deposit a layer of fibrin and result in a captive lung. Even tube thoracostomy is inadequate for complete drainage of thick pus, which usually calls for open drainage with rib resection.
4. Malignant pleural effusions. About 50% of malignant effusions will resolve after complete evacuation with 4 or 5 days of dependent closed-tube drainage.[3] In one report, introduction of sclerosing agents, such as tetracycline, through the chest tube prevented reaccumulation of fluid in about 87% of neoplastic effusions.[1]
5. Following any intrathoracic operation.

CONTRAINDICATIONS

There are no absolute contraindications to this procedure, although it may be prudent to defer it briefly for the reversal of anticoagulation or the infusion of needed components, such as platelets.

■ PATIENT EVALUATION AND PREPARATION

1. Obtain a chest roentgenogram, which should be an upright posteroanterior view, if the patient is not in shock. (Omit this step if a tension pneumothorax is suspected in the traumatized patient; depend on physical signs and the exploratory needle. Time may be vital, and a tension pneumothorax may be bilateral.)
2. Obtain a prothrombin time, partial thromboplastin time, and platelet count. If the patient is uremic, taking drugs, or has a disease known to affect platelet function, a bleeding time should be obtained also.
3. Explain the procedure and its potential complications to the patient and obtain a written informed consent.

■ PERSONNEL AND EQUIPMENT

1. One physician trained in the insertion of chest tubes and an assistant.
2. Principal implements: a chest tube, drainage apparatus, chest trocar cannula, scalpel, scissors, suture, curved hemostat, connecting plastic tubes, and adapters.
3. An antiseptic solution and cup to hold it in, sterile gloves, 4 × 4 inch sterile gauze pads, sterile draping towels and clips, sterile package petrolatum gauze, and adhesive tape.
4. Lidocaine, 1%, 45 ml, 5- and 12-ml syringes, and 27- and 21-gauge needles.

■ SELECTION OF DRAINAGE APPARATUS[7,8]

1. The chest tube can be drained into a one-way flutter valve, one-, two-, or three-bottle systems, or a disposable unit (the most commonly used in the United States). Although suction is generally applied to these systems, they will all function without suction unless there is a large air leak from the lung.
2. A one-way flutter valve allows air to leave but not return

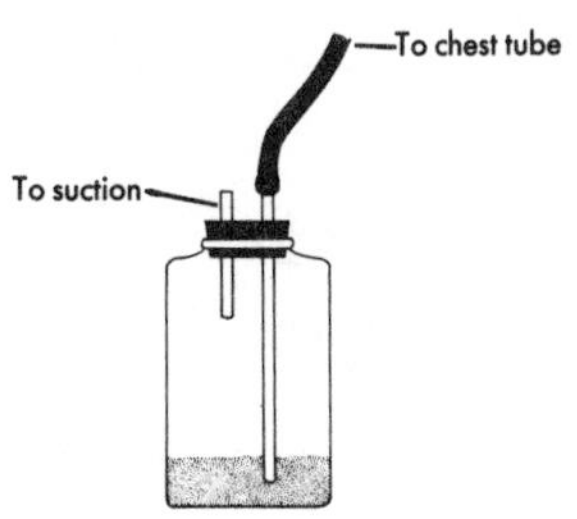

FIG. 41-1. One-bottle system.

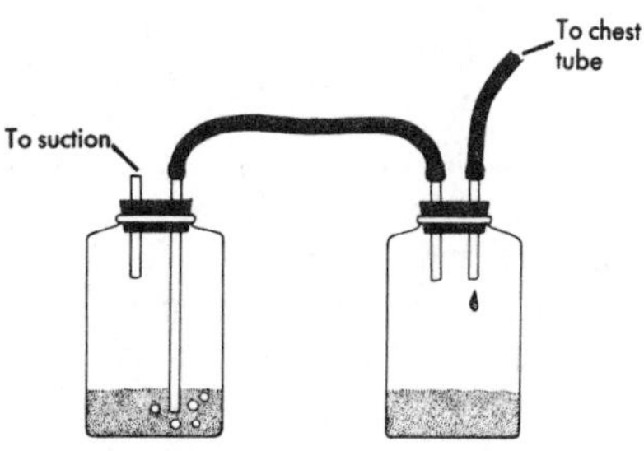

FIG. 41-2. Two-bottle system. Right bottle collects fluid, and left bottle contains underwater seal.

to the pleural space. It may stick when thick fluids such as blood or pus are drained through it, so it should be restricted to use for a pneumothorax.

3. In a one-bottle system (Fig. 41-1) a tube from the pleural space is placed below the patient and opened under water in a bottle. Air and fluid will leave the pleural space and enter the bottle whenever pleural pressure is higher than the pressure generated by the height of water in which the tube is immersed. This will occur during coughing and forced expirations. Fluid or air will be unable to enter the pleural space from the bottle, unless the bottle is raised above the patient. If the bottle were tipped over and the water seal lost, air would enter the pleural space. Large amounts of drained fluid will raise the level and obviously change the water seal or threshold pressure in this system.

4. The two-bottle system (Fig. 41-2) is similar to the one-

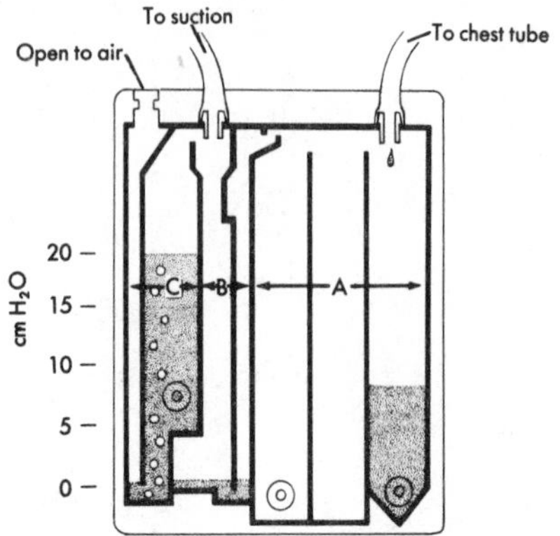

FIG. 41-3. Disposable "three-bottle" system. Section *A* collects fluid. Section *B* contains underwater seal. Section *C* regulates maximum amount of subatmospheric pressure that can be applied to pleural space. In illustration, when more than 20 cm H_2O of subatmospheric pressure (often referred to as -20 cm H_2O of pressure) is applied to suction tube, air will be drawn into port open to air and bubble through section *C,* thus preventing pressure in sections *B* and *A* from falling below -20 cm H_2O.

bottle system, but an additional bottle is interposed between the pleural space and water seal. The additional bottle collects fluid, without changing the depth of the underwater seal. Thus the pressure required to force fluid or air out of the pleural space will also not change.

5. In the three-bottle system or disposable unit (Fig. 41-3)[7] the amount of suction applied to the pleura is regulated by an external tube immersed in water to the desired depth (20 cm). In the disposable unit this is incorporated into a single plastic apparatus. Suction is supplied by an electric pump or a wall suction outlet. The plastic unit can be converted to a water seal by simply disconnecting it from the source of suction.

TECHNIQUE

1. Familiarize yourself with the suction apparatus and then set it up with 20 cm of sterile water in the suction control (or immerse the water seal tube 1 or 2 cm beneath the water level).

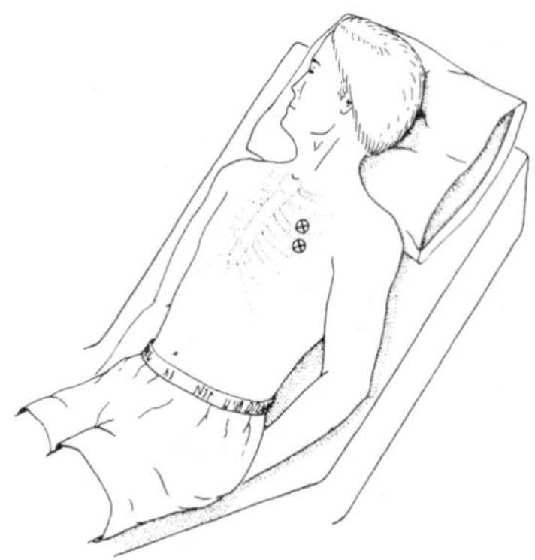

FIG. 41-4. Position for anterior approach to evacuate pneumothorax.

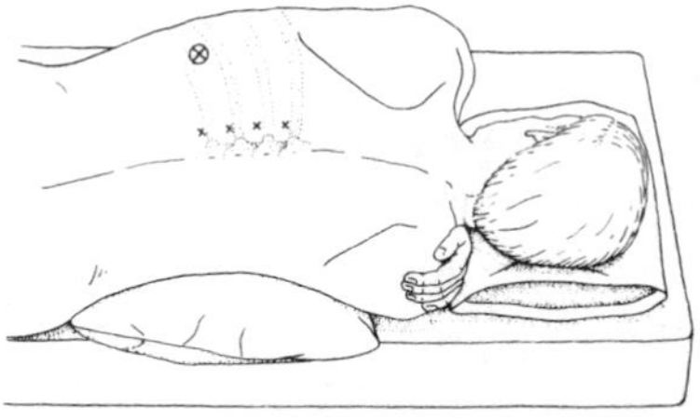

FIG. 41-5. Position for posterior approach to remove fluid.

2. Select an appropriate site for insertion of the tube by reviewing the chest roentgenogram and percussing the patient's chest in the upright position. For a large pneumothorax the anterolateral second or third intercostal space will suffice and the patient may remain on the back for the procedure (Fig. 41-4). For a large effusion the tube should be placed posterolaterally and dependently through the ninth interspace (Fig. 41-5). This will require the decubitus position with the fluid side up. The ribs on this side may be spread apart by placing a pillow under the chest on the down side.

3. Intercostal nerve block.

a. Use the anterior approach for the control of a pneumothorax. After a preliminary alcohol preparation, block intercostal nerves three, four, and five just lateral to the edge of the pectoralis major muscle. The anesthetic solution (1% lidocaine) should be injected upward and backward beneath the lower costal margin with the arm abducted (Fig. 29-2). Supplemental injections are advisable above the upper margin of the corresponding ribs and in the middle of the interspace or the site chosen for insertion of the catheter. Haste is usually not indicated, since full action of the local anesthetic requires 5 to 10 minutes.

b. Posterolateral approach for the removal of fluid.
    1. Locate the tip of the scapula. When the patient's "up" hand is on the "down" shoulder (Fig. 41-5), the tip of the scapula is usually at the level of the seventh rib posterolaterally.
    2. Along a paraspinal line midway between the scapular tip and spinous processes, prepare the site with alcohol and palpate the lower edge of rib seven. With a 5-ml syringe of lidocaine solution and a 27-gauge needle create an intracutaneous wheal 1 cm in diameter, and mark the site on the skin by a cross with the needle. Repeat this over the lower palpable edges of ribs eight, nine, and ten.
    3. Insert the 21-gauge needle (attached to the 12-ml syringe filled with local anesthetic solution) through the skin wheal and advance it toward the center of the rib in a slightly cephalad direction (Fig. 29-2). Move the needle gradually down the rib until it reaches the rib's lower border. Advance the needle 2 mm and aspirate. If no blood is obtained, slowly inject 5 ml of lidocaine, advancing another 2 mm during the injection. Repeat this through the other skin wheals, repeating the alcohol preparation with each. Up to this point you have not worn gloves.

4. Put on sterile gloves and widely prepare the field with the antiseptic solution three times. Select and mark with a crosshatch the site designed for tube insertion and drape the field to expose an extra interspace above and below. At the selected site add supplemental anesthetic to the skin and deeper structures, including the parietal pleura. The exploring needle under suction will often discover fluid, which should be discarded to avoid seeding bacteria or malignant cells.

5. Make a 2-cm transverse incision through the skin at the selected point. Dissect with a curved hemostat down to the pleura (Fig. 41-6).
6. At this point the experienced operator may choose to use the trocar cannula combination apparatus (Fig. 41-7). Insert it at right angles to the skin until the cannula reaches approximately rib level. Then direct it craniad 35 to 40 degrees and carefully push the cannula

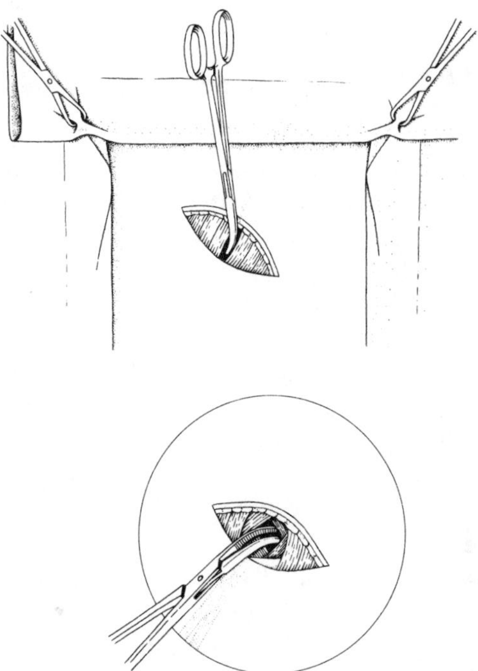

FIG. 41-6. Dissection with curved hemostat to pleura.

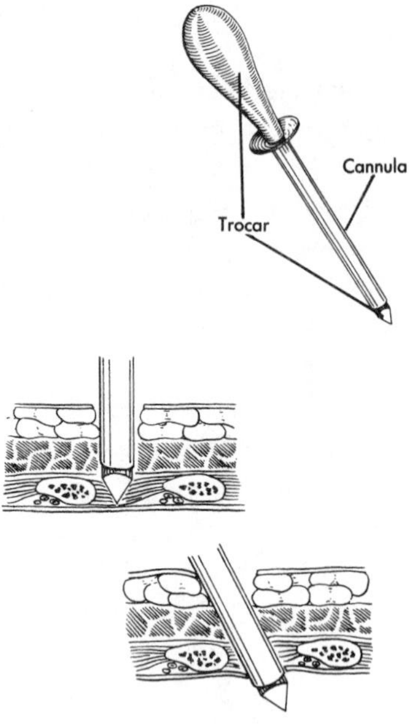

FIG. 41-7. Insertion of trocar cannula into pleural space.

through the pleura. Remove the trocar; a gush of fluid or hiss of air signifies the correct location. Cover the open end of the cannula with your thumb to prevent air from entering the pleural space. Feed in the largest catheter that will pass through the cannula (18 to 28 French) with added fenestrations (Fig. 41-8). Clamp the catheter distally and remove the cannula over it. Then clamp the tube proximally and remove the distal clamp and cannula (Fig. 41-9). Be sure all fenestrations of the tube are well within the pleura.

7. Since the trocar may damage adherent lung or penetrate the diaphragm, spleen, or stomach if an improper site is chosen, the tyro should penetrate intercostal muscles and the pleura with a curved hemostat. After spreading the clamp to widen the opening in parietal pleura, gently explore the pleural space with a finger (Fig. 41-10), and then pass the fenestrated catheter (a number 26 Robin-

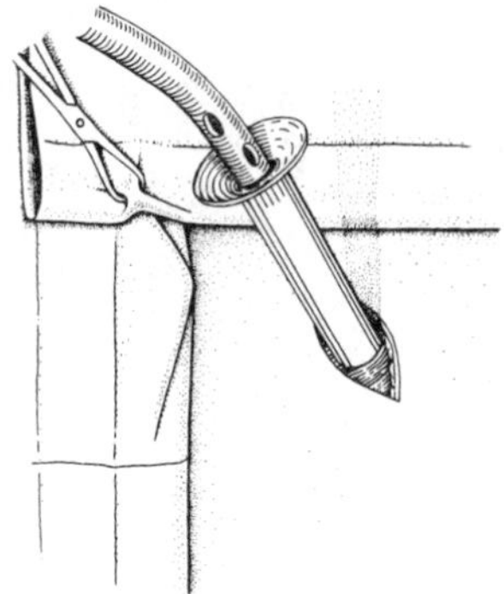

FIG. 41-8. Insert chest tube through cannula.

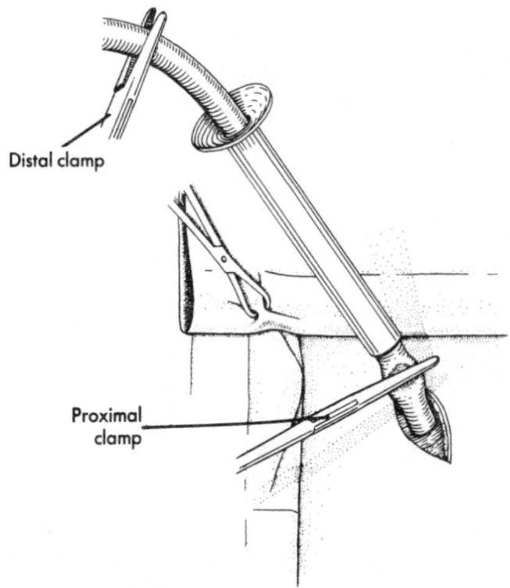

FIG. 41-9. Clamp chest tube distally, remove cannula from skin, clamp tube proximally, and remove distal clamp and cannula.

son or larger) into the space, using the hemostat as an introducer (Fig. 41-11). In either case good anesthesia and controlled force are necessary.

8. Fasten the catheter to the skin with a heavy silk stitch tied around it twice (Fig. 41-12). Place appropriate dressings and secure the connections with tape so that they

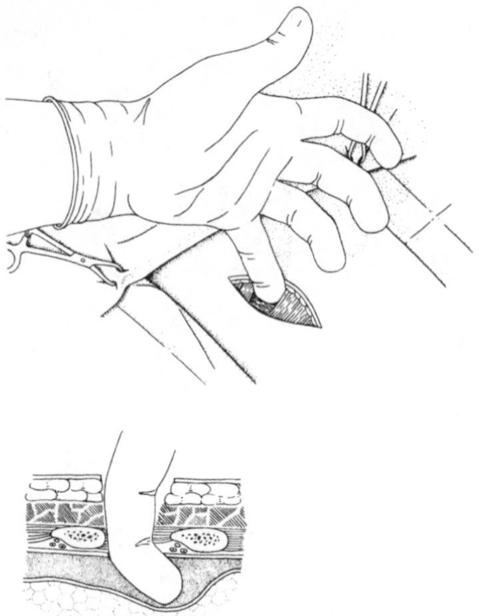

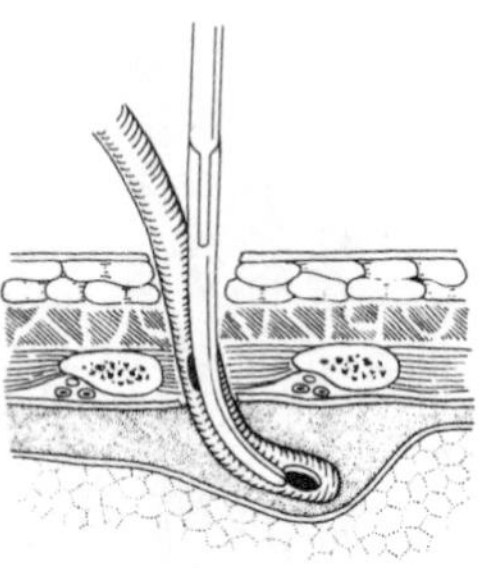

FIG. 41-10. Explore pleural space with finger.

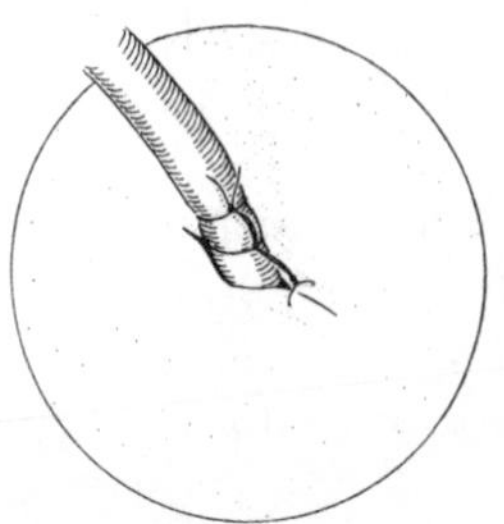

FIG. 41-11. Insert chest tube with curved hemostat.

FIG. 41-12. Secure chest tube with sutures tied twice around tube.

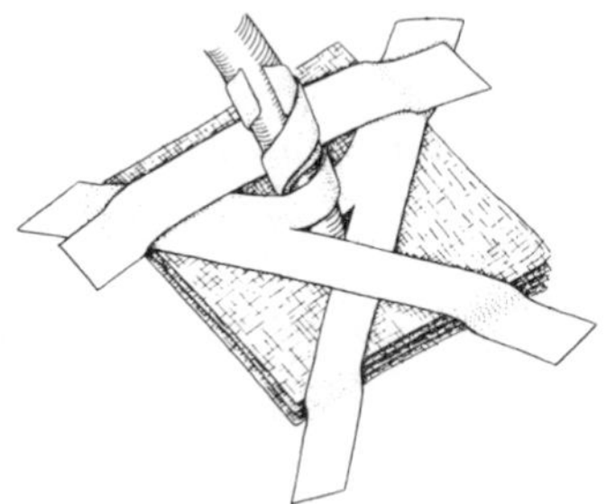

FIG. 41-13. Apply dressings and secure tube with tape.

cannot come apart (Fig. 41-13). Cover the area completely with 2-inch cloth tape.

9. NOTE: Sudden removal of too much fluid may result in syncope due to a vasovagal reflex (intractable cough, bradycardia and other serious arrhythmias, and hypotension) or may be followed by ipsilateral pulmonary edema. To avoid these dangerous side effects, clamp the tube for 15 minutes after incremental removal of each 1000 ml. This is the responsibility of the physician who places the tube, not of the attendants on the floor.

■ INJECTION OF SUBSTANCES INTO THE PLEURAL SPACE

1. Sclerosing solutions are occasionally injected through the tube to treat refractory spontaneous pneumothorax and malignant effusions.[4] Commonly used for this purpose is a suspension of tetracycline, not to exceed 500 mg in 200 ml of saline. Clamp the tube near the skin, insert the solution proximally, and leave it for 1 hour, while the patient changes position often to distribute the solution uniformly over the visceral and parietal pleura, including the mediastinal and apical areas. Since tetracycline is irritating and painful, diazepam or meperidine should be given 45 minutes in advance of instillation.
2. Occasionally a tube placed for a hemothorax or plastic pleuritis may not remove all the clot or gelatinous exudate. In such a situation, uncontrolled studies have suggested that the instillation of streptokinase through the

tube in the manner of tetracycline may liquefy the material in question and allow it to drain.[2]

■ CARE OF THE TUBE

1. The disposable drainage apparatus has a port from which aliquots of fluid may be aspirated for culture and cytologic and other studies. These aliquots should be obtained promptly after tube placement and drainage.
2. A chest roentgenogram should be obtained within an hour after placement of a tube to determine whether tube placement is proper, a pneumothorax has been evacuated, or adequate fluid has been removed.
3. After the local anesthesia has worn off, the patient may need some mild analgesic medication.
4. As long as the tube is draining air or other fluid (or as long as the patient is being ventilated) it is serving a useful function. Daily checks should be made on the amount of drainage and whether the tube is sealed (i.e., Does the chamber in the disposable unit indicate a leak, or does "stripping" flatten the tube? Does coughing fill the stripped and flattened tube?).
5. Stripping is done on a section of soft rubber tube about 1 m in length interposed between the catheter and the more rigid disposable tubing. Proximally, this soft tubing is clamped shut by the thumb and forefinger of the left hand. The opposite thumb and finger rapidly milk, or strip, the lubricated soft tube and then hold it, while the proximal hold is released. Several such maneuvers carried out in succession will evacuate the proximal air and flatten the tubing if there is no leak, that is, no communication between the pleural space and airway. If the patient can cough the tube open, a leak is still present. Reverse stripping may dislodge a clot or inspissated secretion and unmask a persistent leak. Persistent leaks or pneumothorax may be associated with a leaking connection or a tube fenestration outside the skin.
6. When air leaks and drainage have ceased, a tube has fulfilled its function and should be removed. At the end

of a week the point of entrance through the skin should be inspected and perhaps reinforced with petrolatum gauze. All tubes should be changed at the end of 2 weeks. If there is still an absolute need for decompression, a new site should be selected and the new tube placed before the old one is removed.

TUBE REMOVAL

1. If the tube has been in place a week or more, the skin around it will be fixed in the form of a circular opening that will not seal without the placement of one or two skin sutures. The physician should bring, then, the following equipment for extubation: sterile gloves, two sterile 4 × 4 inch gauze pads, two sterile 2 × 2 inch gauze pads, a sterile single piece of petrolatum gauze, scissors, a local anesthetic with appropriate needle and syringe, a needle and suture, tape for a pressure dressing, and an adherent solution, such as compound tincture of benzoin.
2. Remove the dressing, cut the suture holding the tube, apply the pressure dressing, and instruct the patient to exhale. Remove the tube *suddenly*. If needed, a local anesthetic is administered, and sutures are placed before extubation. The pressure dressing is simply two 4 × 4 inch and two 2 × 2 inch gauze pads and the petrolatum gauze firmly held over the tube site before and during removal. The dressing is firmly anchored in place with 2-inch tape.

COMPLICATIONS[4]

1. Empyema, 2.4%.
2. Lung laceration, 0.44%. Lung laceration is said to occur more often in patients with pleural adhesions; in these patients a gloved finger should be inserted to break up adhesions prior to inserting the tube.
3. Diaphram perforation, 0.45%.
4. Injury to stomach, liver, or spleen. This is rare.
5. Subcutaneous placement of the tube.

6. Unilateral pulmonary edema may occur if too much pleural fluid is removed rapidly. Clamp the tube for 15 minutes after the removal of each 1000 ml of pleural fluid to avoid this problem.

REFERENCES

1. Austin, E.H., and Flye, M.W.: The treatment of recurrent malignant pleural effusion, Ann. Thorac. Surg. **28:**190-203, 1979.
2. Bergh, N.P., Ekroth, R., Larsson, S., and Nagy, P.: Intrapleural streptokinase in the treatment of hemothorax and empyema, Scand. J. Thorac. Cardiovasc. Surg. **11:**265-268, 1977.
3. Leff, A., Hopewell, P.C., and Costello, J.: Pleural effusion from malignancy, Ann. Int. Med. **88:**532-537, 1978.
4. Millikan, J.S., Moore, E.E., Steiner, E., Aragon, G.E., and Van Way, C.W., III: Complications of tube thoracostomy for acute trauma, Am. J. Surg. **140:**738-741, 1980.
5. O'Hara, V.S.: Spontaneous pneumothorax, Milit. Med. **143:**32-35, 1978.
6. Roe, B.B.: Physiologic principles of drainage of the pleural space, Am. J. Surg. **96:**246-251, 1958.
7. Van Way, C.W., III. Persisting pneumothorax as a complication of chest suction, Chest **77:**815-816, 1980.
8. von Hippel, A.: Chest tubes and chest bottles, Springfield, Ill., 1970, Charles C Thomas, Publisher.

Index

E

K

L

M

N

U

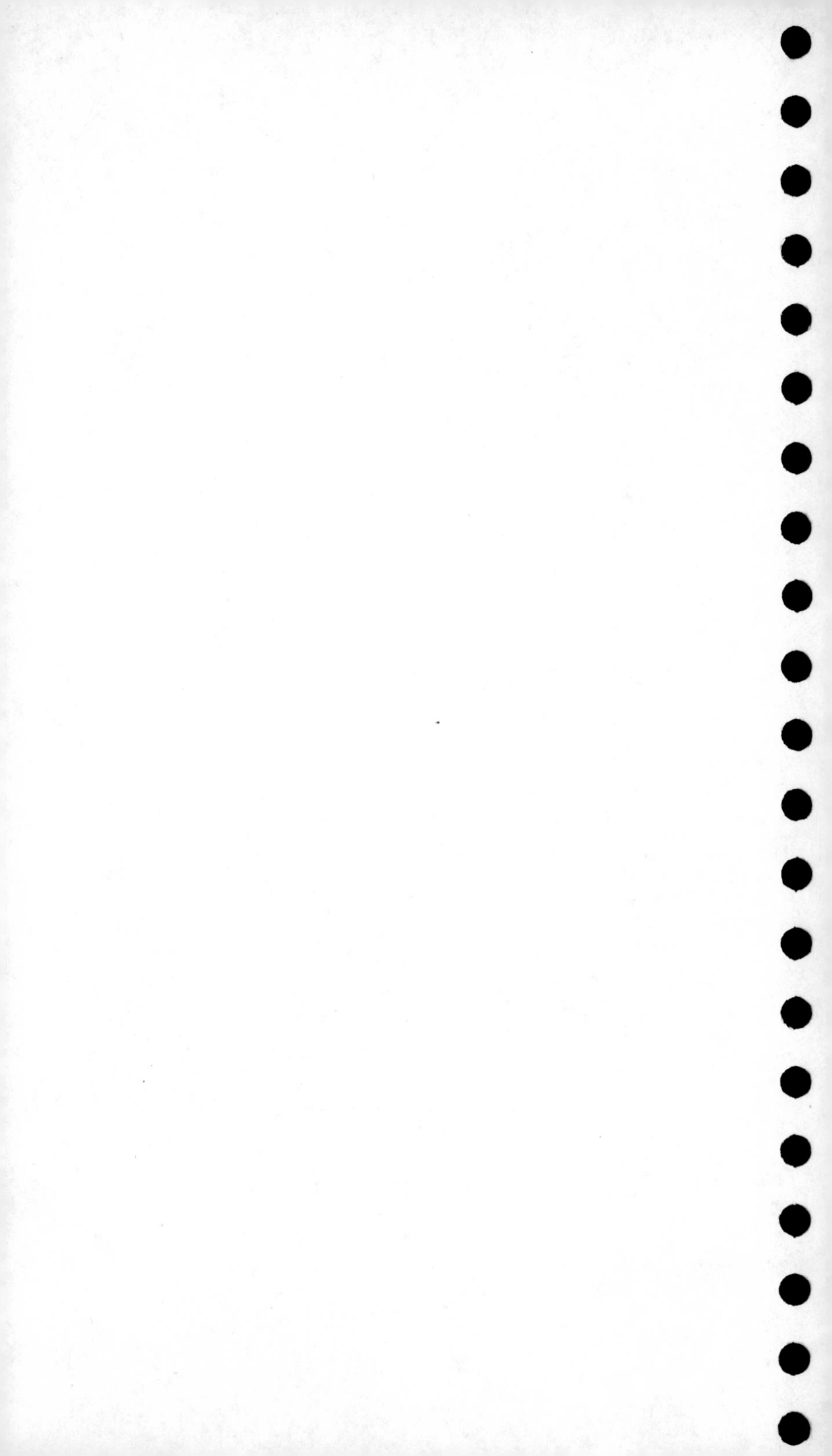